IBS
CHAT

IBS CHAT

Real Life Stories and Solutions

Selections from the online Bulletin Board
of the Irritable Bowel Syndrome Self Help and Support Group

Barbara Bradley Bolen, Ph.D.,
Clinical Psychologist,
Author of *Breaking the Bonds of Irritable Bowel Syndrome*

Jeffrey D. Roberts, M.S.Ed.
President and Founder,
Irritable Bowel Syndrome Self Help and Support Group

www.ibsgroup.org

iUniverse, Inc.
New York Lincoln Shanghai

IBS Chat:
Real Life Stories and Solutions

iUniverse books may be ordered through booksellers or by contacting:

iUniverse
2021 Pine Lake Road, Suite 100
Lincoln, NE 68512
www.iuniverse.com
1-800-Authors (1-800-288-4677)

ISBN-13: 978-0-595-39827-0 (pbk)
ISBN-13: 978-0-595-84232-2 (ebk)
ISBN-10: 0-595-39827-8 (pbk)
ISBN-10: 0-595-84232-1 (ebk)

Printed in the United States of America

For Rhonda, Rebecca, Daniel and Dara, who are there for me each and every day, and to the caring and supportive members and moderators of the IBS Self Help and Support Group community.

Jeffrey D. Roberts, M.S.Ed.

Again, for my boys, and for Kathleen, for all the 'so much more than just chats' chats.

Barbara Bradley Bolen, Ph.D.

Contents

Introduction

LyndaG
Prolific Member

"Blessed is the influence of one true, loving human soul on another."

—George Eliot

From: **Toronto, Ontario, Canada**

Bring up the subject of Irritable Bowel Syndrome in a casual conversation and you are likely to get one of two responses—either a blank stare or "Heard of it? I *live* it!" Therein lays the strange dichotomy of IBS: although its symptoms of severe abdominal pain, urgent diarrhea, and/or chronic constipation, affect 10 to 20 percent of the population, the social stigma attached to bowel problems results in ignorance of the disorder and isolation for sufferers in a way that is generally not seen in other physical ailments. In addition, the fact that IBS is considered a "functional disorder" because no visible inflammation, malformation or tissue damage is generally seen through standard diagnostic testing, has often resulted in a minimization of the havoc that IBS can wreak on a person's life and a lack of serious attention to the disorder by medical practitioners.

As a lifelong IBS sufferer, Jeffrey Roberts has made it his life's passion to advocate for awareness, education and treatment regarding this devastating disorder. Knowing first-hand how isolating IBS can be, he started a web site to try to serve as a means of disseminating information about the disorder. Through feedback from visitors to the site, he realized that there was a desperate need for sufferers to have a place to discuss their struggles and to share information about ways to feel better. Thus, the Irritable Bowel Syndrome Self Help and Support Group (www.ibsgroup.org) was born. The site maintains the goal of providing education and support to IBS sufferers, their families, and health professionals. Over the years, the site has grown to become the world's premier online community for people with Irritable Bowel Syndrome, with over 150,000 visitors each month.

A visit to www.ibsgroup.org clearly illustrates why the site has been so successful in carrying out Jeffrey Roberts' mission. The site contains a Bulletin Board and a chat room where individuals can share their experiences and advice. Links to the most current research findings are displayed prominently. Information is also available to help sufferers to find local support groups, to direct them to other helpful Web sites, and to make sufferers aware of books that offer help in managing the disorder. Additional opportunities for social support include IBS Penpals, which helps IBS sufferers to form relationships world wide, and IBS Blogs, a community of individuals sharing their experiences through personal online journals. The archives of the IBS Self Help and Support Group contain the largest collection of postings about IBS—in excess of 550,000—offering an invaluable resource to individuals whose lives have been affected by this challenging disorder.

Several years ago, in an effort to gain information to help her IBS patients, Dr. Bolen came across the web site of the IBS Self Help and Support Group. The breadth of information offered and the generosity of spirit manifested by members in proffering support and advice to fellow sufferers amazed her. It was plain to see that the comfort afforded by the anonymity of the Internet helped to resolve one of the most vexing aspects of the disorder—the social isolation that contributes to shame, confusion, and misinformation. The quality of the postings on the Bulletin Board of the site inspired Dr. Bolen to approach Jeffrey Roberts with the idea of putting together a book, to provide an alternative method of making available this sense of community and range of information to IBS sufferers and the people in their lives. The result of this collaboration is *IBS Chat: Real Life Stories and Solutions*.

As you will see, *IBS Chat* presents members' posts in a helpful, organized manner, so that anyone picking up a copy, whether they have access to a computer or not, could have immediate access to the wealth of information provided by members of the IBS Self Help and Support Group in the years since its inception. As IBS is a complex disorder, with many facets and numerous treatment approaches, *IBS Chat* is organized in accordance with the various forums of the Bulletin Board, each of which addresses a separate aspect of the disorder. In terms of postings, the best of the best have been chosen, reflecting the most active topics of discussion on the Board. Although posts have been edited for readability, (e.g. grammar, spelling, and relevance) they remain the words of Bulletin Board members who have generously offered stories of their heartbreaks, trials and tribulations, and solutions to the immense challenge of IBS.

You may find that sometimes the suggestion of a simple change, like adding a supplement to a diet, can cause a major reduction in intestinal symptoms and a return to normalcy. Other times, a multi-targeted approach is needed to bring the disorder under better control. In these pages, you will be introduced to an immense selection of possible solutions. We hope that reading through these posts will help you to find your way toward improved health, with the new knowledge that you are not alone.

Jeffrey D. Roberts, M.S.Ed.
President and Founder
Irritable Bowel Syndrome Self Help and Support Group

Barbara Bradley Bolen, Ph.D.
Clinical Psychologist

Forum I: <u>Irritable Bowel Syndrome</u>

"Use this *general* forum to ask a question or discuss your symptoms and how you cope with your Irritable Bowel Syndrome. This forum will help you find answers to commonly asked questions for new members. Post and discuss information that may be helpful to others who suffer from IBS."

The "Irritable Bowel Syndrome" forum is usually the first stop for new members. For some, a visit to this forum is the first time they find there is a name for the symptoms that have turned their lives upside-down. For others, discussing their symptoms openly online is a way to get some answers while waiting confirmation of their diagnosis from a physician. Those who are newly diagnosed find a welcoming place to get questions answered. Long-term sufferers find the company of fellow patients a refreshing change after years of struggling alone. Reading through these posts will provide you with the comfort of knowing that you are not the only one out there dealing with IBS and the assurance that there are plenty of things that you can do to help yourself.

<u>Discussion</u>: Is This IBS? ...

These first groups of posts were written by people who are experiencing severe digestive distress, but have not yet been diagnosed. Members of the Bulletin Board offer support and suggestions for obtaining a proper diagnosis:

1

Topic: Is this IBS? Help!!

Capittm
New Member

I've always had really weird bowel habits. Having C for a week, then D for three to four days. I always have really bad abdominal pain during an "episode". It's sooo bad. I know you all can sympathize!

I've never gone to a doctor about this because, well, I'm a bit ashamed if that makes any sense. Right after both my daughters were born, I had the worst episodes ever!! They've run every test in the book on me thinking it was a "female" problem of some kind. Everything there checks out okay. I just don't even know where to start.

How do you find a good IBS doctor? What kinds of doctors specialize in this type of thing?

I'm really getting desperate for answers … don't know what to do.

Please, please … if anyone has any info on how to find a good IBS doc or any advice for me I would really appreciate it.

Carol

From: **Arkansas**

Jleigh
Very Prolific Member

Welcome to the board Carol,

You need to get to a Gastroenterologist. Ask around about tummy doctors. Ask your Family practitioner to recommend one or better yet, if you know any nurses, ask them who is a good Gastro doc. That is the best way to find out whom to go to. You need to be evaluated and have special tests to be sure it is not something more serious.

Good luck to you and stay around here and post more, read more and heck, even ask if there are any IBSers from your area so you can maybe get pointed in the direction of some good help.

I'm really sorry you are suffering the way you are. Keep us posted.

Jleigh

From: **USA**

Nmwinter
Very Prolific Member

Jleigh had good advice. I just wanted to add that you shouldn't feel embarrassed about this at all—not that I don't understand of course. This is a medical problem you're dealing with—GI docs are used to it. I also wanted to say that your pattern C then D is familiar to me too and not uncommon either.

Once you have a diagnosis of IBS for sure, you and your doc can work out how to treat it. I also recommend arming yourself with as much info as possible including from this site because honestly, I can say I've found more help from this site than my docs.

Good luck,
Nancy

From: **Portland, OR, USA**

Topic: Do I have IBS???

NHLgal
New Member

Hi … I'm new here!!! I'm 28 years old and I'm not sure if I have IBS??? I have not been to the doctor but I am making an appointment. I honestly have been scared.

It's embarrassing to talk about my problems, but I've realized that I cannot make it anymore without knowing what is wrong with me! About 2 months ago I got extremely nervous and stressed, I was literally a basket case! I got severely depressed and noticed changes in my bowel movements, increased gas and cramps. For the last two months my symptoms have been there ... but not as severe ... I have days where I am extremely uncomfortable and others where I am fine! I notice that around my period I get diarrhea a few days before and lower back pains. I usually strain when I go to the bathroom. I have no pains and there is no blood. Are the symptoms of IBS more severe during your period? Do my symptoms sound like IBS? I do not have the cramping that much ... rarely ... just gas with certain foods, constipation, I feel like I still have to go to the bathroom when I am finished going, lower back pain near my butt. HELP! I'm scared!

From: **Burbank, CA**

Lflower
Prolific Member

Sounds very familiar to my IBS. I get more pain/diarrhea before/during my period. I'm mostly diarrhea. Don't put off seeing the doctor though. IBS is very common, 1 out of 5 people get it. There are other diseases that are more serious, but more uncommon, that can have these symptoms. The diagnosis is mostly all on the symptoms, since you can't see it.

Good luck, and RELAX!!

From: **California**

Nmwinter
Very Prolific Member

Yup, it sounds like it could be IBS. But you do need to see a doctor to make sure. If it is IBS, then the good news is that it's not something that can lead to more serious problems. Bad news is that there is no cure though. But there are lots of us out here and many of us have found help through this board.

Now go to the doctor! If you're like me, you're making it worse by stressing over the unknown!

Nancy

From: **Portland, OR, USA**

NHLgal
New Member

Thanks for the support ... I'm just a very stressed out person and I'm scared of getting a zillion tests done! Like I said before ... it's just scary and embarrassing! I'm glad that there is a site like this that lets people talk about it!

From: **Burbank, CA**

Topic: Do I have IBS?

Lily1
New Member

Hi,

I just recently started doing research on my stomach problems, and from what I've read I think I have IBS. I'd rather have feedback from people who are sufferers than go to the doctor who generally always thinks you're complaining for nothing ... anyways ...

My symptoms are the following:

- periods of diarrhea (i.e. 1–2 weeks) alternating with periods of constipation (i.e. 1–2 weeks)
- diarrhea is made worse when I am stressed (i.e. before an exam, before a big event like a dinner party)

- sometimes I get bad cramps like I'm going to have diarrhea, but nothing happens, even after sitting for 30 minutes
- sometimes the urge to go is so bad that I barely reach the bathroom in time (I mean, sometimes it's REALLY close)
- these symptoms (diarrhea) generally get worse when menstruating

That's about it. Again, not trying to avoid the doctor, but sometimes they just don't listen.

Thanks.

From: **Canada**

BQ
Very Prolific Member

Lily, your symptoms sound familiar, however, only a Doc can make a diagnosis and I would urge you to seek one.

BQ

From: **USA**

Kazzy3
Prolific Member

Lily,

Your symptoms do sound like IBS. It is a good idea to see a doctor, just to be sure. IBS is diagnosed by process of elimination. Don't let a doctor dismiss you, if you feel the doctor is unsympathetic to your needs, see another.

From: **Niles, Il**

Shanmari78
New Member

Lily,

Your story sounds familiar. I fight similar symptoms. Only a doc can diagnose IBS, but be prepared, it is by process of elimination, they test for all the "serious" illnesses first (My doc's words, not mine).

Keep your head up, you are not alone.

~~ Shanmari ~~

From: **Chicago, IL**

Topic: And another newbie

Hamster169
New Member

Well I've yet to be to the doctor. My sister works in a clinic and she has asked around about my symptoms and her doctors say I probably have it too. I'm 30 yrs old and first started having problems a couple years ago. I was going through a very bad breakup. Then I was taken to court by this girlfriend, so my stress level was high for months. I could hear her name or see her name on the caller ID and have stomach pain that would put me lying on the floor.

Now the stress is not an issue. My problem is I am fine as long as I'm not really moving around. My job requires a lot of walking. I can be working around the house and not have any problems at all. Once I start moving a lot, the bathroom is calling. There is no holding it!! I sometimes will get a pain in my stomach and will be running to my truck to get myself to the bathroom. The stomach pain doesn't happen every time. An example is yesterday. I was at work and had to walk only about 1000 feet or so. It wasn't a couple of minutes that I walked down there and then I was running back to my truck. Later in the day it happened again. I walked maybe 1500 feet and I was running back to the truck again. The doctors at my sister's clinic said that the activity of exercise can trigger it. Being 30 and living alone my diet consist of mostly fast food ... I know my diet needs to be changed but does anyone know of other stuff I could also try???

Aaron

From: **Indiana**

Ohnometoo
Very Prolific Member

Welcome.

Different things works for different people .... I don't think eating fast food all the time is going to help your IBS ... You should go to a doctor (Gastroenterologist) that can rule out anything else that is the matter. Medication, hypnotherapy, and diet can all play a part in your symptoms being reduced ...

Hang around here and read all the information on the board you can get ...

\-
Donna

From: **Wild Wonderful West Virginia**

Lexi_Con
Very Prolific Member

Hi Hamster,

I have some idea of what you're going through, and you have my sympathy.
In my case, the IBS symptoms started about 10 years ago when I was in a bad relationship.
It wasn't until AFTER I got out of the relationship that the IBS got really bad.

There are a lot of ways to deal with IBS.
For many, the best approach is one that combines treatments.
This combination of treatments can vary from person to person, just as the IBS itself varies from person to person.

There are forums at this site with a lot of information on a lot of things:

Medications for digestion
Medications that deal directly with stress
Dietary modifications
Stress-reduction techniques like meditation, yoga, etc.
Hypnotherapy tapes
Food supplements such as calcium, etc.
Mild exercise as a stress-reducing activity

The "fast food diet" is bound to be aggravating your IBS badly.
I think that it could cause a problem in a person who doesn't even have IBS!
I hope this is of some help.

Take care … from Lexi

From: **Winnipeg, Manitoba**

Topic: Does this sound like IBS?

Notso8
New Member

Hi everyone … I'm 15 (soon to be 16), and in the past month, I have been getting Diarrhea at least once a week. I was like this once before, but haven't been for almost two years (although I did get constipation every couple of weeks). In the past week, I have cut drinking milk and caffeine products, and it seemed to get better, but then I got it again (I think it was due to salad dressing). It didn't start until about a week after school ended. Also, I have pains in my lower RIGHT abdomen …

Any suggestions?

From: **USA**

Jezabel_007
Prolific Member

Well if you're worried, then go see your doctor and tell them your symptoms.

You said you had it once a week, which isn't too often, some people with IBS have said they sometimes go up to 12 times a day. You said you cut out milk and caffeine and were better, so perhaps it has something to do with lactose intolerance? Also coffee is a stimulant, so that could mean something too perhaps …

Here are the symptoms of IBS:

Severe crampy/sharp pain in the abdomen
Constipation
Diarrhea
Alternating constipation and diarrhea
Feeling that you haven't finished a bowel movement
Gas
Bloating, sometimes quite severe
Mucus in the stool
Urgency
Occurs usually after a meal

I'm not a doctor, but it could also maybe have something to do with your diet. Try upping your fiber intake so you become more regular, and eat a lot of fruits and vegetables, and stay away from gas inducing foods as well as junk foods. I went on a diet and since then, my IBS has been a hell of a lot more tolerable than before the diet.

Anyways, good luck, and see your doc if you're worried.

From: **Earth**

Notso8
New Member

Thank you for the info Jezabel ... I think that if it continues, I will be seeing a doctor ... but what was curious to me is that this didn't start until after school stopped ... can something like this just pop out that quickly?

From: USA

Jezabel_007
Prolific Member

I dunno, but I remember my doctor once telling me that IBS can be seasonal, like it flares up only in warm months or cold months. So I dunno, but see your doctor anyways, when you're experiencing symptoms.

From: **Earth**

Darth Do'Urden
New Member

Not to hijack your thread, Notso8, but I thought I'd use this one to piggy back off of instead of starting yet another thread asking the same questions. So here goes =).

I've not seen my doctor yet, as I've just very recently found out about IBS in general, and that it might very well explain why my wife thinks I'm a freak what with all my horrendous gas and frequent bowel movements.

The above list of symptoms all apply to me with the exception of bloating (not real sure what that feels like), and the whole mucus thing.

Some stats:

Age: 27
Sex: Male
Other known issues: Lactose Intolerance; allergy to cow's milk.

I know the classic answer is going to be that I see my doc. I know. As I said, I only very recently considered the possibility that my pains and whatnot are not normal.

Things that noticeably cause immediate cramping and sense of urgency are Chinese, and spicy foods; sometimes coffee tears me up, sometimes it doesn't, and other caffeinated sodas don't seem to have any adverse effect. I have to drink soymilk with cereal or coffee, but it almost always causes me to have a very loose BM (better than the very painful alternative … constipation, but still …).

I haven't tried to alter my diet yet (again, my realization of this whole issue is still in the infant stage … and man, do I really like different foods).

From: **SoCal**

Rocknrolljunkie
New Member

I'm also going to piggy back this topic and give my two cents (well actually my story) so here it goes:

I am a 27 year old female
I am a coffee drinker and a smoker
I have a terrible time going to the bathroom (sometimes I don't go for a week, other times it's three times a day)

My stool is never "normal", as sometimes it is almost like diarrhea, and other times I can barely force it out)

I get abdominal pain, sometimes cramp like but mostly like my insides are going to fall out.
I have not gone to see my doctor about this.
What does it sound like to all of you?

From: **Canada**

Jezabel_007
Prolific Member

Darth: sounds like IBS to me. But a visit to your doc or a GI doc will give you a better idea of what you're dealing with. Plus, it sounds like junkie/greasy foods trigger your upset tummy. And the milk problem too—my GI doc said that IBS can often be mistaken for lactose intolerance.

Rocknroll: Well, first, seeing your doc might be a good idea. Second, you drink coffee and you smoke, not a great combination. What is your diet like? Do you eat a lot of fiber? Maybe you're just lacking the proper fiber intake. You didn't say you had urgency, which is a common IBS symptom. Also, make sure you eat lots of veggies and fruit. I recently lost a lot of weight, and since then, my IBS has been TONS better than before, which I conclude is because of the healthier lifestyle I'm following.

From: **Earth**

Discussion: ... Maybe It's Not.

Sometimes the answer to the question, "Is this IBS?" is "maybe it isn't". Many of the symptoms of IBS are seen in other, often more serious disorders. This next set of posts consists of discussions regarding symptoms that are *not* typical of IBS. Remember, anyone experiencing chronic digestive problems, typical or not, should be seen by a qualified physician.

Topic: Does this sound like IBS?

Cms
New Member

Hello. I'm 25 and ever since I was a little kid I have always had bowel problems such as constipation. I didn't really get it checked out till I was 18. I've been to several different GI doctors and they all tell me it's IBS, but they don't do any tests. I have these symptoms every day: constipation, mucus in stool (no blood), tenderness when I press my upper abdomen, gas, and indigestion. I'm pregnant and I feel terrible. I've told all the doctors about these symptoms and they don't seem to think it's a big deal. They gave me Bentyl to take. I'm scared to death I have cancer or Crohn's or something worse than IBS. Please help if you can relate?

From: **USA**

Kmottus
Very Prolific Member

So far you haven't listed any red flag symptoms that would indicate it might be something else. IBS is the most common cause of these kinds of symptoms, so most people, especially under the age of 60, that go to the doctor with these symptoms are diagnosed with IBS.

Red flag symptoms:

Blood in the stool, especially bloody diarrhea. Small spots of bright blood are almost always hemorrhoids.

Pain that wakes you up when you are fully asleep (more common in other problems, less common in IBS).

Totally inexplicable weight loss. This is to eat plenty and still lose weight like you are fasting.

Elevated Sedimentation Rate (this is something they check when you have your blood tested for stuff like anemia, so it is commonly done, especially in women who are the age to get pregnant).

FWIW, colon cancer pretty much doesn't have any symptoms until it blocks up your rectum so bad every last stool is pencil thin. It is a silent killer. Reproductive cancers sometimes cause GI symptoms, but that would have been checked with the whole pregnancy thing.

Constipation is rare in people with IBDs (Inflammatory Bowel Disorders)—it does happen, but most of the time they tend to have diarrhea 4–20 times a day, particularly during a flare up.

Being sick isn't fun, but the MOST likely thing that it is IBS. 1 out of 5–10 people have IBS. Very few people have Inflammatory Bowel Diseases and very few people under 50 get colon cancer.

K.

From: **NC USA**

Topic: Do you think I have IBS???? HELP!!!

Maryr_32
New Member

I'm new here, but am really glad I found this place. In reading, it seems that I have the same symptoms for the most part as you guys!! OK, here's what's been going on. About six weeks or so I started having this D a couple/three times a day, pretty much every day since then, with a few days of C occasionally. Rarely "normal" BM days since early November. No blood, just frequent runny loose stools, URGENCY to go sometimes, and I feel so much better afterwards!!

My stomach feels like it has butterflies in it …. I've heard it called a 'nervous' stomach … that definitely fits. I've had A LOT of extra stress for the past few months … A LOT!!! I have been put on Paxil CR 37.5mg for anxiety/depression since about October. I'm actually wondering if since I'm on meds now for anxiety, my body has just developed these new gastro ways of dealing with my constant stress????

Any help/comments will be appreciated. Thanks.

By the way, I am a very, very bad hypochondriac (goes along with the anxiety) and am always afraid it's the proverbial "something awful!"

From: **Elizabethtown, KY**

Sabriel
Prolific Member

Hi Maryr_32,

Sorry to hear you have been feeling so unwell lately.

From the symptoms you have described it is possible that you do have IBS, however it is a little too soon to say for sure. Usually, one does not get a diagnosis of IBS until all other possibilities have been ruled out.

Also, in general the symptoms have to have occurred on more than one occasion, over a period of 12 months or more, before IBS is considered likely.

Also, it is not that uncommon for people that don't have IBS to suffer bouts of diarrhea in relation to stress, so it could just be that. I would see how things go when the stressful period for you comes to an end. In the event that the stress is likely to be long term, I would say go see your doctor.

Any kind of diarrhea that lasts more than a few days should be checked out by a doctor. Having a few tests will also go a long way toward easing your mind, which will also reduce the stress and maybe the diarrhea too.

Good luck, hope you feel better soon and let us know how you get on.

From: **Australia**

Nutriqueen
Regular Member

I see you were put on Paxil in October and then developed diarrhea in November. From what I have read, Paxil can cause diarrhea as one of its side effects. Is this possible? If so, mention it to your doctor and see if he can change the dosage or something.

From: **Canada**

Ohnometoo
Very Prolific Member

SSRI'S (like Paxil) for me made my IBS-D worse ...

Donna

From: **Wild Wonderful West Virginia**

Topic: Do I have IBS??? Need Help

Browneyedgirl
New Member

I've been under a lot of stress recently, but I've never experienced THIS because of stress before. Last week I was in a bar, talking to a guy, everything was great. And then …

I crapped my pants. Seriously. It was the most embarrassing thing ever!!! The worst part about it—I was wearing a skirt (with a thong) because this is all new to me. I had no idea it could just … explode like that. It's made me so self-conscious this past week. My diet is suffering too. I mean I can't even eat a French fry! How do you deal with this? Do you just eat in the bathroom? Somebody help me with this, please!!!

I'm glad there are people that I can talk to who won't judge me for my problem.

From: **Alabama**

Boykins
New Member

It could be IBS, maybe you will be lucky and it will be a one time thing (stomach virus). You will know soon enough. IBS is not a one time thing. If it continues, I would suggest you see your doctor.

Good luck.

From: **South Carolina**

Nmwinter
Very Prolific Member

It could be IBS. Before saying for sure though, you really need to get a diagnosis from the doc. If it was possibly a one time thing though, then it could have been from a number of things too—a bug or food poisoning for instance. Although you'd have other symptoms typically.

If you find that it's IBS, then there are thing to help. If you're like me and stress is the big trigger, then there is relaxation, mind body therapies and medications (anti-anxiety, for example) that can help. Personally, I use hypnotherapy and it's been wonderful. There are also things to help and you can learn about them on this board and hopefully from your doc (if you find a good one—my docs have never been that helpful).

Mostly, I'm just saying don't get the attitude that if it is IBS there is nothing to be done. It's a complicated thing to be sure but lots of people have found ways to cope well.

Nancy

From: **Portland, OR, USA**

Kmottus
Very Prolific Member

Poor thing. Accidents are no fun at all.

The first thing is to run this by the doctor to see what, if anything needs to be tested for. Also, they can prescribe things that can help.

For the eat-must poop NOW!!!!! thing, often taking an antispasmodic or anti-diarrheal 20–40 minutes before eating tends to calm that down. Fatty foods are often worse for causing this. The stomach lets the colon know it ate, and that signal appears to be over-responded to in some people with IBS.

Peppermint and Imodium are available over the counter for this, but even if they work you need to check in with the doc. Many antispasmodics are prescription, and for some people antidepressants also work. The nerves of the gut use serotonin a lot and sometimes taking one of these drugs calms down the over-response thing. Stress reduction and things like CBT or Hypnotherapy can also calm down the nerves in the gut.

K.

From: **NC USA**

Topic: Hi I'M NEW—DO I HAVE IBS???!

PTpowwow
New Member

Hello everyone. I'm new to this board and after reading several posts, I'm glad that I've found this site. At first I was surfing out of desperation. Recently for the past 2 months I have been in extreme discomfort. The main problem I have is bloating and discomfort after I eat. I am only able to eat very small amounts of food and I get bloated and feel extremely uncomfortable afterwards for several hours. I have constipation and sometimes diarrhea as well. These problems have made me lose so much weight. I was 189 pounds back in the end of February and now I only weigh 169 pounds. I went to see my primary care doctor several times and he has no idea what the problem is with me. He says I have mental problems and it's all mental. He referred me to a GI specialist and I did an X-ray on my upper GI tract and an ultrasound on my abdominal area. All came out negative. The only thing they said was that I may have excess acid??! But that shouldn't account for my absolute loss of appetite. I mean I totally do not feel hungry at all. And when I eat it feels very uncomfortable. The GI specialist, after seeing my results, concluded that I had nothing wrong and said he could not help me. He said it was caused by anxiety … and I think he's just BSing me … I get very frustrated and one time I went and ate a lot despite my fullness. Later I regretted it. I felt like puking but I couldn't and I felt dizzy as if I was going to pass out. And my stomach was just killing me. I don't usually have severe pains in my stomach area, it just feels bloated and that something is stuck there and it feels extremely uncomfortable; sometimes I have small pains but nothing as severe as the ones you guys describe. Please help and give me some input??! I made my doctor refer me to another GI specialist and I want to get a colonoscopy as well. I did blood tests and they said I have no infection as well …. I'm very lost and in need of help …. Thanks for replying!!

From: **Pasadena/CA**

Watchmedream
Prolific Member

Your symptoms sound EXACTLY like mine. But I do not lose weight—that is a "red flag symptom".

From: Anywhere

Leefromnj
Prolific Member

PTpowwow-

No appetite and regurgitating ... could be Delayed Stomach emptying ... ask the new GI about that. What about GERD? Ask them to do an endoscopy.

—Lee

From: **New Jersey**

Topic: do I have IBS? Help!!

Carrie
New Member

Hi, I'm new but desperate for some answers.

Since I was young I have always had problems with constipation. As I got older, I also got lower tummy pain. My GP told me I had IBS when I was 17, but did not perform any tests. The past few years symptoms have changed and increased, including alternating diarrhea/constipation (can changes three times a day) constant lower pain in pelvic area, sharper pain lower right, very sharp pains top left stomach and under ribs, feeling sick, being sick occasionally, very bad pain in lower back, feelings of exhaustion.

I have changed GPs twice due to moving home and they still said IBS without tests. I recently took a food allergy test and found I was very sensitive to wheat and dairy which I have cut out of my diet. Symptoms lessened, but have since come back even though I have had no wheat and dairy. My new GP said that the wheat and dairy were aggravating my IBS, (still no tests).

I've tried peppermint, high fiber, low fiber, etc., no change.

My mum has Crohn's disease and her sister has Ulcerative Colitis. Should I go back to my GP now that pain and symptoms are getting worse or is it time I accept that I do have IBS?

Please help anyone, I'm in my 2nd year at university and this is ruining my life.

Carrie

From: **England**

A lie
Prolific Member

Hi Carrie, I really think you should get some tests done. Diagnosis of IBS without any tests done is not an accurate one. Since your family has a history of IBD, I suggest you get a colonoscopy, or at least some blood tests to test for inflammation, in order to get some peace of mind on whether you may have UC or Crohn's.

Good luck on your condition and God bless!

From: **Singapore**

Carrie
New Member

Thank you for your concern.

I saw the doctor again, but this time it was a different lady and she was so understanding. She is testing me for Celiac's disease due to the wheat intolerance and also referring me to specialist for tests for Crohn's and Colitis. She was quite angry that I'd not been tested sooner due to family history.

Carrie

From: **England**

Topic: Do I have IBS?

Sartris
New Member

I think I might have a mild case. Once every couple years I'll have a week where whenever I eat I have stomach cramps to the point where I feel like I'm gonna vomit. They last an hour or so and then it's like nothing ever happened. Stomach feels tight, sometimes painful.

I'm going through it right now and it isn't fun at all. Hard to think, concentrate … when it gets bad, the thought of having to deal with it every day is very depressing … sometimes it gets to the point where I'm afraid to eat.

Thanks in advance …

From: **California, USA**

Sartris
New Member

I should mention that I have no problems with BM. I have been going to the bathroom every day with similar consistency as always …

From: **California, USA**

Polly6034
Regular Member

Sartris:

I'm pretty sure that the "diagnosis" for IBS includes a change in the frequency/consistency of BM and that the pain is relieved by passing gas or BM … but with the pain you are describing you should definitely see a doctor!!

Good luck!

From: **Brisbane, Australia**

Sartris
New Member

Yeah, I'm starting to lean towards it being an ulcer … Going to a GE today.

—Steve

From: **California, USA**

Discussion: Newly Diagnosed.

When puzzling symptoms are finally given a name, IBS sufferers begin to focus on what can be done to feel better. Read on as senior members offer guidance to "newbies". Their suggestions can serve as a road map for you on your own journey toward improved health and well-being.

Topic: Can Anyone Help??

Tngirl
New Member

Hi,

I was just diagnosed with IBS and I'm not sure what I need to do for it. I was put on medicine for it, but other than that I am at a loss. The pain in my stomach will not let up. I'm at the end of my rope.

Any information on how to deal with IBS or anything that you can pass on to me would be so very helpful.

Thanks a lot.

Tngirl

From: **Tennessee**

Evelyn Doyle
New Member

Sorry to hear that you are going through this also. I am also an IBS sufferer, not so much with pain, but with urgency. I am trying a grain-free diet at the moment and will let you know if this helps.

I am sorry I cannot offer you anything in the way of helpful advice but commiserate with what you are going through.

Best of luck.
Evelyn

From: **Canberra, Australia**

Sherlock
Very Prolific Member

Tngirl and Evelyn, welcome to the board.

Best thing you can do to start is read, read, read the boards. You'll soon find other posts that are similar to what you deal with personally, and from there you will be able to ask more specific questions about what others have experienced. IBS is for many of us an individual experience, but often we cross paths in all the "fun" stuff IBS has to offer us.

From: **An excursion around the bay**

Jane1721
Regular Member

Hi Tngirl,

Like Sherlock, I recommend reading the board. I have learned SO MUCH here! Take a look at the nutrition board especially, it helped me figure out what foods I should be careful with and/or avoid. Of course, it varies from person to person, so my trigger foods won't necessarily be yours. The two BEST things I have done to control my IBS are cutting out sodas/caffeine/aspartame (all the same to me), and cutting out pain relievers (Excedrin). Both are big triggers to the digestive system.

I also want to recommend a couple books to you ... I know there are quite a few books about IBS out there, but I only bought two. "Eating For IBS" and "First Year IBS," both by Heather Van Vorous. A lot of useful information.

Hope this helps! Hang in there. You are not alone!

Jane

From: **Ohio**

Christy
Regular Member

Welcome TNgirl!! (I'm a Tennessee transplant girl!!)

I have also read the books by Heather Van Vorous and they helped a lot!!

I have so many different meds I take; it just depends on my symptoms at that particular time.

Finding ways to relax yourself is an awesome way to relieve pain. Lots of folks on this board have found ways to do that through hypnotherapy or other means. I use some of the stuff I learned in Lamaze classes years ago to help me.

I wish you luck and send you hugs!!

From: **Tennessee**

Topic: Newbie—where do I start?

Rim101
New Member

Hi all—was diagnosed with IBS about three weeks ago, and I am still trying to figure out what is 'normal'.

In the past two months I have had an upper GI series, an endoscopy and a colonoscopy—none of which indicated any problems. Blood tests show that I have had consistent anemia since April, even with the taking of iron supplements. We have checked for bacteria, occult blood in the stool, and parasites, but have found nothing to indicate any are present.

I have bloating (followed by burping) pretty frequently, but it feels almost random as to when it happens; sometimes even drinking water can bring it on. Just about any time I put my hand on my belly, I can feel it spasm-ing slightly.

Bowel movements go from diarrhea to constipation, and seem to cycle (diarrhea for a few days, then constipation). I do take Immodium for the diarrhea, and a single dose usually takes care of it. Sometimes I have multiple bowel movements per day, but usually it's three times at most. Stool can be black (from the iron), orange, yellow, or green, depending on what I've eaten. Sometimes there's a mix of colors and consistencies. Frequently there is white mucus mixed with the stool. Stool can run from pellet shapes to long snaky shapes to large stools; none are what I'd consider 'normal'.

Right now I have blood mixed in with the stool, although my doctor says this is from the irritation of the rectum and the opening up of hemorrhoids. Blood does drip out when I go to the bathroom and have a bowel movement, but it's not pouring out.

I get pain in the abdomen most days, but not enough to keep me awake at night.

While I seem to be able to digest most things, I often find pieces of vegetable matter in my stool, especially the skins. Lettuce and spinach appear to pass through completely undigested.

Except for a multivitamin and the iron supplements, the only medication I am on is NuLev for the spasm-ing and Analpram to treat the hemorrhoids. I try not to take more than three NuLev a day, because I've heard there can be colon problems from using it.

So here are my questions:

How much of this is normal for IBS?

Are there any tests that we've missed to determine what else this could be?

What should I be watching out for to see if this is getting worse?

What vitamin/nutritional supplements should I be taking to make up for what my body is not absorbing from food?

And are there any support groups that I can attend that you know of?

And any advice for what steps a newbie should take to see if this can be kept under some sort of control?

Thanks much for all assistance—the worst of this is the loneliness of it.

Rim

From: **Forest Hills, NY**

Kmottus
Very Prolific Member

Sounds like pretty normal IBS, as long as the blood is bright red on the surface of stools.

If it is brownish (old blood) and more mixed in that tends to be something else.

If the hemorrhoids/irritation are causing you to bleed enough to be anemic they may need more treatment.

You might want to get a blood test for celiac because of the anemia, just to be sure. It can take six months of high doses of iron … to reverse the anemia. I was on three prescription iron pills a day for a while. With IBS you should be absorbing normally, but anemia is big with Celiac … which is why I suggested that. (Celiac is gluten sensitivity … gluten is in wheat, rye and barley)

P.S. The undigested matter in stool is normal, just more obvious when you have diarrhea. It is a function of how well you chew, and especially if the lettuce and spinach are raw. They need a good deal of chewing so they are broken up enough to digest.

As for the stomach bloating when you eat, sometimes a digestive enzyme supplement with pancreatic enzymes helps (that is more functional dyspepsia than IBS).

Inexplicable weight loss, the pain waking you up at night, or a lot of brownish blood, are all things to watch out for.

Some things to try:

Keep a log of what you eat to see if anything pans out. You might try avoiding the common IBS diarrhea triggers of greasy/fried/fatty foods, alcohol caffeine, sorbitol (or other—ols). Also you might try avoiding some of the things that are only a problem if you have a specific enzyme/transport molecule missing: Lactose (or take lactase with your dairy) and fructose (mostly high fructose corn syrup).

Calcium supplements can firm up stools.

See if different levels of fiber help or hurt.

If you are interested in the sort of "heal yourself" kinda thing, check out hypnotherapy tapes, they are discussed on the CBT/Hypnotherapy part of the BB. Your symptoms are not in your head, but your brain can influence things.

Good luck.
K.

From: **NC, USA**

Soft
Prolific Member

Hi Rim. Welcome. I remember feeling relieved to find others with this "problem". I read the archives and tried a bunch of the suggestions from posts. The only thing I can add to the great advice above is to maybe keep a food diary and see if anything upsets your system.

Best wishes.

From: **Canada**

Rim101
New Member

Thanks to both of you. K, you have no idea what a relief it is to hear the words 'pretty normal' being used with this is! And Soft, I am going through the archives as much as I can.

So far, it has been bright red blood and on the surface of the stools; I will keep an eye out for changes.

We did test for Celiac and it came back negative.

Haven't tested for lactose intolerance yet, but I'm putting myself off dairy for two weeks to see if there's any change.

This is the first I've heard of fructose being a problem (which with the amount of high fructose corn syrup in everything, could certainly be a trigger I'm repeatedly hitting).

The only reason I have been avoiding keeping a food diary is that I have no idea how to interpret what I'm looking at (would triggers hit me in 20 minutes? 24 hours? 36 hours?). Is this the sort of thing you need to speak with a nutritionist/dietician about?

Thanks again for all your help!

From: **Forest Hills, NY**

Kmottus
Very Prolific Member

It can be a pain to analyze, but usually problems show up within 24 hours of eating something, often less.

I would at least keep a log of symptoms (BM time and consistency) and note if you are doing something as a trial for a couple of weeks (like going off lactose, adding some high fiber foods).

Sometimes the memory of how things were two weeks ago vs. now can be iffy.

AND IBS has an annoying tendency to wax and wane, so that doesn't help either.

One other diet thing … Some people do really well with Heather's book, Eating for IBS. And she is a Bulletin Board member so if you need help with her way of dealing with IBS, she is available to answer questions. There is an "Ask the Specialist button" she takes care of the dietary part of that (I'm the miscellaneous person there).

K.

From: **NC, USA**

Topic: Help newbie here!

April Jane
New Member

Hello.

Firstly, may I congratulate you all on a wonderful site.

This morning after years of pain (which has over the last six months got much worse) I was diagnosed with IBS. Knowing why I feel this pain has eased my mind and knowing I'm not seriously ill is a comfort, but I know nothing about it other than when I feel extreme emotion (happy or sad) I feel really bad. Is this common? I know there are other sources available but I wanted to hear from the people who suffer from IBS rather than the doctors. Besides I don't think doctors understand it, my old ones never have.

Love, AJ

From: **Wakefield, North England**

BQ
Very Prolific Member

Welcome April!

Sorry you have IBS, but glad you found us.

I think your feelings sound quite normal under the circumstances. You have just been told you have a chronic illness. That is gonna take some time to adjust to. It did for me. At first, I was angry about it. Then I went on this mad hunt for a quick fix/magic pill, which was a waste of time because there really isn't one. I eventually accepted it for what it is and began to learn all I could about it and how to manage my symptoms.

There may be no current cure, but there sure is symptom management. You sound like you have a good perspective … you are right; there are a whole lot worse things one could have. But truly, I am living proof that one can learn to *have* IBS and not let it have you.

Be sure to check out all of our forums here that seem to apply to you.

Hope this helps!

BQ

From: **USA**

Steve H.
New Member

Hi! Welcome to the club nobody wants to be in! I agree that it's nice to know you aren't "sick", but that doesn't matter much on a bad day. I've been IBS'y all my life (54) and can only conclude that any stress and overindulgence in certain foods aggravates my condition.

I hate taking long drives in the morning, as I know I'll get the jitters and be looking for a washroom! Never fails! And sometimes I'll dive into a tub of ice cream and spend the night reading old magazines while emptying my brains through my bowels.

I've taken Celexa, an antidepressant for a couple of months now, and while it seems to have calmed things a bit, I still get the odd attack and still worry about proximity to toilets. It's just the way I am. Don't let it rule you. Paranoia about IBS is worse than the actual event.

You aren't alone!

Steve

From: **British Columbia, Canada**

Crankypants
Prolific Member

AJ, I have the impression that it is common for high emotions at either extreme to set off the irritable bowel. I know for me, a little anticipatory excitement is one of the best cures for constipation ...

Glad your diagnosis has at least brought years of uncertainty and worry to an end—that in itself is a very positive health development. Now you can feel free to experiment on yourself.

Hopefully you will find some helpful suggestions here. Good luck!

From: **New York, NY, US**

Topic: Newbie with a question ....

Ohiogirl
New Member

I'm a newbie to this board and just recently was diagnosed with IBS. I'm curious ... what causes IBS??

From: **Ohio**

Modgy
Regular Member

Doctors don't know what causes IBS, and they don't know how to cure it.

Possible causes (or more correctly, triggers) are many and various—you should think about any of these possibilities as they might apply to you. Knowing the probable cause can start you on the road to a solution.

These are just some of the possible triggers or scenarios for development of IBS:

- Onset after a gastrointestinal infection
- Onset after long term use of antibiotics
- Onset after an emotional trauma
- Onset after abdominal surgery especially gall bladder removal
- Occurring with autoimmune disease
- Occurring with autonomic nervous dysfunction (the gastrointestinal system is part of the autonomic nervous system)
- Occurring with anxiety disorder/panic disorder
- Onset after an eating disorder e.g. bulimia or anorexia
- Occurring with specific food intolerance or allergy e.g. lactose intolerance, gluten allergy (Celiac disease)
- Occurring with use or withdrawal of anti-depressant medications (alters serotonin levels in the body, and in turn, in the gut)
- Occurring with Gulf War syndrome or other response to heavy or unusual kinds of vaccination

Many more could be added to this list … and not all these causes are agreed upon by the medical profession, but are often supplied anecdotally as reasons why people with IBS think their IBS may have started …

From: **Sydney, Australia**

Discussion: New to Board, not new to IBS.

For those members who have dealt with the disorder on their own for years, the Bulletin Board provides a welcoming atmosphere of congenial support. Sharing experiences and advice can do wonders in terms of minimizing the impact the disorder has on a person's quality of life.

Topic: New to the board

VJD
Regular Member

Hi all,

I am new here and am glad to find I am not alone in all my weird symptoms. I have had chronic IBS for over 20 years. I have altered my diet and followed doctor directions to the letter, and I still have no relief. Any suggestions or maybe just support from people that understand is appreciated so very much. My family is getting tired of me being in pain all the time. Sometimes I try to hide it from them. Does anyone else have feelings of "guilt" for this illness?

From: **California**

Feelinyucky
Regular Member

Hi!

I can totally relate to your post! While my husband is supportive and sympathetic, he does say "you're sick all the time". I hate having to cancel plans, etc. because I am not feeling well. It is also such a personal and somewhat embarrassing problem to have! How much easier would it be to say "I can't go because of my back/foot/head, etc", instead of "bowel problems"!!!

Take care, and welcome to the board, although I am sure you'd rather not have to be here ...!

From: **Portland, Oregon**

Kristyann
Prolific Member

VJD:

Has your doc prescribed any meds for your symptoms? I am so much better since I started using both prescription and natural products.

Kristy

From: **Wisconsin**

WhoaNellie1487
Very Prolific Member

Welcome to the BB, VJD. Sorry to hear you have IBS. Fortunately (yet unfortunately) I think we can all relate to how you feel. I'll be praying for you also ... I really hope you start feeling better.

::Nessa::

From: **Good ol' Virginia**

VJD
Regular Member

Yes I have been prescribed meds. I was given Donnatal, then I was prescribed Bentyl. Neither of those were very effective. My doctor prescribed Levsin for me a week and a half ago, and it is not helping either. I have tried herbal remedies and diet change as well. My doctor has "upgraded" my condition to "chronic IBS" and wants me to see an associate of his once a month that specializes in IBS. I have gone through all sorts of testing including the dreaded barium enema. My doctor said there are still many meds out there we can try, but he wants me to give the Levsin a chance first.

Do you ever feel like you live at the doctor's office???

From: **California**

Lindalu
Prolific Member

Welcome VJR,

quote: "My family is getting tired of me being in pain all the time. Sometimes I try to hide it from them. Does anyone else have feelings of "guilt" for this illness?"

Oh boy, do I know this one. Welcome to the IBS BB.

You are going to learn so much more from here than what your doctor tells you, just from reading other people's posts.

Lindalu

From: **Salt Lake City, Utah—USA**

Topic: HELP ME!!!

Sarabelle316
New Member

This is my first time here. I am 23 and have suffered from IBS for my whole life! I got diagnosed when I was ten but the doctors were hesitant because it is very uncommon in kids. I have missed a lot of work so far this month. I've gone to work only about seven days. I am starting to have panic attacks when I think about leaving my house, especially the thought of going to work. I have no idea what triggers my stomach problems because it always changes! Sometimes I can eat something, then another time it'll put me in the bathroom for a day. Can anyone help me?

From: **USA**

Kel
Very Prolific Member

Welcome. You will come across many people on this forum who are suffering the same way you are. It makes it a little easier knowing that you are not alone.

Hopefully you can read a lot of the posts and start to identify with the people who sound similar to you.

Some of us have found a few things that really help. Most things that you read about will either not help or only give minimal relief—good luck sorting it all out. It can be exhausting.

This illness is baffling.

From: USA

LaVidaCrapa
Prolific Member

Hi Sarabelle—

What Kel said is right on.

This thing is different for everyone, and by reading the board, you can find out what has worked for different people and what you might try.

I'm the same as you. I never know what might trigger a bad IBS day. There's no pattern of foods or events that I can trace.

Stress as a trigger is pretty much a given. Even "good stress" like happy surprises or excitement before an event.

But, it sounds like you may have fallen into a cycle in which the IBS causes you to have stress and anxiety which in turn, triggers the IBS.

I'm not sure which remedies you have tried in the past, but new options always seem to be emerging.

Maybe if you find a remedy that works for you, your stress will be reduced and you can break the cycle.

From: **Cleveland, OH USA**

Nmwinter
Very Prolific Member

Hey, Sarabelle

I can understand completely what you're saying. I wouldn't say I have an anxiety disorder per se, but because of previous IBS issues, there are some situations that scare me (particularly those I don't control).

Like the others say, there is no one way to fix IBS. There is no cure. But there are some treatments that can help, different things for different people mostly because IBS really is different for different people—what works for someone with primarily diarrhea might cause huge problems for someone who is primarily constipated and those of who alternate have to find yet something else.

Best advice is to read around the board and see what makes sense and then do more research and talk to your doctor. Ask a lot of questions, be as specific as you can with your symptoms (remember, we've heard it all before!)

One suggestion for you is to look into hypnosis. Like many people on the board (but certainly not all) I have found it tremendously helpful, not only with my symptoms but also with breaking those thought patterns. It sounds a little out there I know, but there is a lot of research done on it.

From: **Portland, OR, USA**

Topic: New Member

Stuart999
New Member

Hello everyone one, I have just registered as a new member as I stumbled across this forum with the aid of good ole Google.com. Anyway my story:

My name is Stuart; I am 26 years old and live in Southampton UK. I have suffered from IBS for a little over 10 years.

It all started with a blink of the eye "so to speak". I remember one day being at work dealing with the normal everyday stress, then within a few hours I went from feeling "normal" to feeling like I was going to be sick with stomach pains, and it went on like that for weeks. So I went to see my doctor and explained. He just brushed me off, saying that I either had a bug or a virus. So not knowing any better I agreed and went home, but it still didn't go away. Things were getting worse, to the point I stopped eating as it made me feel 100000% worse. So I went back to my doctor many times, even seeing a different doctor, trying to get them to do more. All they said was it could be IBS and sorry, nothing we can do. Not happy with that, I moaned and moaned at them for weeks to get to see a bowel specialist, and they finally agreed. So I had the camera up my backside looking to see what was up, and all they found was some scar tissue on my bowel lining. And a "Sorry, IBS, nothing we can do", from which I understood there is no "cure" for it. But I was left feeling alone from it …

So here I am today, feeling crappy with IBS D, with a touch of IBS C, and for the last few months, every meal I have gives me incredible pain and lots of D. So again, I stopped eating. I know that's the worse thing I can do but I just want the pain and D to go away. The pain gets so bad I feel like I am going to pass out from it. I mean, I don't even drink fizzy drinks, just plain bottled water. I don't drink alcohol, but OK I do smoke.

So I have had enough from it all, my partner is feeling the strain from it all, many times he has wanted to go out for meal and do the "normal" things couples do and I am scared to death of going and don't go. He has gotten to the point where he thinks our relationship is not worth the hassle anymore, and after 7 years of being with him, that's the last thing I need. I really can't see the point in going on, and I don't mean killing my self, but just getting rid of everyone and everything and lead a recluse life. I just don't know what to do anymore.

So I am now on here asking, what can I do to improve my situation?

Stuart

From: **Southampton, UK**

Minimum
Prolific Member

Hiya, Stuart.

Well, I definitely can relate to your experiences with doctors ... they just brush me off too, and give no helpful advice on how to deal with IBS ... just leave me stranded ... the only advice I EVER got from a doctor (from a specialist!) was to eat more fiber like all-bran for breakfast ... well, I followed his advice and I got worse!

Just a question: what kind of foods are you eating?

This IBS thing really does suck, but I must say I'm better than I was a couple of years ago ... I've really been working hard on my stress levels (I'm an extremely tense, anxious person). I don't think stress caused my IBS per say, but I do notice that whenever my IBS is acting up, stress makes it worse ...

Well, do post again and until then take care.

From: **Canada**

Stuart999
New Member

Hello Minimum, thank you for your reply.

I am also a stressed kind of person, due to many traumatic things that happened to me as a child, for which I have had various types of therapy for. What seems to be helping, at the moment, is that I am not eating anything other than plain toast and bottled water. This seems to be the only thing that my bowel seems to take no notice from. But I have tried various diets and eating more of some things and less of others. I even have seen a diet specialist; she was as useful as a chocolate teapot and an ashtray on a motorbike.

It has been the last few months that have been majorly up and down. I have always been bad with IBS, but it did get it under some kind of control, to where it was at a balance. But now all hell has let loose (forgive the pun).

Stuart

From: **Southampton, UK**

Minimum
Prolific Member

Hmmm ... well, for me personally, I find that not only eating too much sets my IBS off, but eating too little (or not often enough) ... so I've taken to eating something at least every three hours ... hard to do sometimes when I'm at work though.

From: **Canada**

Twin24life
Prolific Member

Hello Stuart and welcome. I have been visiting this web site for almost 2 months now and it is a great place to come to. We all here try our best in helping others. I have had IBS-D for almost 3 years now. I hope you find comfort and support here like I have.

From: **Washington USA**

Forum II: <u>GI-related Diagnostic Tests</u>

"Discuss what to expect or how you feel about medical procedures such as colonoscopy, sigmoidoscopy, endoscopy, barium enema, GI series (barium swallow)."

The tests commonly prescribed by gastroenterologists can be invasive and uncomfortable. Dealing with such procedures when a body already feels terrible can be very stressful. The posts on the "Diagnostic Tests" forum provide tips for getting through the ordeal of some of the usual medical tests ordered when a patient describes having symptoms that could be IBS.

<u>Discussion</u>: Colonoscopy.

Topic: Colonoscopy on Mon. VERY nervous! Can you answer some questions?

Irishbuzzer
New Member

Hi,

I have been reading the posts here and they have been very helpful but I have a few extra things to ask.

Basically, I have gallstones (which took ages to find out, before which the doctors had me convinced I was mad!)

Anyway, I met my surgeon on Wednesday, and he said many people rush into surgery for the removal of the gallbladder, and afterwards still have severe pain. In lots of cases the gallstones are hiding something, such as IBS.

So, he wants to do some tests. Well I jumped off the bed when he told me this, and since then I have not been able to shake off my nerves.

He is going to do two tests—all I picked up was a camera was going to go where the sun doesn't shine!

He said he would make me sleepy first. Does that mean I will be out of it or just pain free?

Does the Doctor maneuver you into the position before or after the drugs take?

Do you lie on your side?

How long does the test take?

Will I be okay to dress myself soon after, or do I have to wait around to recover?

How long afterwards can I leave for home?

Sorry for asking really daft questions, I am just so nervous and trying to get my head around what happens.

Thanks for taking a look!

From: **N.Ireland**

Kwatson
New Member

Hello. I had a colonoscopy one month ago and I was also afraid. Actually it wasn't that bad. They give you an enema or enemas until your stool is clear and then they give you an IV. For me, they then took me into another room where they would do the procedure. The nurse told me she was going to put some medicine in my IV and that's all I remembered until I was woken up by the doctor. You will be able to dress yourself but you will need a ride home. The next day I had some stomach pains, although not too bad. Oh yeah, they have you lay on your side, but your gown is covering you, right before you are put to sleep. I wouldn't be afraid if I had to do it again.

From: **6475n.lincoln**

AMC
Very Prolific Member

I didn't have an enema this past time, but I have had one in the past, when I couldn't stomach the prep liquid they gave me. I've had Colitis for 20 years, and I'm only 30, so I've had about four colonoscopies. Believe me when I say that the prep is a lot worse than the actual test. Just keep some magazines on hand, some hand-held computer games, crossword puzzles, etc., because after you drink your prep you will be in the potty for quite a while. My husband even brought the television into the bathroom for me, LOL. I went from the potty to the bathtub for most of the day, because you begin to get pretty raw after having D for so long, and a hot bath is soothing, or at least it was for me. (This is going to sound kinda gross, but I just want to be honest with you … PAT, do not wipe, when you start to feel raw. I know you'll probably be thinking you are not getting clean, but it hurts SO MUCH worse if you wipe … so just pat gently … again, sorry to be graphic, but that is what worked for me!! Also, keep some Vaseline on hand, that helps with the pain too …) I'd say I probably had a good 5 or 6 hours of potty time. I'd be okay for about 10 or 15 minutes at a time, and then have to go again.

The stuff they gave me to drink didn't taste good at all, but at least it wasn't much to have to drink. I believe I figured it out to be about three cups. In the past, I've had to drink the Go-Lytely prep, and that was a GALLON to drink, so three cups was pretty easy to swallow compared to that!! It tastes bad, but just mix it with some 7-Up or Sprite, and drink it with a straw so it goes down fast. And after you drink it, make SURE you are near a potty.

The test itself is not bad. I went in and they put me in this little waiting room, hooked me up to an IV, and let my Mom and my husband come in and talk to me until it was time for my test. Then when it was time, they wheeled me into the examination room, put some medication into my IV, and I was in la-la land, LOL. I could sort of tell what was going on, but didn't care, if that makes sense?? Like I could see my colon on the TV, but I don't remember feeling any pain or anything. They told me that anytime I moaned or made any sort of noise like I was in discomfort (which I don't remember making any noise at all, but I guess I did!!), they gave me a little more of the sedation medication to help me relax. I got through the test pretty easily, and was actually awake while they were wheeling me to the recovery room. I never slept after my test. They said that was kind of odd, because it's hard to wake most people up after those tests. But I have to take sleeping pills at night to help me sleep, and they said that can make the sedation medicine not work quite as well.

You'll be pretty groggy for most of the day more than likely. I'd say plan to stay at home for the rest of the day to rest. I had some D after my test, but NOTHING like the prep. I just remember napping a lot.

I think the worrying about the test is MUCH worse than the test itself. You'll do fine I'm sure!! If you have any questions, don't hesitate to e-mail me. I'd be glad to help answer anything I can!! And good luck with your test!!

From: **United States**

Irishbuzzer
New Member

Ashley and Kathy THANK YOU so very much, I feel calmer already from reading your posts.

I guess I am lucky in a way, as I have the prep to take at home tomorrow. It won't be as bad using my own bathroom as it would be to have to do so in hospital.

From: **N.Ireland**

Topic: Had Colonoscopy! It was a breeze!

Irishbuzzer
New Member

Hi,

Well I have not slept much since I got my appointment last Thursday, nor have I been able to eat much, so the prep was not too bad.

It was stinky, but orange juice helped it a bit. There was a time that no sooner had I left the bathroom then I was running back again, but that soon passed.

I was VERY nervous about today. Luckily my parents are paying for me to go private, which means I went to a small, friendly clinic with the best surgeon doing the procedure.

I had been told by my friends that I would be sleepy but able to follow the doctor's instructions, like hell I was!

They put the drugs into me, then a mouth guard (also had to have the camera put down into my stomach) I remember gagging a bit and then I woke up in recovery.

It was AMAZING!

I swear I would never worry again if I had to have it done in the future.

I was asleep for ages! Probably catching up on all my missed sleep.

I get embarrassed easily, so I imagined my bum being showed off for all to see, but the nurses had my dressing gown draped over me so that I was covered.

Apart from feeling a little dizzy—I would not even know I had had anything done today.

Anyway, just thought I would let everyone know how I got one and thanks for all the support!

Bye
Emma

From: **N.Ireland**

Topic: Colonoscopy prep

Bates
New Member

Is there one type of prep that is easier for IBS folks than others? Which is the least likely to cause IBS cramping? Thanks.

From: **Maryland**

Kselibrary
Very Prolific Member

I cannot do the GoLytely. There is just too much of it. I do the phospho soda and enema prep. That phospho soda is not the best tasting, in fact, well, it's horrid … but I chill it and drink it mixed in as little liquid as possible, so I can just gulp it down, and then follow it with a 7-up mixer, and a swish and rinse of root beer. Sounds insane, I know, but it works for me.

From: **U S of A**

Bates
New Member

But the prep didn't trigger a major flare up of IBS? No major cramps? That's my main concern. I can hold my nose and drink just about anything, and as for being in the bathroom a lot—hey that's pretty much my life anyway.

From: **Maryland**

Kselibrary
Very Prolific Member

I don't know that I would term it a flare-up of IBS. I will say that whatever you take will cause a bit of cramping, it's the nature of the beast. To stimulate good elimination they will have to make the colon MOVE, and to do that you often get cramping. I would call it more of an urgency to GET IN THERE AND GET RID OF IT. A little tip here: the less you have in the colon to move out, the less you have to eliminate, so try a very light diet two days before, and liquid diet the day before your prep.

My husband recently had his first colonoscopy as part of his over 50 check-up. He does not have IBS or Crohn's, in other words, he has normal bowel activity. He did the phospho soda and enema prep [same gut doctor—same prep] and I asked him about cramping. He said he felt mild cramping, but the urgency was he remembers most. That and the taste of that phospho soda.

I don't see what you could take that would cause you no cramping. It's what happens when you are forcing the colon to clear out. The enema alone causes me mild cramping.

If you find a way to do this with no cramping, I'd love to know what it is. I've tried three different ways to do this and find the phospho soda way to be about the most effective and the quickest means to an end.

Karen

From: **U S of A**

Bkitepilot
Prolific Member

Bates, good luck with your testing.

The sodium bicarb (phospho soda) tastes tart, but tolerable. I can't drink it or I get extremely sick with cramps, cold sweats and that sick-all-over feeling, and inevitably I end up vomiting. I can take the GoLytely since it hydrates you with needed electrolytes, which help to stop the cramping and dehydration caused by explosive clean-outs. I take it slowly though. Four ounces every half hour until the gallon is almost gone. Phew, you sure don't raise your rear off the potty for a few hours.

Good luck with whatever prep you choose.

Belinda (queen of GoLytely)

From: **North Georgia**

Kselibrary
Very Prolific Member

The phospho soda is nasty, but there is so little to drink when compared to the GoLytely. I take what I consider to be the lesser of two evils. I still say no matter what prep you take you will have cramping and sweats, as well as that all over sick feeling. It again … is the nature of the beast. The reason you are doing this is to clean you out. To clean you out they must stimulate elimination, which will cause your colon to go into the processes it uses to produce elimination.

Golytely is just so much to ingest that if you are a gaggy person [much like myself], the thought of the sheer amount of liquid to ingest is daunting. Phospho soda is NASTY. I hate it, but it is what I can get down, and keep down, and get the effect needed for a good 'scoping.'

There are also some tablets that you can take, and I have heard varying thoughts on an effective cleaning-out with them. I just figure if I am going to do this thing, I only want to have to do it once. If I took all those pills and then went in only to be told I wasn't cleaned out enough, I would be devastated.

Let us know how it goes. Keep that phospho cold and break it down into small amounts in a bathroom Dixie cup with 7-up. It is a psychological boost to know "hey, that is only a couple gulps, I can do this." Get it down, take a sip or two of a root beer chaser, rest up a sec, mix the next little bit up and go for it again until it is gone.

From: **U S of A**

Dbab
New Member

To me, personally, the magnesium citrate is not nearly as bad as the phospho. You only drink a 10 oz. bottle of mag cit with 8 oz. of water. Then you take your four pills a few hours later and a suppository in the morning. You have to drink about 8 oz. of water every hour but you don't have to drink a lot at one time.

Oh and I almost forgot … ask for the lemon flavor!!

From: **Texas**

Shineon7
New Member

I had the phospho soda prep and I didn't think it was bad at all. I mixed one table-spoon of the 1.5 fl oz. bottle with 8 oz. of apple juice and it tasted fine. It was a little salty because the phospho has sodium in it, but it really wasn't bad at all.

From: **New York**

Mporl77
New Member

I tried the orange Colyte. Nasty in any flavor quite frankly. Just down as much as you can every two minutes. Even I couldn't finish the gallon, I was too full. It took longer than I expected to work, but then I was going quite often.

It still was working two days after my exam. So don't expect to hold down a big meal immediately.

From: **Orlando**

Topic: Colonoscopy prep HELP!!!!!!!!!!!

Stayhomew2
New Member

I am doing the colonoscopy prep right now. Do you have any clues as to how to get this stuff down? I have to force it down, and it is not very fun. I tried flavoring it with Crystal Light like the doctor said, but I am still having problems. HELP!!!!!!!!!!!!!!!! Would appreciate any input!!!!!!!!!!!!!

Stayhome

P.S. I am already so sore that can hardly sit.

From: **Iowa**

Harleighgirl
New Member

What kind of prep are you doing? I've done phospho twice. The first time was hard to get down as I mixed the phospho with apple juice. This last time, I mixed it with ice water and drank it through a straw, and it was a lot better. Some people mix it in Gatorade, or Sprite. Just make sure you don't drink anything with blue or red dyes, it can show up as blood or something during the test. And don't worry about the test—it's not bad at all. Good luck.

From: **Salt Lake City**

Stayhomew2
New Member

Well, the test can't be any worse then this stuff. Having to drink a gallon is killing me, especially since I only weigh 95 pounds. Will let you know how it goes.

Stayhome

From: **Iowa**

Janice 54
Regular Member

Stayhome, yes, the prep is much worse than the test. I'll be thinking of you tonight. Try to relax and know that it will be over soon.

Janice

From: **CA**

Boxgirl73
Prolific Member

Next time, request the Fleet phosphor-soda-it's only a 3 oz. bottle-you drink half at 4:30 PM and the other half at 8:30 PM. Still tastes disgusting even if you mix it with very cold ginger-ale, but there's really no getting around the taste. However, it's much easier than having to drink a gallon of GoLytely.

Glad you're done!!!!

From: **Philadelphia**

OppOnn
Very Prolific Member

Next time also look into MiraLax with 2 Dulcolax tablets. They taste of nothing at all.

From: **New York, USA**

Glenda
Prolific Member

I used the Fleet Phospho soda and it took 12 hours for it to work.

Took it at 1:00 in the afternoon and by 1:00 AM I was on the potty going like a river.

The stuff works well but tastes horrible, like dead road kill.

From: **Washington**

OppOnn
Very Prolific Member

A big trick is to eat very, very lightly at least 2 or 3 days before the liquid day before.

Then, there'll be less to get rid of and a less strenuous time on the potty.

From: **New York, USA**

Fourstars
New Member

Ask for the pills. I have had to have two done in the last 6 weeks and I did the colyte once and the pills once. I REALLY prefer the pills!

Pam

From: **DFW Texas**

Waylock
New Member

I'm scheduled for September colonoscopy and fear the nausea and cramping with the phospho stuff. I still choose pain over nausea but this constant abdominal pain is getting old real quick. Any hints on the prep, or good reports regarding how ya feel, other than an urge to spend night on potty ....

Signed: Apprehensive

From: **Twin Cities Minnesota**

Jane54
New Member

Waylock, I just did my prep last night. I drank one 10 oz. bottle of magnesium citrate (didn't taste bad), then an hour later drank two liters of NuLytely pineapple flavor. I drank all of this through a straw and didn't have any problems. I was entirely finished with the prep and bathroom visits by 10:00 PM and I started at 5:00 PM. I had NO cramping or pain, but a really sore bottom. The actual test was a cakewalk. I don't remember a thing! Demerol is wonderful! Good Luck!!!

From: **Ohio**

Topic: Virtual colonoscopy? Anyone?

Gilly
Prolific Member

Virtual colonoscopy is a type of CAT scan which has just started in Australia. You do need the same prep as before the usual colonoscopy, but no anesthesia, since it is only a scan. The colon is inflated with air. I am being sent some more information. It can visualize the outside of the bowel, also, and in 3-D. The whole process takes 20 minutes. No camera is swallowed.

Has anyone had this test? More or less embarrassing? Is it useful? Thanks.

Gilly

From: **Brisbane Australia**

Kmottus
Very Prolific Member

When I read some detailed descriptions of the studies they were doing on this procedure, one thing I noted that you may need to be prepared for, is that the inflating of the colon can be uncomfortable. A fair number of people who had to do both, because they found a polyp or something that needed a biopsy, found that the regular one was more comfortable because they were knocked out and couldn't feel anything.

I know some people with IBS have more pain with inflation than normal people, so it may be something you want to talk over with the doctor—to see if there is anything they want to do in case you run into discomfort. At the least I would practice some relaxation techniques, since any CAT scan can be claustrophobic, and anything that helps relax you will be useful.

K.

From: **NC USA**

OppOnn
Very Prolific Member

My understanding about the virtual colonoscopy is that while it is good, if they find polyps, you will still have to have the classic colonoscopy anyway, in order to take them out and to get a biopsy.

Since I had a polyp with my last colonoscopy, I don't think I am a good candidate for the virtual colonoscopy. If one has no polyps that one knows of, I guess one has to make a decision whether to risk the virtual colonoscopy or not.

From: **New York, USA**

ERBadger
New Member

This is pretty much brand new in the U.S. also. One of my friends works in the radiology department of a hospital here and said they just got it set up. What I have heard is that this is not a replacement for the regular examination; however since it is a significantly less invasive test, people can have it done more often. If they do find a polyp, they still have to do the real test, but for someone who is not at high risk, this is a great way to have your self checked!

From: **Wisconsin**

Rose
Very Prolific Member

I was told the main downfall of the virtual colonoscopy is that it is possible that it will not detect some of the smaller polyps that a regular colonoscopy would. As long as you have to do the prep anyway, I would opt for the real thing, so any polyps that may be found can be removed right then and there.

From: **Massachusetts**

Discussion: Colonoscopy with Endoscopy.

Topic: COLONOSCOPY AND ENDOSCOPY THE SAME DAY-EARLY MORNING 7 AM

IBSulcerandmuchmore
Regular Member

Hey guys, I have an endoscopy and colonoscopy scheduled together. Are there any pros and cons of having these tests performed on the same day? Will these tests show whether or not I have Crohn's? How good are these tests and what are they are capable of showing? How painful are these tests? I have a prescription of "NuLytely" which I must have before the day of the procedure. I would really appreciate if you could help me find answers to the above mentioned questions.

Many thanks.

From: **USA**

NancyCat
Very Prolific Member

I had an endoscopy and colonoscopy, scheduled one right after the other. For me, the benefit was that I was sedated just once and the doctor was able to tell me right away what he saw from the scopes. They are both done with highly sophisticated fiber optic equipment and if they find anything, e.g. a polyp, etc, it can be removed right then and there. Often they take random biopsies of tissue in there. At the place where I went, they gave me a color printed map of both tests with findings pointed out, and also two pictures. I'm not sure exactly what diseases these scopes can pick up, I think it shows if you have any inflammation or abnormalities which might point to a specific disease. I believe that both tests are considered the gold standard for seeing inside the colon and stomach these days. I was also glad to have both of them over at once. I had a slight sore throat from the upper endoscopy, which is normal, and I passed a lot of gas from the colonoscopy. I was sedated and didn't feel a thing.

Nancy

From: **MA, USA**

Discussion: Endoscopy.

Topic: First Endoscopy—Scared

Irrational enigma
New Member

I'm new to this and slightly uncomfortable. I have an endoscopy soon and I'm a little scared. So:

*I have a big fear a vomiting (insane, I know.) I was wondering if anyone had nausea or vomiting with this procedure. Possibly from being under sedation?

*Any other complications I should expect?

*Will this actually help in diagnosing IBS, (suspected problem) or will I need more tests?

I would really appreciate any response, even though I may be worried for no reason.

Thanks!

From: **Kentucky, USA**

Heather83
Regular Member

Hey, I had an endoscopy done a year ago.

I didn't vomit or get nauseous. They don't put you totally under. It just kind of relaxes you, makes you sleepy, and makes you forget the procedure happened.

The thing that hurt the most for me was the IV, but I hate needles.

They'll hook you up to all kinds of machines. I think it was a blood pressure cuff, a heart monitor, and something else. They give you the meds through your IV and then within seconds you will be sleepy.

They ask you to swallow and you do even though you won't remember them asking or you doing it. I remember feeling a full feeling like there was something big in my tummy. But it didn't hurt ... just a weird feeling. You're in a dreamlike state anyway. The doctor took some biopsies and I was done. The actual procedure didn't take very long. It's the waiting and anticipation that gets you.

Afterwards, there are no restrictions on what you can eat or drink. You might have a sore throat afterwards. I did.

Overall, this test was the easiest for me other than an ultrasound.

I'd rather have another endoscopy done than do the barium swallow (an upper GI with a small bowel follow through) again.

If nothing is found in the endoscopy, they may have you do the barium X-ray or the dreaded colonoscopy ... but I've heard that the prep is the worst for the colonoscopy and that the procedure is easy.

Good luck ... and just remember to take deep breaths ... it relieves the anxiety ...

From: **Illinois**

Stedwell
Prolific Member

I'm a real baby with tests and this one really was fine. I hardly remember anything. The worst bit was when they used the throat spray to numb it before they gave me the sedation. Don't worry!

From: **England**

Luna
Very Prolific Member

For a GI test, an upper endoscopy is a breeze! No prep other than no food or drink after midnight (or whenever your doc tells you the cutoff is) and you get nice la-la land drugs during the procedure.

I felt kind of queasy because my blood sugar was low, but that was it. They numb the back of your throat with a spray so you won't gag. My throat was scratchy for a few hours after the drugs wore off but before the irritation wore off.

An upper endoscopy is generally done if you have acid reflux (GERD), suspected hiatal hernia, etc. It cannot diagnose IBS, which is more of an intestinal problem.

If you are having an upper endoscopy, make sure your doctor takes a culture to test for h. pylori in your stomach. The doc probably was planning on it anyhow, but doesn't hurt to ask. It's a lot easier for them to get the culture now than later, and blood tests for those bacteria can give a false negative.

From: **Ohio, USA**

Kate C
Prolific Member

Endoscopies are easy. I used to say they were fun … come on, you miss school to get fun drugs … what could be better? LOL

It can't diagnose IBS. IBS is not a condition that can be detected with any test, all tests on people with IBS come back normal. The tests are done to rule out other diseases (Crohn's disease and ulcerative colitis, GERD, colon cancer, etc.)

How many tests you want to have should be something you take up with your doctor. Some people feel better if they have every test possible, just to rule out any small possibility that it could be something serious, and some people would rather just be diagnosed based on normal blood and stool tests, and skip the really expensive, invasive testing.

Good luck … you have nothing to worry about.

Kate

From: **Illinois**

Topic: Endoscopy

IBS4me223
New Member

I have to get an upper endoscopy! I'm VERY, VERY nervous. Can anybody tell me what it is like and the possible after-effects also?

If you can, reply, and thanks a bunch!

From: **Ohio**

NancyCat
Very Prolific Member

I had two of them and they were really no big deal at all. I had a very light general anesthesia because I had had another different procedure under "sedation" and had a bad reaction to it. There is NO PREP other than nothing to eat or drink after midnight the night before. You will have an IV with some medication to relax you. I had to bite on a rubber dam sort of thing with a big hole in the middle (like a donut on its side with a big hole in it). I thought this was so you don't break your teeth biting on the scope, which sort of looks like a long black tube. I remember seeing it on an instrument table. My husband is an operating room nurse and he said you bite on it so you won't damage the equipment. LOL. I vaguely remember hearing people telling me to swallow, I think.

When it was over I was put in a recovery room and they checked my vital signs a few times, and then I was given discharge instructions and left. You can't drive or do anything potentially dangerous afterward for 24 hours, you also shouldn't cook, because some of the medications can make you forget things. In my case I was awake and alert and dressed, and ready to leave in 20 minutes, which is really fast, but that's how I react to medications. Many people are a bit sleepy afterward and most facilities ask that you have someone to come and drive you home. The beauty of this procedure, in my experience and opinion, is that your DR will tell you what he/she saw on your endoscopy before you go home, so you do not have to wait for someone to read an X-ray. The place where I had my test gave me a color print-out of a picture of my stomach with a coded map of the structures.

You might have some excess upper abdominal gas (I believe they put in air to better see the structures) and you could burp a bit. You may have a sore throat for a day or so from the scope. I went with a friend of mine for her endoscopy last year (at a different hospital) and she said had to swallow some blue liquid that didn't taste good. Maybe I had to also but I don't remember. I had a polyp in my duodenum which was removed at the same time and in my case I had to have liquids for the remainder of that day, next day regular food as tolerated. Don't be nervous, it's really a very easy procedure and I am the queen of nervous wrecks.

Hope this helps.

Nancy

From: **Massachusetts**

Discussion: Capsule Endoscopy.

Topic: Capsule Endoscopy

StormTrackr
Prolific Member

I am having this test done on the 17th of this month. I have to use the Magnesium Citrate Prep which is no biggie. I know I should ring my GI's office on this question, but I am going to ask it here as well. Do I really have to shave six inches above and below my navel? Also, the instructions say no smoking for 24 hours prior to the exam. Not sure if I could do that; but reckon I have to try so the test is as accurate as possible.

From: **Taylorsville, KY USA**

Vipers
Prolific Member

I had the test about a month ago and I was not told to do any kind of preparation, except for not eating after 12:00 the night before. Also, if you are hairy in that area you definitely should shave because it will hurt very badly when pulling the applicators off after the test. Pulling the applicators off I guess you can compare to waxing, because it will pull off all the hair.

From: **Fresh Meadows, NY, US**

Jleigh
Very Prolific Member

I had the test in September and was told not to eat the day before after noon, and clear liquids after that until midnight and then "nothing". I also had to drink the magnesium citrate. I survived the mag citrate but I didn't like it.

The actual test was a breeze. If you are male and hairy, yes … you would want to shave. The probes are put around on the abdomen and are very, very sticky. I guess that is why they want you to shave.

Jleigh

From: **USA**

Discussion: Sigmoidoscopy.

Topic: Sigmoidoscopy? What is it?

Jondoe
New Member

What is a sigmoidoscopy exactly? How much of the colon does it examine? Is this better/worse than other tests?

Kmottus
Very Prolific Member

It is a scope they put in your colon from the anus that looks at the rectum, the part of the colon that bends (sigmoid) over from the side to the rectum and the descending colon (the left side).

It is less invasive, but less complete than a colonoscopy (which is a scope that looks at the whole colon and the end of the small intestine), and is often done without the sedation that is typically given for a colonoscopy.

Depending on your symptoms there may not be a need for the full colonoscopy, but enough that they want to do a sigmoidoscopy.

K.

From: **NC USA**

Nikki*
Very Prolific Member

Sigmoid isn't that bad, but it isn't nice either. Apparently it doesn't "hurt", but it's uncomfortable. Having anything shoved up your back passage isn't too nice really (unless you are into that kind of thing).

They blow air into you as well. That feels weird. I didn't like that bit! I haven't had a colonoscopy so I can't compare them. Sorry.

From: **UK, London**

Topic: Totally confused + scared—sigmoidoscopy?!

Ama
Prolific Member

Please can anyone advise??

I've had IBS for years—had a colonoscopy five years ago, all clear. It was painful (very) but they increased the sedation and now I don't really remember it. I had a good doc do it. He said I have a very tortuous and long bowel, which makes it even more likely gas gets trapped.

Anyway, I am now booked for a sigmoidoscopy in ten days time, different doc, but a good one, who does lots of these, I'm told. I asked his secretary about sedation, etc., and she said they didn't give any!!! And no preparation to empty the bowel either!!! I thought sigmoidoscopy always needed both!? What should I do/ think? Is this normal? I'm so scared that it will be a) painful and b) messy!!

Any advice or info? I'd welcome anything you can suggest/tell me!

Many thanks,

Ama

From: **UK**

Boxgirl73
Prolific Member

Don't worry-a sigmoid is a test that everyone over 50 has to get—so, it's nothing! (You may not be 50 but I'm just trying to say that it's very common). I have had three of these prior to my colonoscopy. It's not a big deal—but I was told that I could have sedation if I wanted. I am one person that does need it—can't stand the pain of the air! No prep is usually needed as long as you go to the bathroom in the AM. It's not messy. You'll be outta of there in five minutes.

From: **Philadelphia**

Ama
Prolific Member

Many thanks for your help! It does give me some peace of mind—and I'll check out the possibilities of sedation as I'd really like that too!

From: **UK**

Jupiter119
Very Prolific Member

Hi

I had a sigmoidoscopy last year. Was sent an enema in the post from the hospital to use an hour before appointment time.

It wasn't painful, just a bit uncomfortable. No sedation was offered at my hospital (UK). Only took 10 minutes or so. The worst bit was that I was scared I'd need the toilet while they did the test, as had been 'going' so many times prior to it. Was reassured that it wouldn't happen.

From: **UK**

Topic: Sigmoidoscopy

Christywisty
Prolific Member

I'm having a sigmoidoscopy done on July 10, and I've never had one before. I've read some of these posts about people being given some drugs?? As I recall, I'm not going to get a bit of medication. I know it's only supposed to last 6–8 minutes, but I'm already in constant pain (from other diseases), so why am I not being offered any medication?

From: **NC**

Betagirl
Very Prolific Member

Hi.

I had a flexible sigmoidoscopy to check out my lovely fissure. I received no medication; it was done in the doctor's office versus having to go down to the GI lab where the colonoscopy and other fun tests are done. I'm not going to lie to you, it's uncomfortable. They have to make this turn to flip the camera around, and that's probably the worst part. It's not the worst thing I've ever had done, but if you have low pain tolerance you may want to ask for a mild sedative that they may be able to give you in the office.

Good luck!

Crohnie

From: **Chicago, IL**

Christywisty
Prolific Member

Thank you so much for your reply. I guess I'm just nervous about it. I think if my endoscopy hasn't killed me yet, I will probably manage the sigmoidoscopy just fine. It's certainly not going to be the most pleasant morning of my life … but it could be worse. I don't look forward to the Fleets, though …

From: **NC**

Discussion: Barium Enema.

Topic: Concern about a Barium Enema

Cigarello
Prolific Member

Hi, I saw my GI doc and described my symptoms. He feels a colonoscopy would be good but we settled upon a barium enema. My question is this, with my type of constipation (only a little comes out and only in the morning no matter what I eat or how much fiber I take), I am concerned because after the test you have to expel the barium; I honestly don't think I will be able to expel it because I can never ever, ever expel more than a couple ounces at any given time of poop. Thanks for your input.

From: **Farmington Hills, Michigan**

Hyacynth26
Prolific Member

To tell the truth I'd do the scope. You have to cleanse anyway, and they drug you for the scope. You'll wish you were drugged for the BE. If they find anything or don't they will probably want to do a scope anyway. In my opinion BE's are nearly obsolete. They can do a lot with scopes, take biopsies, remove polyps and see a lot of the colon.

From: **USA**

Cgd21
Regular Member

I agree with Hyacinth26. Barium enemas are becoming obsolete. Insist on the colonoscopy. I had one on Monday and he removed a very small polyp. I never expected to have one as I don't do anything that might cause one, i.e. drink, smoke, sedentary, family history, eat meat and I always eat vegetables and fruits.

I'd forget the BE and go with the scope.

From: **New York**

Weener
Very Prolific Member

I don't usually post on this site, but when I saw the subject I thought I would. I would have to agree the colonoscopy is more thorough of the two. If something is to be found, the colonoscopy will find it. I've had both done. They sedated me during the colonoscopy and I didn't really feel or remember much. With the BE, I was not sedated. The secret to the BE is to try to relax and breathe through the procedure. I am also IBS C and I didn't have any problems getting rid of the barium. You are cleaned out the day before, and when you go in for the procedure the barium will flow into you and air is added as well. So when you are done, the first thing you want to do is pass gas, that's when I had to run to the bathroom and get rid of some of the barium. Try to be near a toilet that day. I'm sure it will come out. I'm sorry if I was too graphic. Good luck.

From: **Wellandport, Ontario, CANADA**

Victoria01
Regular Member

Hi. Can't imagine why you settled on a barium enema. What the others wrote about the colonoscopy is right on target.

However, responding to your question, you do need to expel all the barium or you may find yourself being treated in the ER. Don't hesitate to ask your doctor what's best for you. Our systems aren't all alike. When I had a BE, I was given a laxative to take after getting home and ordered to drink water for the rest of the day. After prepping for two days, I couldn't stand to take any more laxatives, and my bottom was soooo sore. I took a very warm enema with a lot of Vaseline on the tube to get the rest of the barium out, and it worked.

With all due respect, it sounds like you need to take charge here. This is your body, not your doctor's. If you want the colonoscopy and are afraid that you won't be able to evacuate the barium, talk to your doctor again. I think the colonoscopy is better for diagnostics, anyway.

Good luck.

Victoria

From: **Glendale, CA**

4WillieC
Very Prolific Member

Add me to the list ... no way I would do that BE ... strictly old hat now ... only thing good about them is that they are cheaper ... but regardless of cost, why not just do the scope? Like was said, you prep pretty much the same, there is usually no pain or even any memory of the procedure at all, and if they find anything in the BE, you can bet you will have to do the colonoscopy anyway ... so why not just cut to the chase? My two cents ...

From: **Sweet Georgia**

Vikee
Very Prolific Member

Does anyone think a barium enema would be better than a colonoscopy to see if parts of the colon are twisted or show spasms?

I don't think a colonoscopy would be good for that. My GI Doctor doesn't seem concerned about a twisted colon since he says people without IBS could have that.

And from symptoms, he feels I do have spasms and seeing it would not help in treatment.

He wants a colonoscopy for cancer screening. I'm more concerned with a colon that may be better off with parts of it removed. Of course I'm no expert but can tell a certain part of my lower descending colon is the main problem relating to spasms and should be removed. (I know the spasms may start in another place.) I could never tell him this, he'd think I'm nuts, and he would probably be right!!

Any thoughts?

Vikee

From: **PA, USA**

4WillieC
Very Prolific Member

I would think that if you had a twisted colon (volvulus), there would be a significant amount of symptomatic evidence for the physician to suspect such a condition. Plus, you can usually detect a volvulus from a clear plate X-ray. I would think that after thoroughly explaining your symptoms to the GI doc, I would go with their recommendation for a diagnostic modality.

From: **Sweet Georgia**

Vikee
Very Prolific Member

Willie thanks!

I needed to hear your words. I agree with you.

Sometimes I get carried away with IBS visions!!!

Vikee

From: **PA, USA**

Topic: Barium Enema Help—Please

Nic D
Regular Member

I'm due to have a barium enema soon and am not looking forward to the laxative you have to take first, as I have a fissure which is painful and D makes it worse. I was just wondering how often this stuff makes you go and whether it causes much abdominal pain.

Thanks everyone.

From: **UK**

Brenda2
New Member

It depends on what you are taking. I drank a bottle of Magnesium Citrate and had results in about an hour. I think the most tiring part was getting up off the couch to run to the bathroom!

Cramping was mild.

I have also used Dulcolax. Three tablets provided results in about 90 minutes. I think three trips to the bathroom is all it took to clean me out.

From: **PA**

Gizzyluver
New Member

When I had this test done, I had to use three types of laxatives in a 16 hour period before the test. What seemed to make it as fast and painless as possible was drinking a lot of water, which they suggested to do. In the first six hours of prep, the first laxative worked almost right away and I only had to go maybe twice … and very mild cramping. I had the test at 8:00 AM and started preparing for it at noon the previous day. It was annoying, but I had a better experience (if you can ever call a barium better) than some have had … good luck.

From: **MA**

Joe 90
New Member

I can't remember the name of the stuff I took. It came in sachets which you mixed with water. I started taking mine the morning before the enema, but it wasn't until lunch time that it took effect. When it did though, I was back and forth to the toilet all the time, even up until the examination. Don't think the cramping was too bad though.

From: **S Wales, UK**

Topic: Barium Enema Pain?

ColonDragon
New Member

Just a question about the BE exam, which I just had. I knew it would be uncomfortable, but it was one of the worst pains I ever experienced. It was wicked stomach cramping, far worse than anything I ever experienced, and I just don't feel "right" afterwards. The radiologist didn't seem to be put out by it. Anyone else ever experience this?

From: **Canada**

Desirae
Regular Member

I had mine a few months ago and it hurt like hell. I was in tears the whole time. I was lied to actually by my mother telling me that nothing would go inside my butt and it wouldn't hurt or be uncomfortable. I guess she knew that if I knew that then I wouldn't go. So I went in thinking it was just gonna be like having your leg X-rayed. It really sucked. And then when it felt like I needed to go, the radiologist was just in there taking 300 pictures. I kept crying telling her how much it hurt and she was just like "you're fine" and would even leave me in there for like a few minutes! Alone! I was like "no!" It was horrible. I was all right afterwards, just my butt was sore and I was a bit constipated, but other than that I was okay.

What exactly do you mean by you don't feel right??

From: **Dallas, TX**

ColonDragon
New Member

By "don't feel right" was just as you said, feeling kind of constipated, but my lower abdomen is still a little sore as well. I think it was also because the pain was so unexpected.

I understand they usually insert a balloon and inflate air into you to assist the procedure, but I didn't have that done, they just went ahead and "injected" the barium solution.

From: **Canada**

Desirae
Regular Member

Oh really? That's weird. I wonder if there's a difference in pain or anything.

Yeah, they told me to drink LOTS of fluids to help with the constipation.

From: **Dallas, TX**

YJ01
New Member

I totally know how you feel. I had mine a couple of years ago and right after they well, "inserted" the thing up my behind, I started panicking. I was in pain, feeling numb, and couldn't respond to the doctors. Fortunately afterwards everything was fine, or it just went back to how it had been (which was the reason I had the exam in the first place.)

I'm having a hard time understanding this procedure, considering barium can be taken orally, of course it's nasty … but I think I'd take that over an enema just about any day.

Hope you've been feeling better!!

Y

From: **Berkeley**

Boxgirl73
Prolific Member

I had it and didn't have any pain during it (uncomfortable but not painful). Except when the doctor blew up the balloon to keep the fluids from coming out! OUCH! Cried during that, but the rest of the test was surprisingly painless! Gassy afterwards and white BMs for a couple of days due to the barium!

From: **Philadelphia**

GX600
New Member

I had a barium enema last Monday. I was surprised at how painless it was. I walked into the hospital at 15:20 and left at 16:00 all done, including 10 minutes waiting at the end. The worst bit was taking the laxatives the day before. The only bit that caused me any pain at all was when I had the tube inserted. I was just looking through the forum and thought I would add this to show people who may be concerned about having this procedure carried out that it doesn't have to cause any problems.

From: **UK**

Discussion: Upper GI Series (Barium Swallow)— Small Bowel Follow Through.

Topic: Small Bowel Follow Through

Firedancer
Regular Member

Anyone ever have a small bowel follow through? I am scheduled for one tomorrow and would like to get a little info about it. Any info would be greatly appreciated. Thank you.

From: **Arkansas**

BQ
Very Prolific Member

Fire,

If you are IBS D type with urgency, make sure you let them know, as that may affect how long they wait between follow through X-rays.

I found it to be a fairly benign and non-intrusive type test. Except, when I told the guy I had urgency and the nurse suggested only a 15-minute wait for the follow through X-ray, he just ignored her and me. Of course the barium was well past the "upper" portion of my intestines in the typical half hour wait that he thought was best.

So they didn't really get all the pictures they wanted. He was an egotistical twit. The nurse was wonderful though.

It is a snap to do the test. For me, I had to be near a bathroom the rest of the day, as the barium that I drank had an evacuation agent (read: laxative, probably LOL) in it, to help it clear out of the body. No cramps or anything, though. So I would plan on just relaxing at home when it is over.

I'll be thinking of you.

BQ

From: **USA**

NancyCat
Very Prolific Member

I had an upper GI series with a small bowel follow through many years ago. From what I remember they just took more X-rays for a longer period of time. Hope this helps.

Nancy

From: **Massachusetts**

Sues
Prolific Member

I just had one done recently, I was given white barium with lots of ice, (made it more palatable) and I was given a small glassful of barium several times during a two hour period, then had to wait 15 minutes, then X-rays. It was painless. I am IBS-C, so I had to drink lots and lots of water after and I have to take enemas for relief and I needed to after that. Nothing to this test, just time consuming, take a magazine or book to read.

From: **Texas**

Topic: Feeling better after small bowel follow through

J9n
New Member

This is the strangest thing. On Tuesday I had a SBFT, drinking barium. It gave me watery diarrhea for about 24 hours, but no cramps or pain. I have not had any cramping or pain or diarrhea since! What's up with that? I have gone from daily drop on the floor pain, to normal. I even tested myself by eating Mexican fast food (lettuce and refried beans, but not a lot). Nothing! I am sure it is going to come back, but I am a bit stumped by this. Any thoughts?

From: **California**

DirtBikJ
New Member

J, Take it slow. Don't let yourself think you have IBS whipped or it will come at you again. Chill out all the time if you can. I have my IBS pretty much under control, but last evening I let my guard down and ate a trigger food thinking I could handle it. It got me today. Had a small case of D.

Good Luck.

From: **Utah**

Bkitepilot
Prolific Member

Barium coats the intestines and makes it all feel better … but only for a little while. After the protective barrier pushes through, it will all go back to usual. Sorry.

From: **North Georgia**

Joanofarc
Very Prolific Member

Barium is constipating—which could be helping you since you have D and pain primarily. Could you take other constipating things? Have you tried antispasmodics?

From: **USA**

Kare_bear88
Regular Member

I've had 2 upper GIs with SBFT and a BE, and each time I was told to be careful because the barium is constipating. However, I found the opposite to be true; all of these tests caused me to have severe D for a few days after. I guess this could have been just because of the stress involved with having the tests though, or the lingering effects of the prep.

From: **Windsor, Ontario, Canada**

Laurenalexis
New Member

I feel for you. I recently had an upper GI, but instead of making everything better for a while; my bowel movements started decreasing and the color changed (which they tell you about barium). That stuff was so gross, though, that I never wanted to eat yogurt again, because that's what it tasted like.

From: **Atlanta, GA**

NancyCat
Very Prolific Member

I'll never have another Pina Colada ever again. I had an abdominal/pelvic cat scan and had to drink gobs of barium and Pina Colada was the flavor. It gave me such terrible gas too.

Nancy

From: **Massachusetts**

J9n
New Member

Yes, it does taste terrible, and my symptoms are now coming back, but I would gladly drink it again, just for that one week of relief!!

From: **California**

Joanofarc
Very Prolific Member

Gosh, I think you should order some of that stuff—acacia root—as it's chalky, fills the colon, has soluble fiber which is known to soothe the digestive tract, and slows peristalsis in folks with D. I'd really give it a try and see what happens. You could also try supplements that make one more C—is it calcium or potassium, I can't remember, or iron? It's one of those.

From: **USA**

NancyCat
Very Prolific Member

It's calcium. There's a lot of it in Caltrate in the pink bottle (I think). It has helped a lot of people on the BB with D.

Nancy

From: **Massachusetts**

Topic: AFTER THE BARIUM SWALLOW … NOT GOOD.

Sparkle*
Prolific Member

Ugh. I was hoping I'd be back to 'normal' by today! I had my barium meal/follow through X-ray on Thursday, and have managed to poop a lot *argh* but it's very white *eek* and I'm so bloated and crampy!

It's like having the worst wind ever, and I'm getting feelings of urgency (like when the runs wanna hit in) except it's solid *yum*

I was in the bathroom at half past two this morning for over half an hour, and I'm still not better.

Sorry to be so graphic, but I dunno what to do with myself. I did drink a lot of water afterwards, and I have a quick metabolism, so no C but this gassy, bloated, white, pooing thing is not fun.

Maybe I'll go hit the Milk of Magnesia … again.

I'm not sure whether the scan showed anything as over in the UK, doctors play 'hard to get' with results. I think they would've told me if it was anything really bad.

Is it usual for them to prod your stomach during the scanning? My doctor guy poked around on the right hand side of my stomach as he must've seen something, and it hurt all along where he pressed so ...?

I'm baffled and windy.

From: **London/Kent**

Stedwell
Prolific Member

When I had my barium swallow, they placed a medium squashy ball between my stomach and the X-ray machine, and pushed really hard in lots of different places. I even had to hold it in place a couple of times. They said they needed to press down on the stomach to flatten out the intestines, to get a better view of what is inside. It was uncomfortable. I guess that may be why they pressed down on your tummy.

From: **England**

Sparkle*
Prolific Member

Aw, thanks, Stedwell—I was kinda confused by the prodding.

(Oh, and the test I had was a barium follow through X-ray where I had to swallow a jug of chalky white slop and have scans at regular intervals to check my digestive tract. Think it was an upper check as I didn't have an enema)

Feeling a little better today after taking some Milk of Magnesia and drinking stacks of water last night.

How I long for a normal colored pooh! *ugh*

From: **London/Kent**

Barbara_in_blue
New Member

Ugh, I'm having bad barium flashbacks (like there's ever a good barium flashback?).

I had to drink three large glasses of orange-flavored snot that they kept calling barium for a CT scan (I'm pretty sure that's what it was, it definitely wasn't an X-ray and I don't think it was an MRI, but I could be wrong—after a while, all the big humming machines look alike). I had white poo for a week and a half, which I guess is not normal. I was told it should only last a few days at most, but mine just went on and on and on. They never warned me about the white poo thing, imagine my reaction when I saw my BMs had gone albino!

From: **Wisconsin**

Baby B
Very Prolific Member

Be glad it was the orange. I had to drink the berry flavored. I had a CT on Thursday. The tech didn't poke around but the ultrasound lady did. I was gassy afterwards, but the barium wasn't coming out. I was C for two days. Finally got rid of some of it yesterday. I was in the bathroom all morning today, losing the last of it. I got the urgency and stuff but it was solid. Hope your feeling better and less gassy soon.

From: **Wisconsin**

RHJPC
Regular Member

Yeah, white "poop" is not really comforting.

I drank A LOT of water and took my fiber and ate butternut squash with a little garlic on it (always helps me go more) and within three days the white stuff was gone!

From: **Colorado**

Sparkle*
Prolific Member

A week on, the white has finally gone, but my insides are buggered.

I'd had my symptoms under control for about a week before the test (that's as good as my IBS gets) and ever since I've been uncomfy and hobbling back and forth to the loo. I just hope it settles down soon, 'because it's so frustrating!

I've got a colonoscopy to look forward to in a week or so *great*. Thank God they'll pump me full of loony drugs because I'm dreading it.

From: **London/Kent**

Auroraheart
Very Prolific Member

Wait a sec … When the heck did they get FLAVOURED barium??! Damn … why does everything come here last?!!?

From: **Ontario**

Topic: CT Scan w/o IV Contrast

KimmiAnn
Regular Member

I went for my abdominal CT scan this morning. When they found out I am allergic to iodine they did not give me the IV contrast. I did have the barium. Will the test miss anything without the IV contrast?

From: **Maryland**

RitaLucy
Very Prolific Member

I find this interesting because when I had my CT scan a few months back, I had to insist that they not give me the iodine because I am allergic to shellfish. They even tried to talk me into it, saying it will be okay. I finally called my doctor from the hospital and his nurse said not to have it. I was told that the CT without contrast will show almost everything maybe except the venous system to the organs etc. The main organs still show up very well.

From: **Houston**

Magicjenjen
Regular Member

I had the CT with the iodine and am not allergic to it, but whew, what did you miss?? Thanks goodness the tech told me first, it feels like you urinate all over yourself for about a minute. Really strange sensation, even though I knew about it ahead, I really did feel like I did, and turned beet red in the face!!

From: **Houston, TX**

Paul yyz
New Member

Hi,

I've worked in CT for 10 years. IV contrast is given during a CT scan so that an optimal image can be obtained. It enhances everything including all the organs and also the bowel wall. Depending on the diagnosis, more or less contrast can be given at higher or lower rates. For example, for a liver scan, you may be given 4cc/sec for a total of 150cc of contrast. With this, the liver can be imaged in three phases.

Many lesions and such can be missed if contrast is not given. Routinely contrast is not needed to see kidney stones, common with a lot of GI patients including myself. Rectal contrast (barium) is given to delineate the bowel. IV contrast also delineates the bladder, which sits on top of the bowel.

As for allergies, most people are not allergic to non-ionic contrast. Ionic contrast has a much greater reaction rate than the non-ionics. I go into respiratory arrest with ionics, but get just a major flush with the non-ionics. We no longer use ionics at my hospital, or most hospitals in Canada, because it is felt that using it, knowing the high reaction rate is a liability, plus patient comfort is of the highest concern, and we want to provide an optimal image for interpretation.

In the US, it may be a different matter, depending upon the institution and the insurance. Ionics are very cheap compared to non-ionics. Generally non-ionics cost $1 per cc.

As far as shellfish go, at one time when we used ionics, we would not give IV contrast to someone who is allergic to shellfish, because of the iodine concentration in the fish and the fact that IV contrast is an iodine compound. Now with the non-ionics, it is no longer an issue.

Hope this helps and was not too long-winded.

Take care,
Paul

From: **Toronto**

Topic: Problems after Barium Swallow

Vicam
New Member

Hello,

I'm having a lot of problems following a barium swallow. I've had severe diarrhea for over 24 hours, with cramping and pain, and it's still white. The nurse said that I couldn't take an Imodium or anything because the barium needs to get out of my system, but I'm concerned because it's very uncomfortable and doesn't seem to be stopping. Has anyone else ever experienced this?

From: **Ontario, Canada**

Bkitepilot
Prolific Member

Vicam, you need to keep cleaning out. Yes, I've had cramping with loose stools after a barium swallow. But I also took Milk of Magnesia and Pericolace to keep it moving. I've had four barium swallows this last year. Plus two gastrographing swallows.

I had barium in me for a three month period this last summer. Not good for it to linger.

From: **North Georgia**

Discussion: Other Procedures.

Topic: Tests coming—anal manometry and defacography

Amj
New Member

I am scheduled to have an anal manometry (inflated balloon test) and a defecography (a form of X-ray) in two weeks. The point is to determine if I have a partial obstruction in the very bottom (anus) of the digestive tract that may contribute to non-stop constipation. Anyone ever had these? How does it go?

From: **Texas**

Honeybee
Regular Member

Hi Amj,

I have had both tests, the anal manometry is not bad, they put a balloon in the rectum and fill with water and you tell them when you feel it. They try it in several different locations; also they have you bear down and check pressure measurements. I was tested for Hirschsprung's disease with this test. For me they found that my anus didn't relax when bearing down and would tighten instead.

The defecography is another story; you should be cleaned out for this test. I did it three times and had to clean out each time. It is not actually painful (some parts hurt me due to hemorrhoids) but somewhat embarrassing. You will be sitting on a toilet in front of an X-ray machine and they will take pictures as you push out the paste that they have packed into your rectum. They used a 5/8 diameter tube to put in your rectum with a caulk gun attached and pushed large amounts of this paste into the rectal cavity, you might feel like you will burst. Also I had to drink barium and they did a vaginal contrast so that all the parts would show up on the

X-rays. They will have you do several things like squeeze your buttocks and then push and then stop pushing and hold, all the while taking the X-rays. This is the test that showed my docs what was going on with me (found four different things wrong with me, that all needed surgical repair, previous to this test I was always being told "Oh you just have IBS"), an excellent test!!! Be glad that you are getting it. Also a little hint for you, when they go to put the tube in your rectum, bear down, it is much easier to take the tube that way. I had this test done in Toledo and also at the Cleveland clinic twice, same size of tube both places, so I assume yours may be that big too.

Good luck to you, I hope they figure out your problem. Any questions please feel free to contact me.

Honeybee (Melissa)

From: **Toledo**, Ohio USA

Topic: LACTOSE INTOLERANCE TESTING

Kim P
Prolific Member

Hi Everyone,

Wondering if any of you ever had a lactose intolerance test done??

I know it has something to do with consuming a beverage made of lactose sugar …

I am a little worried about if I have to take off work for the day, that sort of thing.

Any advice would be appreciated.

Thanks,
Kim P

From: **Scarborough, Canada**

Flux
Very Prolific Member

The LI test is technically a test for lactose maldigestion/malabsorption. That is, it tests for a measured effect and not symptoms. Basically, you drink a huge quantity of it and breathe into a bag periodically, for a few hours. It measures the amount of gasses the gut bacteria make in response to how much lactose is available for them to consume. The less well you digest it, the better they do and the more bacteria gas in the breath.

However, that alone doesn't say much because many people who have an abnormal test result aren't bothered by it, based on studies done in recent years (implying that LI is largely a medical myth). However, if you have severe symptoms during the test and it says you are malabsorbing it, then you really are intolerant.

From: **NY**

Kellina
Regular Member

The test itself is easy! Drink some nasty stuff and breathe into a bag every hour. It takes FOUR HOURS though—you will have to miss work. Bring A LOT of reading material. I was so stinkin' BORED! And I turned out to not be intolerant anyways! UGH!

From: **Rochester, NY**

Topic: Gastric emptying study

Melanie31
Prolific Member

Hi, I have to have this done next Friday. Can anybody tell me what it is and what they do and what happens if my stomach doesn't empty right? I am so happy I have finally found a doctor that is willing to do some more tests on me to find out my problem. Thank you.

From: **Michigan**

Marriah
Prolific Member

Hi, I just had this test done Monday. Assuming they do the test the same way ... they asked me if I prefer oatmeal or scrambled eggs. You choose, and they add a certain radioactive isotope to your food, and a different one to a glass of water. When you're done eating and drinking, they just have you lay on a table with the scanner over you. It takes about an hour, not including your meal.

As I was lying there, I watched the screen with the scans on it. I noticed three different images, and asked the technician why so many. He explained that the first is a picture of the isotopes from the food, the second of the water, and the third is a combined image of both.

As far as testing goes, this one is great. I went in expecting to have to drink a gallon of barium or something equally nauseating. Instead, I got a free meal! All right, the meal wasn't that great, but it could've been worse!

Please, let me know if you have any other questions.

Marriah

From: **Tennessee, USA**

Melanie31
Prolific Member

Thank you so much for the information. You are right this one doesn't seem so bad. I thought I would be drinking that nasty stuff too. What a relief. Thanks again.

From: **Michigan**

Flutter
New Member

So what does this test do? Scan to see where the excess gas comes from?

From: **Australia**

Melanie31
Prolific Member

This test makes sure that your stomach is moving the food through properly and fast enough. I had my test done today and boy, was it a breeze. It only took two hours. I ate my radioactive eggs and they took a two minute X-ray and I sat for a half hour and they did it again. They did that three times, and then the last time I had to wait an hour. The tech said the doctor should have my results back in a couple days. It was so cool to see the images on the machine.

From: **Michigan**

Topic: Hepatobiliary Scan (aka 'hepa scan')

Marriah
Prolific Member

This is the last in a long line of tests. It's not one I've ever had. Can anyone tell me how it's done? Is there an I.V. used? I understand it's to test your gallbladder. If your gallbladder is not functioning well, does it cause you any pain?

Any answers are appreciated.

Thanks,
Marriah

From: **Tennessee, USA**

Sillyface
Prolific Member

Are you sure it's not a HIDA scan? I'm getting one of those, to check my gall bladder too. Maybe in the states they call it a HEPA scan, short for Hepatobiliary Scintigraphy. Okay, here's what it is. It tests the function of the liver, gall bladder and small intestine. You are given a radionuclide injection through an IV. The liver picks this stuff up and they can watch as it goes through the gall bladder. If they cannot visualize the gall bladder within an hour or two after injection, it means the cystic duct is blocked. So anyway, serial images are obtained over an hour. If nothing is seen in the first hour, they take more images in four hours. Then they give you a fatty food and then they watch the size of the gall bladder to see if it can drain. This looks for blockages in the gall ducts.

Since I'm getting this too, I was wondering what symptoms you are having.

Karen

From: **Saskatoon, SK**

Marriah
Prolific Member

Karen, thanks sooo much for taking the time to reply.

I guess it's the same as a HIDA scan. Hepatobiliary Scan is what is on my registration sheet, but I heard someone refer to it as HIDA.

Anyway, my symptoms … episodes with intense vomiting/retching, uncontrollable D. Each time lasts about 12 hours, but has been getting a little longer. It normally happens in clusters, multiple times for a couple months, and then I will go a long time with no sickness. I have been in the ER too many times to count. Nothing will stop an attack. No prescription med my docs have prescribed over the years has done a thing, either preventatively or in halting an episode.

I have found no relation to food, environment, medication, etc., that would show a 'trigger'. My GI is leaning toward severe anxiety, that I internalize my … everything. But we are doing the tests to just make sure. I'm grateful he's being so thorough, but goodness, it's a pain.

My latest doctor is a friend of ours, and he will stick with me until we figure this out.

So what is the total time it will take to have it done? Do you keep the IV in the whole time, or do they take it out when the medicine is injected?

I'll be having it done this coming Thursday. (I was supposed to have it this past Friday, but I was too stressed out and didn't have a car.)

Marriah

From: **Tennessee, USA**

Sillyface
Prolific Member

They told me to plan to be there all day. You go in the morning and they do the first scan, and then they send you for a fatty food, and then they do it again. If they have trouble visualizing anything, then they have to do it again in four hours.

Karen

From: **Saskatoon, SK**

RitaLucy
Very Prolific Member

I had this test. It is a painless test. I didn't have stones either but I did have chronic cholecystitis and I had my gallbladder removed about two months ago.

I am still having upper right quadrant pain and spasms and pain. Also, now on my left side and under my left shoulder blade as well. I could have some sludge or a stone maybe in the common bile duct. I am so mad that my surgeon did not check this duct while I had the surgery. He said they don't check that duct unless the liver enzymes are elevated and mine were not. I could also have SOD. I have been medicating this week with Bentyl, Nexium, and Librax. Today I have been so groggy and it has barely taken the edge off. I see my Doctor on Monday ... I wonder now if the saga will ever end.

Don't be afraid of the test … it is an easy one to handle. Be thorough and careful though in your decisions after you get your results. If you don't have stones on an ultrasound, you could still have stones. (I have heard plenty of gallbladder stories like that). You might just have a low functioning gallbladder like I did. Mine was functioning at 15%.

Let us know how it all goes.

From: **Houston**

KimmiAnn
Regular Member

RitaLucy,

I had my GB out six months ago. I still have the RUQ pain. My common bile duct was checked during surgery and it was clear. I never had stones. Mine was detected on the HIDA Scan with a fraction rate of essentially 0. What I have found that has eased the pain is to totally avoid dairy. I have been using Lactaid milk, it is lactose free. The pain has pretty much subsided. Except for when I hit the bag of Halloween candy over the weekend. The pain came right back. My GI doc suggested I may be lactose intolerant without my GB and to try giving up dairy. So far it seems to work.

Kim

From: **Maryland**

Sillyface
Prolific Member

I'm finally getting my HIDA scan tomorrow. I'm nervous and excited, because I get to eat a fatty food so they can see what it does to my gall bladder. Painful, but I miss fatty foods. I think I'm going to have a cheeseburger and fries. Anyway, I'll let you know how it goes.

Karen

From: **Saskatoon, SK**

Andies76
Regular Member

Hello,

This all sounds too familiar. I had my gallbladder removed about six years ago after the HIDA scan showed a non-functioning gallbladder. Basically all I had was a shriveled up prune in me. Prior to removal, I had EXTREME pain on my right side under my ribs and back. Vomiting and bad D.

Unfortunately, one thing the doctors don't warn you about when having your GB removed is the onset or worsening of IBS. I have now suffered with IBS D for almost six years. Coincidence?

From: **Toronto, Canada**

Sillyface
Prolific Member

Hi Marriah.

I talked with my surgeon about IBS being worsened by removing the gall bladder. That's why he's been waiting so long, he wants to be sure I need it taken out before he does it. Anyway, I have constipation. He said if it's not my gall bladder, it is IBS, or I could have both. I have never had a problem with D, so he thinks if I did get it removed, it might be okay. But there is a significant risk. He said in theory the biliary ducts take over the function of the gall bladder, but sometimes they can empty too quickly, and then you have D. So I'm not sure what I want to happen. All I know is that I can not live with this pain much longer. The tech who did my test today can't tell me my final results, but what we do know for sure is that my gall bladder is slow to fill, and that when it does fill, I have pain. So that could indicate some inflammation. I get the results from my doctor in a week. I think being on Naproxen has really helped with the pain, which makes sense if my gall bladder is inflamed. But I can't stay on it forever. So I just don't know what I want to have happen. Thanks for your story though. It's a tough decision.

Karen

From: **Saskatoon, SK**

Andies76
Regular Member

Hi,

Well hope things go well for you.

I know what a PAIN *literally* it can be.

From: **Toronto, Canada**

Forum III: IBS-Diarrhea (IBS-D)

"Use this forum to discuss any issues related to IBS with diarrhea (IBS-D)."

Coping with chronic diarrhea can affect every aspect of a person's life. Anxiety, shame and embarrassment become constant companions. Activities that others take for granted, such as going to work or having a meal with friends, require careful foresight and planning. This forum allows those with diarrhea-predominant IBS (IBS-D) to commiserate, discuss what helps and hurts, and even find some humor in the issues that they face.

Discussion: Living a Life with IBS-D

Topic: Do you have the same problem I do?

Shuree
New Member

In my IBS life, I seem to only have a liquid-type of diarrhea life. The only time I have any consistency is when I've taken anti-diarrhea pills and I'm coming off of them. That only lasts for a day, if that. I call my trips to the restroom, "fire hose episodes". Why is it that I only have this kind of problem? Sometimes I just sit in my "other home" and cry because I have no control over what is happening. What's worse is that medical people along with naturalists all have different opinions as to what kind of diet we should have. This is the first time I've written about this because my husband and family don't want to hear about this thing that has stolen my life for three years now. I appreciate any help or support. Thank you.

From: **Phoenix, Arizona**

Goldy
Regular Member

Hi Shuree,

I know exactly of what you speak. Funny how other people just can't handle the truth about what IBSD'ers have to contend with on a daily basis. I have suffered over 20 years now and although I was able to function to a great degree as a normal person for a number of those years, it is a lonely place to be when you have no control and not much more understanding of what is happening to you daily. I have seen specialist after specialist and have taken countless remedies, and the answer is always the same. IBS is not curable and there may be some therapies that will help with the symptoms at times, but nothing can fix the syndrome, yet. All we can hope for is a little understanding and an ear to listen when we are not feeling tiptop. I think that try as they may, a non-IBS'er just cannot grasp the magnitude of symptoms and anxiety we live with daily. Maybe science can come up with a cure or something to alleviate some of the symptoms for the majority at some point. I prefer to think that IBS should be more open for discussion among families and the medical community, but as we are dealing with a highly personal subject matter, I don't think that is in the stars for us just yet. Maybe a little public education will make it easier for those who come after us. I do wish you well and am glad you found a place to be heard.

S.G.
Regular Member

Shuree, believe me; I unfortunately understand all of what you are saying. I'm IBS-D, and I have BIG problems in getting out to go to work, and going out ANYWHERE! This is VERY depressing, and it's true that non-IBSers don't really understand. Like me, it's good we found this group, to know we are not the only ones like this. It does help me be less depressed, and I get many good ideas from other people. Welcome here.

S.G.

From: **N.J., U.S.A.**

C. Webber
New Member

Hi Shuree: I am new to this web site. I thought I was the only one out there with this embarrassing problem. Thanks to you and everyone else who have written messages, I realize I am not alone. I have had IBS-D for many years. It comes and goes, as my stress levels change. The only thing that helps me is Imodium when I am going out. Always have Imodium with you. Exercise is helping me, as well, with the stress thing. I am now recording everything that I eat and the kind of BM I have that day to see what triggers my IBS. So far I know that pasta really gets me running. Also, apples. Hopefully you will be able to control it with diet changes and exercise.

From: **British Columbia**

Hostage
New Member

I have never posted a reply, but I have watched the bulletin board for quite awhile. I have had IBS-D for 30 years. It has affected my life in so many ways. Basically, it has really held me back from living life to the fullest. It is an incapacitating, embarrassing situation that causes me to shy away from my career, causes me to be a loner, and on and on. The only thing that I have found that helps is to take a double dose of Metamucil after breakfast, within an hour or so, and the same thing after dinner. This has helped remarkably in the last couple years, and, if I do it religiously, I can pretty much lead a normal life. It tends to overcome anything you eat. I have no idea what my triggers are, although I've tried to figure it out. But it has to be a heaping teaspoon-and-a-half (sugar-free type) minimum to work.

From: **Colorado**

Kelseyk
New Member

Shuree: I am a new member and I feel your pain. I know my husband is clueless. He wants to bike around the lake—I panic. We recently went away for the weekend to a friend's house to go to this huge outdoor flea market. What an ordeal! If you don't eat there's "nothing to lose"—constantly making sure you know where the bathrooms are—hungry, anxious—can't go for that beer or the boat ride—making excuses—everyone thinking I am anti-social. The pain in my side that makes being a wife impossible. The fact that a few minutes ago I was trying to sign on to this site and he was hovering. I went to double over in pain and couldn't because he was leaning toward me and I snapped. The times we are riding home and I can feel it and he won't stop because he thinks it's "all in my head". I will start a food journal and try the Metamucil again—just reading other people's posts has helped me. I always knew I wasn't alone but I feel that sharing this with people who will nod their heads in understanding will really reduce the stress. Thanks!

From: **Illinois**

Scoop
New Member

Kelseyk ... . I'm so understanding of your situation!!!!! My husband has always said, "It's your nerves" ... ... and I hate, hate that!!!!! He can eat anything/everything (don't we wish we could?) and I'm sure it's hard for them to comprehend what it's like for us! And since I don't want this to rule my life—I just don't eat when we do things. He knows it, as do my closest friends—and it works—it's just not fun—but compared to embarrassment—I'll go without eating anytime!!!!! Thanks for sharing and welcome!

From: **Illinois**

Topic: Embarrassment—living in the "lie"

Arakadnil
New Member

Was wondering if anyone else does this, it makes me feel like a heel. Someone asks me to go somewhere with them, on a long trip or not, and instead of admitting I can't go because I have tummy troubles I say that I have a headache, the baby has a fever, the basement flooded, anything else but the truth. Why is it so embarrassing to admit that it is bathroom problems? It's hard to know that I'm considered unreliable for events because the panic of knowing there won't be a bathroom near keeps me away. My sister, whom I love dearly, has begun to think I don't care for her anymore because I've stalled on and cancelled so many meetings. I've suffered from this illness since I was about 15 and am now 28.

From: **Maryland USA**

Bara
New Member

I know exactly how you feel. My husband would often say things about how we never can go anywhere because I didn't like driving very far in the car. He thought I was afraid to drive. In the last month I have finally told him what my problem is (we've been together for nine years) and he said I should have just told him in the first place and he would have understood. But like you, I was embarrassed. Now we have gone away once and are planning more trips because I know if I say PULL OVER he isn't going to question it. He even says "I'll love you, even if you do poop in the woods" (cute). But on the upside, I have started taking Caltrate for my D and it works! I haven't had any D since I started taking it two weeks ago. Good luck and stay strong.

From: **Fort Erie**

SmileyFace
New Member

I know how you feel! I avoid things like meetings and parties. I really have a hard time at holidays because it seems we live in a society that loves to eat! And what does our family do at a get-together? Why they eat of course, and then I have the D the rest of the day. I avoid the work Christmas party every year. I am sure everyone thinks I am a snob. I would Love to Go! If my friends (what friends I have left) go shopping I can't even go in the car, I make some excuse to meet them there. And of course they always want to go to lunch. So I continue to make excuses and people are gradually starting to leave me out more and more.

I have one close friend that I have told. She tries to make it okay when I'm with her. But I still feel embarrassed and like I'm being a big pain. But it does make it easier. My husband tries to be understanding but I can tell that I ruin a lot of our plans by always having D after we go out to eat and during movies. Everything always seems to revolve around my stomach problems, so I try to keep it a secret so as not to ruin our time. But he knows (probably because he is always standing around by himself waiting on me while I'm in the toilet). I am trying the calcium thing and have had four days without D. I hope it works! I wish the rest of the world could be as understanding as the people here.

From: **Missouri**

Maloo
Regular Member

Time to start being honest with people and go to the parties and just not eat the food and enjoy yourselves! I am very honest and if I can go, I go and just don't eat what is there. If I don't feel well then I don't go! People know and they are very understanding. It is better to be honest and then people will not think you are blowing them off. Don't be ashamed of what you have! Laugh about it! That is what I do, in fact I call my D cha cha's and now when friends and family get it they call it cha cha's too! It's all good!

From: **NY**

Kitten33
New Member

I 'SO' know where you guys are coming from ... I've missed out on great day trips because of the fear of being stuck in a car for a few hours, especially long weekends when the traffic can be at a standstill ... that sets off the panic and then of course the 'need' to go to the bathroom ... I don't care if its real or psychological ... IT CERTAINLY FEELS LIKE I NEED TO GO!!

BUT the past two weeks I've been taking calcium citrate and had NO cases of D ... its like a miracle ... I know on this site a few people have told me to be careful of the magnesium in citrate BUT its not affected me and I've been going out all over the place and NOT thinking about where the bathrooms are ... its amazing and I can't believe its taken so long to find something that helps ... I've had IBS-D for approximately seven years so this is a wonderful find, as is this site ... I feel close to everyone here and can fully sympathize ... so I'm saying TRY THE CALCIUM ... it might not work for you all, but what harm can it do to try?

Cheers.

From: **Ontario**

Trudyg
Prolific Member

I just tell people that I have a 'bad stomach'. They know what that means—and you'll be surprised how many people will then tell you they have it too! Some worse than others, but at least they see why you don't help yourself to the donuts that they bring in, etc. One of my coworkers about falls over her own feet trying to get to the break room when she hears there are cookies—she is fat and I'm not! Ha ha on her!

From: **Huntsville, AL**

Twocups424
Prolific Member

Boy, I don't know who you all are interacting with, but the people that understand how I feel and why I can't do things are VERY FEW AND FAR BETWEEN!!!!!!!!!!!!! It's very hurtful. First you have to deal with this crummy disorder, then you have to deal with people's snide remarks and misunderstandings or worse yet, they understand and believe and blame it on you for being SO UPTIGHT OR LETTING THINGS GET TO YOU!!!!!!!!!!!!!!!

From: **PA**

Maloo
Regular Member

TwoCups, I am really sorry to hear that! It sounds like you are surrounded by a bunch of jerks! You have all the support you want here! We all understand! No one should treat you that way. Sounds like they need a good hearty dose of D for a few weeks to straighten them out!

From: **NY**

UnluckyMe
Regular Member

Arakadnil—Would it really be so bad to tell the truth? Especially with your own family? You don't have to say the word IBS, just say you've come down with digestive troubles, or even an anxiety disorder (that's how I describe it to friends—since IBS is triggered by anxiety, it's not a lie, just a little spinning of the facts). Good luck to you.

From: **Somewhere**

Twocups424
Prolific Member

I don't agree that IBS is triggered by anxiety. I think we get anxious because we have IBS!

From: **PA**

Maria_del_Carmen
New Member

Wow, this is a great bulletin board! I can so relate to all the things you are saying! I hate going to restaurants because it is expected that you eat, but it seems that eating out is the worst I can do for my IBS. Either the food has too much fat, or I overeat because I feel I have to finish my food, or it is simply impossible to avoid all the trigger foods. My former roommate and still very good friend can just not understand why I never want to "just grab dinner!" I'll "grab dinner" at home where I can eat something small and manageable and be close to a nice bathroom! Also, going to clubs and discos totally freaks me out. I can't drink because of my IBS, which everyone has to comment on ("Oh, just have a small drink! A beer won't hurt!"), and then the restrooms tend to have looooong lines.

While I am rambling—I am going to school in Southern Europe in the fall and I am afraid ... I love that part of Europe but I'll miss the nice restrooms here in the US! Wherever you go, be it the grocery store, Target, or a gas station, you can count on there being a decent bathroom. I guess I'll just have to map out all the McDonalds there!

One more thing while I am here—since I am skinny, most people who don't know me assume I have an eating disorder if they see me decline food. My friends know that I can eat like a horse when I am doing OK, but others will constantly comment on my weight and the stress of that doesn't make my IBS any better! And yes, maybe IBS could be called an eating disorder—we get sick when we eat! It is hard to gain any weight when I already have a high metabolism, and fats and sugars makes my IBS act up horribly.

From: **California**

Princess Purr
New Member

I make up stories all the time. I have a headache, an ear ache, I have to study. I always try to have a plan. And if I have to go somewhere, I try to make it clear I can't stay long. It would be sooooo nice to take a road trip! But unless my hubby gets the RV running well, there is no way. No potty, no me!

From: **NJ**

Arakadnil
New Member

Twocups, I am inclined to agree that my IBS causes the nerves and not the other way around. If I didn't have to go to the bathroom all the time and after every little thing I put in my mouth, I wouldn't be afraid to go places.

BTW, I have told my sister about it, and she doesn't get it. She just says, "Doesn't your doctor have medicine for that?" And rolls her eyes if I say I have belly troubles.

From: **Maryland USA**

Teriehart
New Member

I must be blessed. I have found that all of my friends with the exception of one (we'll get back to him in a second), are very understanding and accommodating. Sometimes, I will take two bites and ask for a doggy bag. That's just how they know me now. I find it easier to "come clean" with people and then you won't have to explain every time or come up with excuses. I just started a new job three months ago, and none of my new co-workers know, but when I get to know them better, I will confide in them. Some of them anyway. If your friends can't be understanding about an illness, they aren't being very good friends.

About my one exception friend, I usually put a curse on him, hoping that he would catch it for a week. But I usually say something smart like, "someday there will be a pill that will cure this for me, but I don't know what you can do about being ugly!" (We've been friends a long time!)

From: **Wisconsin**

WindyCityRich
Regular Member

It is hard for other people to understand this whole thing called IBS. I tell all my friends and family about the condition, and they are very accommodating. Whenever I go to dinner with them, they ask me to pick a restaurant, or they suggest a restaurant and ask for my approval; they give me "veto power" over where we eat. Same thing for going to dinner at their place. They usually make something special for me if the main dish they are having is not something I can tolerate. But every once in a while, someone will say they cannot understand why I can't eat a certain food that they think is harmless; they think I'm being overly cautious or paranoid about eating stuff. I politely tell them, "trust me, I know what I can and can't eat", and tell them "You don't want to see me what happens to me when I eat that!"

At work, it's a bit tougher till you get to know and trust people. My boss now asks if I'm OK with the food when he is taking us to lunch, or having a company meeting with food. He doesn't know all the details, but enough to know that I can get really sick from eating the wrong foods. He himself has an allergy to nuts, so he is quite understanding. Lots of people have food restrictions for one reason or another.

The more people you can tell, the more helpful and understanding people will be of your condition. Trying to hide it, or eating something you really can't eat for fear of being impolite or embarrassed, should not be an option.

Rich M

From: **Chicago, IL**

Desirae
Regular Member

Even though most of my friends know about my IBS, I still end up making up something, just so I don't have to go somewhere with them in fear that I'll need to go. I often, as someone else also said, feel like a pain in the butt when I'm with my friends. Always having to stop if I need to, rearrange plans and what not, so that I'm okay. I am very fortunate, though, to have a boyfriend who happens to be my best friend and who understands it all. He's never once complained about the fact that I'd rather go get food and eat at home, or rent a movie instead of going to one. I'm so lucky to have him and lucky that he's as understanding as he is. It's made dealing with this a lot easier and we can even joke about it. It's great, but it does suck that sometimes I end up lying to my friends to avoid going somewhere with them. I'm just a lot more comfortable with my boyfriend so I don't need to lie about it to him.

My mom goes back and forth from being supportive to almost acting like she doesn't get it. She'll ask me to run an errand after I've just eaten something that I KNOW will give me D and when I say no, she gets mad and acts like I'm making this all up. But other times when we're in the car going somewhere and I have to make a stop she's really sympathetic. She confuses me.

Oh well. Anyways, I love this board. I LOVE reading about how you guys are feeling and it just happens to be how I'm feeling. It brings a sense of closeness even though I don't know any of you. This web site is wonderful.

From: **Dallas, TX**

WindyCityRich
Regular Member

Desirae—

You're so lucky to have a boyfriend that knows all about your condition and is so considerate and accommodating. Sounds like a prince!

One of the really tough things about this condition (as if there weren't enough already), is that it's hard to date and meet new people due to the limitations. The usual first-date places—dinner, going out for pizza and movies, can be really difficult and it's hard to explain this all to someone new; hence, we avoid even trying to meet people. Once they get to know you, and like you, it's a lot easier.

On the issue about going out with friends, I'd say you shouldn't worry so much about being a "pain in the butt to them", or ruining their fun. If they like you and want you around, they'll be more than willing to deal with it. The times they are with you, they might have to avoid going to places they normally would go to—but they can always do those things some other time.

Lots of times I'll go out with friends, even to a place where I can't eat, so as not to ruin their fun. I eat before we go out, and then join them at the pizza place; while they eat pizza, I eat plain bread or pasta, salad, or whatever. That way, I feel like I'm not ruining their fun, and still can feel part of the group (not an outcast). It's very important to keep the social life going, and maintain the support of friends. By avoiding going out with them, they may feel you don't want to go out with them. They will be a lot more helpful and accommodating than you might think.

Sounds like you're doing well, and not turning into a hermit due to this goofy IBS!

Rich M

From: **Chicago, IL**

Topic: How do you deal with accidents?

Karen P
Prolific Member

I'm so panicked about having an accident. I've never actually had one but the anxiety is always there. I'm always thinking "I've been too lucky; it's got to happen sometime". I was thinking that if I got a better understanding of how people handle them, it may help me feel that it's not such a big deal. I know it won't kill me, but its sooo scary. There is such a stigma attached. Any ideas/input?

From: **Mississauga**

Greeen
Prolific Member

Hi Karen P—I suffer from anxiety-induced IBS-D. The last time this happened to me was after I went to a restaurant with my family and ate the wrong things. On the way home we hit traffic from construction ... I panicked because I felt my tummy boiling and knew I needed a bathroom right then. So what saved me was totally calming myself down, almost shutting myself down on the inside. I have trained myself in these situations of almost-accidents to put myself in an almost meditative state and it has calmed me enough to make it home.

From: **NJ**

Countrygirl
New Member

I hear ya Karen, I worry about accidents too. When I have to go, I have to go now! And I'm so worried I won't make it when out in public. So far I haven't had any in public, but have had some at home, because, as I mentioned in an earlier post— one bathroom, five person family. Once when someone was using the bathroom I had to go so badly that I ran out in the backyard (thank God we're rural, LOL) It was dark, and I went out the next day to clean it up, because I didn't make it any further than the bottom of the deck steps

Another time, I was in my son's bedroom, bending over, picking up toys (not a good thing to do with IBS-D, LOL) and had such a sudden urge (bathroom was occupied again) that I had to grab one of his diapers, pull down my pants and go right there on it.

So anyway, I hear ya, I feel your pain, and I have no solutions, sorry. But you're not alone.

From: **Ontario**

Jeanne2
Prolific Member

Hey Karen,

Certainly, that is all of our biggest worry when we have the D part of IBS. Keep reading on here, and you will find things.

I have had a couple of bouts ... and decided to wear protection when I am at work, etc. I buy Depends ... and others here do too. They fit pretty well. I wear underpants or tights or pantyhose over them. I'm not overweight so it doesn't look bulky ... but I wouldn't let that stop me anyways!

Or, have a back up plan at your house ... keep a bucket with a heavy duty kitchen bag in it ... and use that if the bathroom is full! I bring change of clothes, plastic bags, and wipes in the car with me whenever I travel. I have never had an accident in the car ... but when my kids were young, we had a big van and I put a porta-potti in back … we had a curtain attached to the ceiling of the van. I used it maybe twice in all those years … but it gave me a lot of piece of mind …

Also … I too have had pretty good success with trying to calm myself … doing deep breathing until the urge passes, especially in a car, just to get me to a bathroom. I keep telling myself that the urges are contractions that will come and go, and they do. Of course, there are those times that it just explodes, I know that too … but for me they are rare.

Good luck … be creative.

Jeanne

From: **Michigan**

Chamuca
New Member

Newbie here—Boy can I relate! For a while I was using diapers every time I went out, but I find that I get diaper rash almost right away and am very uncomfortable. Once I was at an Aunt's house (who I had not seen in over 35 years!) and slipped on her stairs—the bump caused me to lose control and whoooosh. My dear husband was standing next to me and he just squeezed my hand in support. Two of my cousins were right there too and they sort of faded away. I walked into the nearest bathroom and right into the shower. It was horribly embarrassing—but I survived it and love my relatives even more for being so understanding.

Usually when that terrible insistent urge comes, I try to clench everything and wait for the contraction to subside and then duck-walk to the nearest bathroom. I keep changes of underwear all over the house—that idea of a plastic bag when there is no bathroom available is a very good one—from now on I will stash a few where the underwear is! Lining a waste basket with one could be a life saver! I also take Imodium when I go out, but it does not always work.

Sheila

From: **Middle of Mexico**

Sassymoon
New Member

Hi, newbie here too. After a couple of accidents in the car (by myself, thank God), I get quite worried about it happening again. I know every gas station on the way to work. I know how much time it takes to drive to the next one. I always note in malls, etc. where the bathrooms are. Makes me feel more prepared, just in case, and like Jeann2 says, stay calm. Anxiety is the worst.

I wear panty liners, make me feel better in case one passes gas and has a little oops.

Good luck.

From: **Canada**

Careena
Very Prolific Member

Since my husband started taking Questran, he doesn't have diarrhea anymore. He's a mailman so he is not near a bathroom. He'd go in his mail truck. Thankfully, there are no windows in those things. LOL.

Anyway, he used to carry around a bag with emergency things in it. We had one in the car and he had one at work. He had a pair of pants, a pair of underwear, a small container of travel baby wipes, a garbage bag, and a jacket or sweater of some type.

You could carry these things in a slightly bigger purse or backpack if the situation warrants. The object of the sweater or jacket was that if he did have an accident, he could tie that around his waist (in a somewhat fashionable statement) and make it to the bathroom so that he could change his clothes, and it would mostly hide the accident.

Once he made these little emergency packs, he didn't ever have to use them. Just knowing he was prepared for anything calmed his anxiety quite a bit.

From: **South Fork**

Kelli_from_Cali
New Member

Hello Karen,

I really understand your feelings, and once you have an accident it gets much worse. Even though I do take medication, I still have sudden attacks of diarrhea. I have a great Doctor that suggested that I try wearing protection (diapers), and gave me several to try, and at first I felt really weird wearing them, but only someone that has had an accident understands the peace of mind. Whenever I leave my house, and when I sleep, I must wear a diaper.

Here is what works for me when I have an accident. Make sure to always have extra diapers and baby wipes with you, and you are "good to go". Because I have frequent accidents I take Nullo pills because it takes away the odor, and it gives me time to change.

As I said before, I refuse to let the diarrhea control me.

Good Luck

From: **Southern California**

Fancy_pants
Regular Member

Hey Karen … newbie here too, but I have found what greeen said to be helpful. In those cases where my tummy starts going, I try to take my mind off of it and blast the a/c in my car (which sounds weird, but my palms get all sweaty and I break out in sweats and for some reason, it works). Luckily, the only time I ever had one was the day after I had gotten out of the hospital and my friend was staying with me (and luckily sleeping), so I snuck my stuff out to the washer. Sometimes I think worrying about it and focusing on it makes things worse …

From: **South Lousiana**

Jeanne2
Prolific Member

We are creative aren't we? As I read other posts, I realized yes, I too wear skirts more often … easier to pull up if you have to go … AND I also bring something to tie around my waist, just a light jacket or cardigan.

I did think of one other thing … not only plastic bags you may need to use to actually "go" in, but one for the seat of your car if you do have an accident. When I had my first big accident, my pants were soaked, and I was NOT prepared. You'd sure want to keep your car seat dry until you could get cleaned up.

Also, thicker pads when I don't want to wear the full diaper thing, and except around home, I don't ever go out anymore without a pad or diaper.

People with normal GI tracts would never believe the things we go through would they?

Jeanne

From: **Michigan**

Discussion: Mornings

With IBS-D, it is fairly common to find that symptoms are worse in the morning. The following posts offer suggestions on how to start the day off in a better frame of mind and body.

Topic: I hate mornings …

Mamamia
Prolific Member

Dear friends:

Aren't mornings the worst? You can't leave the house until you've cleaned out. Then you have to eat some breakfast and that's usually where the trouble begins. The body has been nice and calm all night and now digestion has to start! Nausea usually arrives at this time too!

However, I have finally found a breakfast that really gives me the minimum amount of symptoms: Life Cereal with Vanilla Soy milk, half glass of orange juice, tea. I will eat this every morning 'til the day I die. I'm even bringing it with me on vacation.

Anyone else hate the AM????

Love, M—

From: **New Jersey, USA**

Tamgirl21
Prolific Member

Mornings are my worst, too. I eat plain waffles and peppermint tea and that usually makes me go, and I'm okay for the day. If not, watch out, I'll be a mess for the rest of the day. I'm going on vacation next week, and I am praying mornings won't be so bad.

From: **New York**

CrystalOne
Regular Member

Mamamia, how right you are. Mornings are my absolute worst, too. Every morning, same thing, up at 6:00—toilet till at least 7:00. This is very frustrating. I'm sure my kids (ages 10 and 7) are wondering what I've got going on in the bathroom. I'm also one of the few that gets woken in the middle of the night with terrible pain and explosive D. Those of you that have jobs that allow you to work from your homes are very lucky. I'm desperately looking for something I can do from home. I don't want to become scared to leave home, but I'm slowly moving that way. Believe me, Mamamia, when I say you're not the only one. Anyone have any answers for these terrible mornings?

From: **USA**

Mikala1
Prolific Member

Mornings SUCK!! Thank God I recently starting freelancing and my schedule varies, so I no longer have to be out the door every day by 8:30.

The only advice I have is to make sure you have enough time. For me that means no less than an hour and a half.

I also try and think of it as purification rather than severe diarrhea. Corny, but it does help my state of mind when I'm running to the bathroom four or five times before I can even attempt to leave the house.

From: **Austin, TX**

Kitty19HasIBS
Prolific Member

I understand I have to get up at 6:00 AM for my 10:00 AM class and I live five minutes from school. I have to have time to try to eat a few crackers and then be sick. I hate how my friends can get up 45 minutes before class. Wow, it would be so nice to get up at 9:00 AM instead of 6:00 AM. After I finish school, I will be counseling people, so there is a good chance I can do that inside my own home or somewhere that I will have my own restroom. Then again if I marry my BF, I think I will just be a stay-at-home mom.

Kitty

From: **I live around New Orleans**

IBSBC
New Member

I, too, hate mornings!! Sometimes I can feel the cramping even before my eyes are open! That is the worst feeling in the world!

Thankfully, the number of mornings like that is fewer! I have changed my diet a lot (no dairy, no red meat, little fat and lots of peppermint tea).

I am taking 650 mg of calcium twice a day to make sure that I don't lose my bones, but I find that it makes me nauseated. Any thoughts on which supplements are less hard on the stomach?

From: **Maple Ridge, BC**

Becks
New Member

I'm right there with you all!! My stomach "wakes" me up around 5:00 AM and then it all starts. I "go" from about 5:00 AM to 7:00 AM. Probably about six or seven times before I feel like I can go anywhere. It is so frustrating, especially when I am visiting someone or traveling. I can't figure out why the morning is such an awful time for us all, especially because it's not like I've eaten anything to trigger it prior to the attacks.

Becks

From: **Beverly**

Reinnil
New Member

So, I am not the only one who is afraid to leave the house before the dreaded BM. I have to get up at the crack of dawn so I can complete eliminating before I take my pills. The minute I hit the floor, I have to make a bee-line for the bathroom. I can go from normal to water in half-an-hour. The pills usually take a half-hour to work. I daren't take them before, as that will constipate me. Yes, mornings are awful! You have my sympathy.

From: **Venice, Fl. U.S.A.**

Katz
Prolific Member

Oh my GOD, I'm so not alone out there! My mornings really are the PITS! I wake up and usually in about a half an hour (if I'm lucky) I have to haul it to the bathroom or ELSE (you know)! I really wish someone would tell us why in the hell this happens! I heard it has something to do with some kind of nerves in the brain that are "overactive" in IBS-D people in the mornings. I work on an assembly line and just pray for a relief person to be around when I need them! The bad thing is when I need them for three or four times in a half-hour, ya know!

From: **Ohio**

KrissyC
Very Prolific Member

The only thing that's ever worked for me is to set my alarm, take a Xanax about an hour before I have to "get up", and then go back to sleep.

You wake up groggy, but it helps a lot. You might have a BM, but it's not painful, and it's quick.

From: **Texas**

Kristian
Very Prolific Member

Hi All,

I just wanted to say that I loathe mornings as well, but not for the same reasons. I am generally crampy (but no D) in the mornings and I'm very gassy. What I hate is wondering every morning if today is going to be a good day or a bad day. Some mornings I do have a BM before I leave the house, but that's rare. Mostly, I have stuck to the ritual of not eating anything (maybe having some water) in the morning UNTIL I get to my office. My doctor agreed that this was a decent temporary way to deal with my D fears in the morning.

Has anyone else done this? If so, do you think it's a sane way to handle the situation?

From: **New York City**

BQ
Very Prolific Member

It is just what your Doc said, a good *temporary* way to handle it. For me, the better long-term solution was to just think it was going to be a good day. And believe it or not, positive thinking has helped me. I expect to *not* have problems. I'm prepared if I do, but I really try to see things positively. I am currently having trouble doing this because I'm grieving a loss. These problems I am having, (increase of symptoms) are natural for a person like me who is evidently a very sensitive gut responder. When the grief eases a bit, and I am able to once again think more positively, I am certain my symptoms will wane again. So, even though it sounds trite, positive thinking can help some of us.

BQ

From: **USA**

Cristina21
Regular Member

I TOTALLY AGREE!!!!!! MORNINGS R THE WORSE!!!!!! THEY SUCK!!!!!!!!!!!! (and that's all I have to say).

From: **Central America**

Bronzee
Regular Member

I have really bad cramping after I eat breakfast, it doesn't matter what I eat. I am bent down, tummy is cramping and hurting … its getting to point I don't want to eat anymore in the morning. So, my mom keeps saying suck on peppermint candy after you eat … it will help, but I needed something stronger. So, I went to a health shop and purchased this stuff call peppermint spirits … its a little brown bottle with a syringe in it to dispense drops …. I takes two drops before I eat … you can take it with water or put the drops in your tea, coffee or any other drink. It has some alcohol in it about 82% … but its two drops. It doesn't bother me … Its the second day now and both times I had this I haven't have any stomach cramps … the gas just shoots right through me … now I hope this continues to work for my body … I wanted to let everyone else know about this … and it only cost me about $2.00. Sometimes the simplest things are out there for us … and it takes a lifetime to find.

Good luck and sweet blessings to you.

Lora
New Member

It's nice to know that I'm not the only one. Mornings are really bad for me. First thing is awful bloating and gas, and then the D hits. It's awful because I'll think I'm okay and my husband gets in the shower and then I've gotta go. I often wake with very painful D, and it usually lasts quite a while on those really bad mornings. I cannot eat breakfast because I either throw up or it goes right through the other way. I am so miserable. I'm just trying to see a light at the end of the tunnel.

From: **Anaheim, Ca, USA**

Pisces65
Regular Member

Same here for the morning. I usually do not eat at all because I'm afraid I will have a problem while driving to work. When I get to work, I sip tea. It stinks!!!! The only time I eat breakfast is if I'm going to be home after I eat. Mornings are always the worst part of the day for me.

From: **NY USA**

Crisstee
New Member

Hi everyone, I'm new. It is nice to know I'm not alone, although I do not wish this suffering on anyone. I, too, have bad mornings. Cramps wake me up, in the bathroom forever; my kids are even late for school sometimes because I can't get out of there!! It is horrible, the pain is so bad sometimes that I feel dizzy and get cold sweats. I often feel like I'm gonna have to call 911. I just started taking Bentyl and had a great weekend, but first thing this morning, I had the cramps and big D again. I thought the Bentyl would make the cramps stop. I can't figure out if certain foods are bothering me, or what else might be causing this, it just came on so suddenly!!

From: **Torrance, Ca.**

Mamamia
Prolific Member

Dear friends:

If you can do this, please try (I know for some it's impossible.) CHANGE YOUR WORK HOURS. See if you can come in 10:00 AM to 6:00 PM instead of 9:00 AM to 5:00 PM or something.

I work 11:00 AM to 7:00 AM because of NJ traffic and my health troubles. I commute by car 50 miles one way. My boss is cool with it.

I never schedule any appointments for the morning. I just freak too much at that time.

You may think your boss will not understand, but it is worth TRYING. It could really change your life.

Much love and light to you, Michele—

From: **New Jersey, USA**

J Risio
New Member

I also agree that mornings are the worst! But I have been trying something that seems to be working for me; maybe it will work for others. I don't have a real big dinner, and try to stay away from foods that aggravate me, and I know everyone knows what aggravates them. So right before I go to bed, I take a packet of Metamucil with water, and 500 ml of calcium + Vitamin D.

In the morning I mostly have one or two BMs, but after that I feel good to leave the house. I also take an Ativan and a NuLev before I leave for work. I have been doing this for about four months now. It has helped me, I used to have between three & five BMs every morning, and I was always running late to work. So I hope this may help someone, if it makes you feel worse, I'm sorry! Good luck.

Joe the trucker

From: **New York**

Topic: Morning D

Grrrl-aghast
Prolific Member

I saw that I'm not the only one here whose stomach/D seems to be worst in the morning. Does anybody know why? This is really annoying, because I usually can't tell if it's gonna be a bad day and I should just take a sick day, or if it's just the usual morning tummy and will even out later on. Does anybody have the same problem, and if so what do you do about it?

From: **NYC**

Jenn24
Regular Member

I know exactly how you feel!

Every morning I go through the same thing … should I take a sick day, or will I be better in an hour or two? The way I deal with it is that I get up about an hour earlier than I have to. If I feel uneasy an hour later, I take an Imodium. If it is really bad then I call in sick.

I hate calling in sick because of D. I would rather save my sick days for when I am "normal person sick" (i.e. the flu).

Good luck,
Jenn

From: **Canada**

LJones
Regular Member

My D was really bad in the morning when I wasn't used to getting up early, but it's a little more under control now. I've been getting up two hours earlier than when I have to leave. I take Imodium about every other day though; I don't think I could survive without it!!

From: **California**

Grrrl-aghast
Prolific Member

Well, I'm glad I'm not the only one ... kind of (meaning I wish **none** of us had this problem, but you know what I mean.)

Ugh, getting up an hour early doesn't really sound too tempting, since I'm already not getting enough sleep. But I guess it's the lesser evil in this case. I don't think I have any sick days left, but luckily my boss is very understanding about the whole thing and will let me leave or come in late if I have to. But then, of course, if I take time off I won't get paid for it either.

I've been trying not to get hooked on Imodium, but once again, it's the lesser evil I guess. Maybe I can bring myself to try getting up early ... it'll take a whole lot of convincing myself first—LOL.

From: **NYC**

Trudyg
Prolific Member

I get up two hours earlier than I need to, eat, take Imodium and finish getting ready, and then I crash in the recliner until time to go. I catch a nap when everything's set for the day and leave enough time in case it goes bad on me.

From: **Huntsville, AL**

Yarnie
Regular Member

Mornings ... Ugh. I always felt it was the nerves of a new day, plus not having been to the bathroom all night which caused the problems. I normally find that I am better if the house is empty when I get up, so I know nobody will steal the bathroom, and I also have always found that my ritual of taking a bath/shower and washing and drying my hair helps to calm me down or preoccupy me to keep the nerves away. Try not to eat too much rubbish food before bed too.

From: **London, UK**

Maki
Regular Member

Everyone on this post sounds like me. Yes, I too get up two hours earlier, have breakfast, get ready for work, (and between this time) make numerous trips to the bathroom. Then we know if it's an Imodium day. When it's time to leave, hopefully, there's nothing left … … … What a way to live.

From: **New York**

Redspruce
New Member

Mornings are worse for me as well, but seem quite mild compared to some. I have had better AMs by changing my diet, I avoid milk products in the AM and high fiber foods. For some reason I can eat some of these at suppertime or later with no ill effects but definitely not in the AM.

From: **Brenton, NS, Canada**

Homebound
Very Prolific Member

Oh yes, mornings can be rough for me also. Seems like the earlier I get up the worse it is too.

Now I'm not sure, but I believe that what I read is that it's because our bowels tend to "sleep" when we sleep, which is why most people who just have IBS don't have a lot of attacks that will awake you during the night. So when we wake up, so does our guts, and for me that means spasms and more D. If I wake up early needing to rush out the door and go somewhere (like my doctor appointment was last Friday) forget it! I'll be incredibly sick. I really try not to do things TOO early!

From: **USA**

Boston_Britt

I only seem to get it in the morning, I seem to wake up feeling hungry and then have a D attack which makes me even more tired and hungry … it sucks! I don't feel like I can be productive at work until a couple of hours after I get there. I also frequently feel hungry during the day. What is the first thing that people eat/drink in the morning to help get energy back?

From: **Boston**

Colestid
Regular Member

Mornings are bad. I found eating breakfast was not even an option. I would skip it and hope by lunch-time I would be more "stable".

I am taking Colestid now, which really seems to help the overall experience. Now the mornings are only the scheduled time for a regular movement, instead of a painful attacking one. I highly recommend asking your doctor about it. The medicine is prescribed for cholesterol, but I was given it for the side effect of con- stipation, which in my case makes me normal, per se.

From: **Columbus, Ohio 43082**

Rbrzan
New Member

Wow. I just found this site today and it's already been a gold mine of information. I, too, have attacks of D in the morning. By the afternoon, my system seems to mellow out. I've changed my diet over the last two months, avoiding caffeine, chocolate, onions, fast food, and fatty food. I've also slowly increased my fiber intake, taking psyllium. My doctor just prescribed Dicetel, although it doesn't seem to do much of anything yet (anybody else taking this??). After all of these steps to a hopeful improvement, I still wake up about one to two hours before I have to go anywhere and am still worried about having to make a pit stop on the way to work (one hour away). A very stressful way to live!!

From: **Balderson, Ontario, Canada**

Angel V
Very Prolific Member

I know everyone probably hears this all the time, but have you tried exercising in the morning? I used to have the Daily-D every morning, but once I started working out when I first got up, it seemed to help. That and the calcium supplements, and stress reduction, and watching what I eat, and … ….

Boy, IBSers have the self-discipline thing down don't we?

From: **Florida**

Topic: Morning Symptoms

Gastron
Regular Member

Friends,

I'm curious if there are others out there whose symptoms (i.e. episodes of diarrhea) are most pronounced in the mornings. What typically happens to me is that I'll wake up with an urge to have a BM. The first time I go everything is rather normal. Then I have to go again, and again, etc. Each time I go the consistency seems to be waterier. This all happens within an hour (or two). After that I won't have to go for the rest of the day. Can anyone identify with this?

This is my first posting. I was just given a tentative IBS-D diagnosis today after having lots of other (and scarier) things ruled out.

Thanks!!

From: **Planet Earth**

S.G.
Regular Member

Yes, Gastron, mornings are really bad for me too. I really, REALLY, understand. I am always late for work, because of this. Yes, it's so depressing!

I have a doctor's appt. tomorrow. I started taking calcium three times a day, because quite a few people write that it really helps them. Perhaps you should try it, too. It can't harm you, and will be good for your bones, too! S.G.

From: **N.J., U.S.A.**

Maxson
Regular Member

I have the same exact symptoms, what is it with mornings? I get nervous about waking up because I know what will happen and then being nervous only makes it worse! Good grief. I'm going to try the calcium too; it is worth a try that's for sure. Also, taking a mild tranquilizer when you get up can help, but you don't want to have to do that every day either. I also started drinking peppermint tea, as soon as I wake up, to help settle my stomach, it helps a little. Too bad we couldn't skip the mornings and just start the day with afternoons.

From: **Illinois**

Inafog
Prolific Member

Calcium has worked for me. I've only had one episode of D in five weeks.

I've had the morning problems, but usually my D hits me without warning at any time during the day. I've read that not eating anything after 7:00 or 8:00 at night will help with the morning attacks.

Kathy

From: **Way to go Ohio**

Jellster
New Member

I know what you mean about mornings! I dread waking up because it all starts. I couldn't even let the dog out and feed the cat before I had to hit the bathroom. I did start calcium three times a day and it really helped. I went on vacation and didn't bring it with me and what a mistake. Now that I'm home I've started again and am starting to get some relief. Try it, I do think it works. Good luck!

Jellster

From: **Middlesex, NJ**

Trudyg
Prolific Member

The morning D is because your system is 'asleep' at night, then you wake up and everything gets moving again. Just like you are wide awake first thing, so is your system. (Hah! I never feel rested or wide awake) Then, the 'after you eat' D is because of the natural way your system works. Eating sets in motion the entire digestive system, moving it all right along. IBSers just move along lots faster than normal folks. I get up at 5:00 AM and don't have to be at work until 8:30 AM, just so my system can get over it. I eat only pretzels while at work, even though rice or rice cakes work pretty well. Those foods are bland and expand in your belly to make you feel like you ate and your tummy won't growl, you just don't get any energy from them. I also eat lots of peppermint lifesavers (sugar as well as peppermint to soothe). Hope this helps.

From: **Huntsville, AL**

Safety
New Member

Mornings are (or were) the worst for me. I would immediately go to the toilet with severe D and vomiting. And like you, my first movement was not too bad, but afterwards they got very watery up until mid-afternoon. I think I have now found somewhat of a solution. I have been taking calcium with Vitamin D twice a day and four ginger tablets (for bloating) for about five months and along with many fruits and vegetables (oranges, nectarines, apples and carrots), I have had some success. I can actually wake up and have a smoke before going to the toilet, without the mad dash. Stay with this board—the information is so helpful and hopefully you will find something that works for you. Good luck.

From: **Calgary**

HereIam
Prolific Member

Even though my D is "under control" using Questran, mornings are still a problem, and sound just like yours. First BM is normal then it goes downhill for two or three more BM's, all urgent. After that, I'm okay for the day.

I never take an early morning flight or ride and get up two to three hours before having to leave the house. Am living with it this way. I remember the days in my 20's when I used to hop buses, trains, car pools, whatever, early in the morning to get to work in the city and I can't even remember being that person. Now, it's a sweat just to drive the kids to school in the morning!!! At least the rest of my day is "normal", thanks to Questran.

From: **Massachusetts**

Les T
New Member

It's been about a year since my symptoms began, very similar to yours.

My doctor suggested Metamucil, morning and night. Within a week, I was down to one BM in the morning. Still not a normal BM, but the D is mostly gone, (unless I miss the Metamucil). I couldn't believe how much an over-the-counter changed my life.

If you haven't started to take the Caltrate yet, you should. Chances are you'll be avoiding dairy, and that can lead to other problems if you don't replace the vitamins.

Occasionally I eat something that throws me off for a few days, but it's not nearly as bad as it used to be.

Best of luck!

From: **USA**

Kirksbunny2
New Member

Well it must be true, misery loves company. I too suffer in the mornings with bouts of D. It is not uncommon for me to make five or more runs to the bathroom. On occasion I will suffer with it in the afternoon but usually it starts in the morning and usually when I'm in the middle of eating breakfast. I've had this now for five years and am used to eating a cold breakfast!

I've never heard of trying calcium until I joined this site, but will have to try it. I think if road kill helped I'd even try that, LOL!

From: **USA**

Fjp2k3
New Member

For me, I can get D any time of the day or night. As I mentioned in another post that I would, I have tried the calcium and I noticed improvements. I went three weeks straight 100% normal. I've had a few bumps on the road, but very few (maybe two or three in the entire month) as opposed to two to three a week.

So far, I've only tried calcium two times a day (i.e., two 600 mg tablets). Imodium cuts any D I get at any time. I use it before trips and it helps. I'm not sure I'd like to use it every day, though. I'm still looking for a good combination of medicine/supplements. I now believe that calcium is part of the equation, thanks to this newsgroup.

The important thing is to not lose hope and NEVER, EVER give up on fighting this s**t, literally!

From: **Pennsylvania, U.S.A.**

Discussion: Public Restrooms

Out of necessity, people with IBS-D are quickly forced to become experts on the topic of public restrooms. You will certainly relate as members share their horror stories and express their wishes for easy access to clean, private restrooms.

Topic: Public Restrooms

Lora
New Member

I was wondering if I am strange or if there is someone else that hates to use public restrooms because of the embarrassment. I sometimes am in the middle of a panic and I really gotta go and I know that by the time I get there it is gonna be very noisy and I dread it so much. Public restrooms are the worst for me and the employee restroom at work.

From: **Anaheim, Ca, USA**

Tattoo
Prolific Member

Do you mean you have a *choice* of when/where to go??? LOL

But I have been known to just sit in my stall and wait until everyone else is gone before I emerge.

While I'm griping, one of my pet peeves is when people are sitting in stalls and having business meetings. Hey, I don't go potty in your meetings; can you show me similar courtesy and not have meetings in my bathroom???

(Hey, do ya think I maybe feel a bit proprietary about the bathroom because I spend so much more time there than anyone else?)

From: **Uranus**

Mrsmason
Very Prolific Member

Tattoo, you never fail to make me chuckle.

Though I must say, it is a serious topic, I agree about that. I don't think *anyone* enjoys having an attack in a public restroom. But sometimes you gotta do what you gotta do! As Tattoo mentioned, we don't always get a choice. One thing I like to do is scope out the number of bathrooms around that are "one at a time" bathrooms. You know, the kind where it is just one commode and a sink. Those provide a bit more privacy, but it still is no fun. Shoot, I don't even enjoy it when it happens at home! LOL

From: **Indiana, USA**

Bre
New Member

Are you kidding??!! I won't go places where there is the one-at-a-time bathroom. If I do, I am a nervous wreck anytime I see anyone heading in the direction of the bathroom. Then I panic because I think I am going to have to go and there will be no vacancy. I just think with the public multi-person restroom, "Hey, by the time I get out of this stall the people that were in here when I was stinking up the place and making lots of noise will be long gone". And besides for the most part you will never see any of those people again. As for the employee restroom, it may be less embarrassing to come clean and tell others about the problem verses worrying about having to use the employee toilet. Good luck bathroom worriers—I can relate, but my biggest worry is not having a public bathroom where I am at all. That is THE worst—I think.

From: **New York**

Jeanne D
Very Prolific Member

I do not like public restrooms and I try to avoid them as much as possible, but if I absolutely have to use them, I do. I often hope that they are empty, but if they aren't, I do a lot of flushing as I am going.

It's embarrassing, but sort of silly in a way. Let's face it, everyone does the same thing. We all go to the bathroom, and we all make noise at some point. It's not as if we are doing something "unusual". I try to look at it that way.

Jeanne

From: **USA**

Trots
Prolific Member

Jeanne, I understand not wanting to be heard, but when you flush, tiny particles become airborne. If you're sitting there, guess where they're going. I mean germs from other people, yuck. Just hide out for awhile, until it's safe to come out, then flush.

Now I have become somewhat of a freak in public bathrooms. I flush with my foot … last week when I tried to raise my leg up after too much exercise, I knocked down the metal tampon receptacle. Not embarrassing at all.

From: **New York**

Marcel
New Member

The Turd Burglar:
Someone who tries to open your bathroom stall door while you are still in there.

The Pre Flush:
Clean out the bowl before you go (gets rid of most of the germs).

The Courtesy Flush:
Flushing the toilet as you explode (works well).

I totally understand your bathroom woes!

Marcel.

From: **Canada, ON**

Jane1721
Regular Member

I never, never, never use a public restroom for D. ESPECIALLY at work! Actually, at the job that I had when I was first diagnosed I was the only woman there. So it was no problem! The job sucked, but for that reason and that reason alone, I miss it!!

I have taught myself to hold it (which, BTW, is not always a smart move ... I'll be holding it all day at work and can't wait to get home so I can GO ... and by that time I am constipated!) Actually, I think I taught myself that a long time ago, way before IBS, because my mother always told me that it was impolite to do #2 in a toilet that wasn't yours! So for many reasons, it is a darn good thing I live alone and have my very own bathroom all to myself!

Jane

From: **Ohio**

CrystalOne
Regular Member

I fear public restrooms too. What I don't understand is how you guys say you can hold it. When I have to go—I have to go NOW. There's no holding it.

Also, I have to wonder about what Jane1721 said about how she grew up thinking it was impolite to go #2 in someone else's restroom. I grew up with that kind of mindset too. Also, passing gas was impolite and something you just did not do in the presence of others. I wonder if holding it all those years has anything to do with IBS. I just have to wonder about that.

Anybody else have thoughts on that?

From: **USA**

Michele
Prolific Member

I agree with Bre. I love public restrooms with tons of stalls! OK, not that public restrooms are so wonderful, but I love having a restroom available when I need it and not having to worry that all stalls are full or that people are waiting for me to get out of the only stall so they can use it. I especially avoid restaurants with one-person-only stalls. I end up spending the whole meal with one eye on the bathroom so I know if it's available.

From: **Texas**

Bikerfish
New Member

The bit I really hate in public loos is when you have someone on either side of you who is waiting for you to let rip and there's this strained silence as you all just sit there listening to each others shuffling.

If any of those shufflers are reading this ….
STOP IT, or my bowels WILL explode!

From: **Worcestershire, ENGLAND**

Nmwinter
Very Prolific Member

My fear is NOT finding a public bathroom when I need it! I can't hold it very long when the D is coming (although much better since learning some relaxation techniques). I also do a lot of flushing as I go—takes some of the smell with it.

Of course now I'll be thinking about other people's germs coming up to greet me—thanks a lot, Trots.

Nancy

From: **Portland, OR, USA**

NANCY588
Regular Member

I will do whatever I have to do to avoid public bathrooms!! The sounds, odor, etc. are always embarrassing. However, my biggest concern when using a public toilet is … what do I do if I find myself having one of those episodes that just keeps on going with no end in site? You hope you're through … start to get up and WHAM … the cramps start up and you have to sit back down … quick! I've not eaten for days in anticipation of air travel. What do you do if you're in the midst of an 'explosion' and the pilot announces it's time to return to your seat to prepare for landing? I've also sat on many a runway at O'Hare waiting to take off, feeling that awful impending attack about to hit—just as the pilot announces we're number 15 to take off (14 planes ahead of us)!

So many of you talk about using public bathrooms—or wearing adult diapers. You must have the kind of movements that run their course and end within a short period of time. Am I the only one who often gets stuck on the toilet for an hour or more at a time—unable to get up? Sometimes this can go on all day … fine for an hour and it starts all over again. And the volume is sometimes enormous. Hard to keep up with the flushing!!

From: **Chicago, IL**

Sunny
Very Prolific Member

I am more worried about having an accident than someone hearing me. Cleaning myself up in a public restroom is the worst thing that can happen. And what do you do with the soiled garments???? I'm glad that doesn't happen to me very often.

Sunny

From: **KANSAS USA**

Bre
New Member

I agree Sunny!! I would rather use a nasty stinky public restroom then have an accident. A few months ago I was on my way to my mother's house (about a 45 minute drive) and I had to go. Held it, held it ... finally pulled into a fast food bathroom and while having to get my daughter out of the car it started coming. Well, I had overalls on and trying to quick get them undone and off, the straps fell in the toilet and then got on my shoe. Trying to clean up in a restroom (and hold a baby) was not fun. I had to get back in my car and deal with the mess the rest of the ride. So the moral of the story is ...

If there is a potty around just go. It is better to stink it up then clean it up.

From: **New York**

Audrey F
Regular Member

I sure wish I could figure out how to hold it. When I have to go, it is NOW. I thank God when there are public restrooms with multiple stalls. I die when there is only one for a restaurant (I usually won't go back again). My problem is when I have to go it usually isn't a quick trip. It usually is 30 minutes to an hour. I thank God when I can make it in time. I've taken to wearing a dress when I travel in the car in case I have to pull over on the side of the road. That way I could drop my drawers and go with a bit of cover (so far haven't had to do so but it makes me feel a bit better) It is nice to know others share the same crazy worries. I scope out toilets wherever I go just in case. Lots of times I find I would rather not go out than have to deal with bathroom issues. Then I take a breath and tell myself I refuse to let IBS totally run my life. I dread looking for a new job as most everyone here knows my problem and covers for me but my job ends before the end of the year and I have to figure out what to do. Seems to be always something. In the vote of toilets, I say yeah for public restrooms, stinky, dirty and all.

Your pal in misery,
ALF

From: **Houston, Texas**

Reinnil
New Member

If anyone out there can tell me just how you hold it, I would give anything to know! When I feel the urge I have to make immediate tracks for the bathroom … any bathroom. One time I was in a public state park and I just made it in time but made the mistake of breathing in! Moments later I was losing it at both ends! I came out to a queue of people. I was madly apologizing but they were pretty unforgiving and called me disgusting. I fretted over that for weeks. Dear God I wish I could hold it!

From: **Venice, Fl. U.S.A.**

Kristian
Very Prolific Member

Hi All,

I just had a few thoughts, incidents to contribute to this thread. I would much rather go in a public bathroom than risk an accident and I've become very adept at figuring out where they are. I loathe the idea of using one and always have. But about a year ago, I had an incident where I didn't make it to the bathroom. I had left the office and was about three blocks into my six-block walk to the train when it started. I thought I could hold a bit and turned around and started walking back to my building. After a few steps, I had to stop walking and was trying very hard to hold it, but the D started coming and I couldn't hold it. (Luckily, I had on a ¾ length leather jacket and took it off quickly; I mean I was in the middle of Wall Street at rush hour.)

So I walked back to my building and shut myself in the handicap stall and threw my undies out. Luckily, I remembered that one of my closest friends lived a few blocks from where the incident happened. So I was able to go wash up and borrow some clothes. Some people are so cool about this stuff.

Another rather bad incident happened when I went out with my then new boyfriend to meet his oldest friends (a couple). Well, we had dinner and the cramps started and we went to this bar where I spent the next 30 minutes disappearing and emerging from the bathroom. I was soooo embarrassed but told them that something we had at dinner didn't agree with me. (I had already shared my tummy troubles with my beau.)

I will say that since I've been taking fiber supplements (Metamucil, mostly) that when I get the urgent cramping, I can hold it much better than before, but do suffer from massive pain when I do.

I do think that the fact that I was totally averse to using public restrooms until I was an adult may have had some effect on my IBS. I remember spending tons of times as a kid, holding it in and then not being able to go when I got home. I'd really like to know how many other people have a similar history. Maybe it does have something to do with developing IBS later in life.

I just have to add that I love this board and was just telling my BF that it's so great to be able to interact with people who have the same problem.

Good luck to all.

From: **New York City**

Sabriel
Prolific Member

Oh, I can so relate to this topic!

Especially the comments by Bre and Marcel. I, too, dread the possibility of a bathroom not being available when needed more than it being too public.

Marcels comment about "Someone who tries to open your bathroom stall door while you're still in there" was something else I could totally relate too. Like DUH, if the door is closed or locked, of course there is someone in there!

Embarrassing enough being stuck in the loo and not able to leave but do we really have to put up with people who don't seem to understand that a locked door means there is someone in residence?

Aargh! I have lost count of the number of times now that someone has tapped on the loo door and gone "Is someone in there?" That really drives me crazy!

From: **Australia**

Pat..
Very Prolific Member

I remember seeing a TV program about a year ago and it was on in Japan. Apparently in some places they now have these loos that have air suction around the rim that draws away any smells, etc. They also have music to cover any noises. Sounds like absolute bliss to me. I expect when we are all long gone this might be the norm for everywhere. I carry a small bottle of Neutradol in my handbag. Although the smell of it is not great, it does tend to neutralize smells rather than cover them up which is worse. Just having it with me helps the anxiety. I also carry a plastic bag and some tissues just in case. I think I'd rather "go" behind a bush in a bag than use public toilets. Know it sounds daft, but I prefer to travel at night so if I did have to go I would have less chance of being seen. Sad, eh?

From: **England**

Audrey F
Regular Member

I think the bottom line is through sharing of feelings and ideas we will all realize that we are not alone and others have the exact same issues and problems. I am new to the board and have found it extremely helpful to know I am not a nutcase. Thanks to everyone that participates.

From: **Houston, Texas**

Reinnil
New Member

Hello everyone!

I love this site! Lots of company and lots of advice. The humor is wonderful. If you can stand another 'it happened to me story' … here goes. I was in Home Depot with my daughter. Suddenly the urge was upon me and I had no idea where the bathrooms were. My daughter gave me instructions but they proved wrong. Now I am starting to sweat … I ask someone the directions, got the general direction but starting to feel as if it was already too late. Panic was setting in; running like a knocked-kneed ostrich and dribbling all the way … I finally found the restroom … empty!! What heaven! I madly cleaned up before anyone came in. Luckily, I was wearing a loose skirt so nothing was obvious, but from then on I ALWAYS inquire for the loo first, no matter where I go. My name was Wadham, so my family calls this 'The Wadham Curse'. Every time anyone gets diarrhea they say 'I have the Wadham curse'. It's gotten to be a family joke! Still, we have to keep our sense of humor, right?

From: **Venice, Fl. U.S.A.**

Theba77
New Member

Wow, I love this site. I just want to say that it is such a relief to know that I am not alone. The whole public restroom thing is totally me. I get nervous if I go out to eat at a restaurant that I know does not have dual stalls. This kills me. I get nervous sometimes at home. I live in a one bedroom, one bathroom apartment with my fiancée and when people come over to hang out or for a party, I freak out. Even though I know I can go at anytime, I still cramp up. Sometimes, I can't go out and have any fun because I get nervous. It seems like I am always on the sideline when it comes to going out. No matter what I do, nothing seems to work, except for not eating and filling up with Imodium, two things that won't help in the long run. But if I didn't have such a supportive fiancée, I don't know what I would do. You know, we should come up with some sort of IBS dating service. It would probably make millions … just a thought.

From: **Home**

Sabriel
Prolific Member

Hi again,

I just thought of another 'addendum' if you will to this topic.

Don't ya just hate if you go into a public loo and there is no paper??? Especially when you have the D really bad. I have been carrying a supply of facial tissues around with me in my bag for YEARS for just this reason.

I usually check for loo paper first, but sometimes you don't have the time for that luxury and thank goodness for my bag of tissues. Certainly has gotten me out of some literally 'big messes'!

From: **Australia**

Jeanne D
Very Prolific Member

I do the same thing, too. I always make sure I have some Kleenex in my purse, just in case there is no paper.

To go into a public restroom is bad enough, but to find out there is no paper is adding insult to injury.

Ah … the challenges we face with IBS.

Jeanne

From: **USA**

Poeticalms
Prolific Member

As far as public bathrooms are concerned, if it flushes I will use it. My mother recently visited me in NYC, and I told her we needed to walk down Broadway because there is a Starbucks every few blocks, in case I needed to use the bathroom. Needless to say, I have tried several Starbucks bathrooms, they flush and have toilet paper, can't ask for anything else.

From: **New York, NY**

Dom
New Member

I envy all of you who can hold back the 'D' till an appropriate time. I sometimes only have seconds to hit the toilet and have had my share of accidents as a result.

I carry the wet wipes and a small can of deodorant spray like Lysol around with me, and keep towels and a change of clothes in my car. I have gas-propelled 'D', so noises are unavoidable.

I've had IBS for over 30 years and nothing stops it. I've just learned to live with my limitations which is hard to do for some of you, especially those of you who work outside the home.

Dom

Debra M
Regular Member

Oh yes … I know what you mean. If I have to use a public restroom and someone is in there too … I usually sit and wait till they are gone. Course you know sometimes you can sit there forever!! Then, oh my gosh, if someone comes in while/after I am going … oh, I wait till they leave so they won't know who the person was who tried to kill them in the next stall!!! My husband says to me, "Just go Deb, who cares, like they are ever gonna see you again anyway?" Geez … no way I tell him. If I am having big-time flare-ups, I just don't go out. Rather stink up my own "library" than go out. And most times there is NO way I can hold it. Like at work, I just told them I have this thing, and just make sure we have plenty of TP and air spray. Better to not hold it in, my doc says, causes even more problems … so everyone just knows I'll be camping in the bathroom and make sure I am well armed … LOL ….

Debra

From: **Acton, CA, USA**

Topic: Public Restrooms

CatPurrson
New Member

Hi! I'm new here, and I'm sure this question has probably already been asked, but how do you handle public restrooms? I have diarrhea-predominant IBS (okay, completely dominant ...) and I HATE using public restrooms. Invariably there's always a rude child (or an even ruder adult) who has to comment. "God, it stinks in here!" "What crawled up her b* and died?" All my friends tell me that I should just ignore it, but that's a lot easier said than done! It's not bad enough that I'm miserable; do I have to be humiliated too? Do people expect me to become a hermit just because I have IBS? Any help/suggestions would be most appreciated!

From: **SC, USA**

Blackcat
Prolific Member

I have a hard time with pubic restrooms. Sadly my body shuts itself off until I get home (especially traveling) which actually causes more and worse problems. I'm trying to work with my body to just do what it needs to do, when it needs to do it. If I am in a public restroom, I usually think to myself that I am really never going to see these people again. That usually relieves some of the anxiety that goes along with public restrooms. Also you can do the whole flushing when making noise thing. That can always help, as for the smell well, just be proud???? Remember these are normal bodily functions, and our bodies seem to need a little more attention, but we are great, strong, unique individuals. Hope that helped in some way!

Love always
Amanda

From: **Orange County/Santa Cruz, California**

CatPurrson
New Member

Thanks for the help! One of my bigger problems, though, is at school. I go to a small college, and using the restrooms there can be quite mortifying ... I know what you mean about trying to hold it! I've done that a few times. I think another reason public restrooms bug me so much is the idea of being away from a "safe" place. Especially when it's REALLY bad, I get cramps, nausea, cold sweats ... Just the thought is causing a few threatening rumbles! I do like the flushing idea. Have tried "coughing" or clearing my throat ...

Thanks again!

From: **SC, USA**

Michele
Prolific Member

Ooh, I was so mad the other day. I had my husband stop at McDonald's because I really needed to go. One stall was locked without anyone in there, so I went in the other. Someone came in and tried both doors then knocked on mine. (You couldn't see feet because of the way the stall was made.) I said "Yes?" to let her know someone was in there. She waited about a minute then left and I heard her say to someone (before the door swung shut), "There's a rude sh***er in there." I am now wishing a nasty case of food poisoning on her.

From: **Texas**

Christi
Regular Member

HI,

I hate going in public restrooms ... they are usually dirty and disgusting ... I was very proud of myself the other day. I was at Walmart with my sister shopping ... Then all of the sudden I started having severe pains ... I knew if I did not use the restroom I would be in big trouble ... Thankfully I made it stay in there for a while ... I put a lot of toilet paper on the seat ... and here is what I do, I know it may sound weird but I close my ears with my hands and shut my eyes and pretend that I am in my own bathroom ... Plus I don't care who is talking about me because I can't hear or see them ... It was the first time I ever did that and it seemed to work ... . I don't know, maybe you should try that, it might work ....

Good luck.
CHRIS

From: **Philadelphia, PA**

Skye
Regular Member

I may have to try that shutting my eyes/blocking my ears thing! I too, hate public restrooms and usually try to hold it till there's some privacy … which, as was stated before, always makes things worse.

From: **Florida**

Auroraheart
Very Prolific Member

I absolutely HATE stall washrooms. Whoever coined the phrase STALL was so right. I know I should not, but at work I often use the wheelchair washroom b/c it is its own separate room. Sometimes I flush when a big "spurt" comes out and let it all go until the flush noise stops.

From: **Ontario**

Karen P
Prolific Member

I can't believe people in washrooms can be soooo rude! What do they THINK goes on in there? Do they think their @#$% doesn't smell!!! Now that I've vented, when I have an attack and I have to use a public washroom, I just keep saying to myself "everyone gets D sometime in their life" and it makes me feel better. I also flush a lot to dull the noise.

From: **Mississauga**

D-gasblaster
Prolific Member

Public restrooms suck! When I have to use one, I try not to touch anything. I see people come out of the stall and then leave without washing their hands. This is disgusting and it makes me not want to go in there at all. I don't think too much about taking a s**t in there when other people are around, because I don't know them. Bathrooms are for sh***ing, and that's that! When I have to go, I have to go!!

From: **Here, In The USA**

Jay
Prolific Member

I have gone to many horrible bathrooms since my IBS started (about three years now). Once however, I went into a bathroom stall in a restaurant outside NYC and the stall had sh*t on the seat and the floor. This sounds horrible but I actually decided I would risk having an accident (which is what ended up happening) rather than use that facility. I figured better to sit in my own sh*t than someone else's.

From: **Canada**

D-gasblaster
Prolific Member

Speaking of public toilets ... ... what about those disgusting portable toilets they have in campgrounds? I usually opt for the friendly tree or bush instead.

From: **Here, In The USA**

Mamamia
Prolific Member

Dear D-gas:

As far as port-a-johns go, the woods rule!!

Port-a-johns are the absolute worse, as if you weren't feeling ill enough already ....

Love, M—

From: **New Jersey, USA**

Maki
Regular Member

Had the same experience as Jay. I didn't know if I was going to make in my pants or throw up from the smell, really. I got so nervous and ran out. Thank God that one time it subsided till I got to a restroom next door.

From: **New York**

HereIam
Prolific Member

I think I've said it here before, but I say "any potty in a storm." I really don't care where I go, as long as it ain't in my pants or behind a small tree. I have many phobias; luckily, public toilets ain't one of them. My girlfriends are always appalled at the "disgusting" places I'll place my big old butt if necessary. Have had too many accidents in my pants to worry about this one. Port-a-potties, gas station bathrooms, men's rooms, girl's rooms, I really don't care.

Been this way for years and am happy to report that I've not caught any diseases from my disgusting behavior.

From: **Massachusetts**

Bobo
Prolific Member

I cannot believe I actually have a good experience to share about public restrooms! And believe me; I've had my shares of using public restrooms that were lacking.

At the grocery store the other day, I felt that urgent need (ugh). Went in the ladies' room and they had decorated it! Fake vines draping the stalls, baskets full of fake fruit. But the best thing was—it smelled like bushels of apples in there! Bushels and bushels of apples! Even though I had a bad attack of D, there was NO lingering overwhelming smell. I was the only person using the facilities, but it made me feel so much better mentally.

Everyone poops. Why can't they pay more attention to ventilation and such in public restrooms everywhere?

From: **USA**

Discussion: IBS-D and Work

The need to have quick and easy access to a bathroom can be in direct opposition with the need to be at a job at a certain time. Read on to find out how others get to work on time and tell bosses and co-workers what they need to do in order to keep themselves comfortable.

Topic: To all working people ....

CDG1228
Regular Member

What kind of work do you do and how do you handle the bathroom issues that you have?

From: **North Carolina**

Engine23
Prolific Member

I have two jobs .... My paid job is in IT and I go whenever the heck I feel like it!

The other is as a volunteer firefighter. I usually respond to about three hundred calls a year and when the true emergency need hits, I knock on doors until someone lets me in, find a tree, or go in a burning building ... whatever it takes.

From: **Houston, TX USA**

Mandsu815
Regular Member

This is a good topic … I am currently a college student and work in an office part-time, so right now it is not a problem. I am studying to be a teacher and am very worried about what I will do when I have 30 students to watch. Yikes!

From: **California**

CDG1228
Regular Member

I work in an office (8:30 AM—5:00 PM) and am able to go whenever I need to, but it's embarrassing. There are eleven people and two bathrooms, but they are in a bad location. And, of course, no one else here has any issues AT ALL. Just me! No one has ever asked me any questions, but I'm sure there have been conversations (or e-mails).

From: **North Carolina**

LifeLongIBS
Regular Member

I'm an Occupational Therapist, work in a town that is about 50 miles away from my house. My main problem is the drive, rather than when I get to work; as I have previously posted, I have had to pull off the road before …. We have two restrooms in the outpatient clinic and not much privacy, so that is not great. I also sometimes have to do some home health and therapy at a nursing home, as the hospital I work for contracts with several other entities. Since I have been off of my acid-reducer, the uncontrollable "D" has been a lot better, almost having more trouble with "C" now … and always have the gas, pain, bloating. Thank goodness I usually wear elastic waist scrubs to my job. I have had to let the elastic out, though.

Take care everyone,

Kandy

From: **Texas**

PrairieAngel
Regular Member

I work in a retail store that luckily has a large bathroom in the back room. And luckily, we usually have enough staff on that I can "discreetly" leave the sales floor should I need to. But the biggest help was that I was totally up-front with my co-workers. I said "I have a condition called IBS. When I say I need to use the washroom, I REALLY mean it." Everyone was pretty cool about it. We always buy lots of air freshener. It helps too that my boss' husband has Crohn's, so she understands.

From: **Manitoba, Canada**

Linda C
Regular Member

Mandu, I am a teacher, and yes, sometimes it's a challenge when you're stuck in a classroom with 30 kids. What I have found helpful is just privately explaining my situation to the principal and vice principal. That way, if I need emergency "coverage" I can call down to the office and they will understand what's happening. Also, if you have a friendly teacher working next door or across the hall, you could ask them to keep an eye on your class. Of course, this depends on the age of your students. Technically, you're not supposed to leave the classroom, but if it's a true emergency, what can you do? You'll be surprised at how understanding most people are if you just explain the situation.

From: **Toronto, Ontario, Canada**

Maxdenq
Regular Member

I'm in IT and can displace myself anytime. Once a month, I'm on call for a week at nights, which works out really fine because even if I'm not on call and hanging out with friends, I can always say "got to take this call" and disappear for a couple of minutes.

From: **Toronto/Canada**

Trudyg
Prolific Member

I'm a clerk in a public office, bathroom down the hall. Not a problem unless we get real busy—some customers don't understand "I'll be right back" and you don't show back up for 20 minutes! My coworker is okay with it most of the time, but she's getting old and cranky, so who knows. There are several people with the same problem in the downstairs part of my office (only one toilet on that entire floor for 18 people in the office!) but they seem to understand. The ones without IBS go to the basement bathrooms, probably because the rest of them stink up the other one.

From: **Huntsville, AL**

Kimmie
Prolific Member

I quit my job five years ago, but I worked as a hairstylist and all the girls I worked with knew about my problem. They were okay to my face, but I always felt some of them talked behind my back. They thought that I could just take an antidiarrheal and be fine. But I was lucky, my husband made enough that I was able to quit and be a full-time Mom to my two kids. Nothing was worse than being in the middle of doing someone's hair and to feel an attack coming on. Plus we only had one toilet and it was across from our supply room!

From: **Ohio**

Whataboutmen
New Member

I manage a web site, so I can work from home and go to the office when I need to. Although I had to tell my boss about the IBS because I was going to be out for a colonoscopy, I haven't brought it up to him again. He hasn't said a word about me coming in late or not being around all the time, so I haven't explained that I was working … just from home. Do you think it is wise to talk to him about it again and make sure it's okay to stay home or go home early some days? I'm worried that he will take it the wrong way and I just need to try harder to get the IBS fixed.

From: **North Carolina**

LifeLongIBS
Regular Member

Whataboutmen,

Do you get the feeling from your boss that he has a problem with the way you are working your schedule? I guess I would gauge what I am sensing from him and go from there. How about if you do decide to talk to him, get some info about IBS that explains it is not curable but manageable, and give it to him? Don't know if you are comfortable with that, but maybe it will help. I think there are a lot more of us with this horrible IBS than I ever realized until I found this board.

Good luck,
Kandy

From: **Texas**

Grrrl-aghast
Prolific Member

I work in a small company making fake tattoos and special FX makeup for movies (The Mummy, Blade II, X-men ...). My boss has been pretty cool about my IBS (letting me leave early/come in late), but of course she can't pay me if I'm out of sick days and have to stay home (which really hurts financially) ... so it's still a problem. I'm also taking web development classes, and Saturday mornings are usually pretty bad for me. I can only miss up to 24 hours off school without getting in trouble, plus I can't really afford to miss that much without falling behind. The school stress doesn't help my symptoms of course, but I'm trying all I can to keep up and attend. Hopefully I can tough it out until February (that's when I—hopefully—graduate), but then I'll run into the next problem: having to find a new job and being able to keep it, despite the IBS troubles. Maybe one day I'll be able to freelance from home ... that'd be the ultimate!

From: **NYC**

Carlowrower
New Member

I have IBS w/D. Very bad D lately. I work in a restaurant as a waitress and bartender. The other bartenders know about my issues, they have similar problems. It is pretty easy to escape. It is hard when you're at a table and the people want to ask a million pointless questions and I can feel an attack coming on. I actually finished school to be an art teacher and am supposed to be substituting but have been holding back for fear of attacks while in class. I am going to the doctor soon to ask about prescription medicines to (hopefully) help.

From: **Pittsburgh**

LaVidaCrapa
Prolific Member

You all know it's true: that when looking for a new job, if you have IBS-D, it figures into your job search.

At every interview, by necessity (interview jitters) or just to know, I usually would check out the bathroom situation as best I could.

Having a good bathroom situation at work is crucial! My job is in an office setting. There are a few jobs that I interviewed for that actually gave me concern because of the way the bathrooms were set up. (One place had a bathroom for everyone that was located just off someone's office! So you had to pass through there every time you had to go! Plus it was a single toilet for about 30 people! I'm glad I found a different place!)

At my current workplace, we have men's and women's restrooms down the hall, which we access with our own keys and each has at least two toilets in it. I can sneak off to the bathroom discreetly with no one to notice.

It certainly helps my confidence level during the work day. I've been in workplace situations with less favorable conditions and a bathroom crisis would weigh on my mind all day.

From: **Cleveland, OH USA**

Julianna
Regular Member

Oh my goodness! This issue is SO important! I work in a hospital, my boss is about 15 miles away, and I have very little contact with patients. When I need to go, I take off. If there's someone in the bathroom, I either go to another floor's bathroom (if I can make it) or try to hold it until they leave. I know all the bathrooms in this hospital well!

My previous workplace featured one bathroom for like 25 employees, both men and women. Also, there was some kind of acoustical phenomenon going on with that bathroom; you could hear EVERYTHING from the nearby hallway. That seriously factored into my decision to leave.

Julianna

From: **Southern CA**

Twocups424
Prolific Member

OMG, I am so glad that I haven't had to have a full-time job while suffering from IBS-D all these years. I have managed to raise three children and keep a house going and keep it relatively clean and even do some refinishing, wallpapering, painting and staining. I have had a part-time job at Christmas quite a few times. That was enough. I DON'T KNOW HOW ALL YOU WHO HAVE IBS-D MANAGE A FULL TIME JOB!!!!!!!! God Bless You!

From: **PA**

HereIam
Prolific Member

I am a pediatric social worker in the emergency room of a community hospital. Bathrooms all over the place and they are clean. The stress can get thick and there are many situations I can't just bolt from because my stomach's knotting up. I think this has been good for me though, as it's taught me to ignore a lot of the false signals my gut sends out. I work three twelve-hour days and then do four hours of administrative work on my computer at home each week. The twelve-hour shifts were tough on my diet at first, until I finally figured out that it was important to stick to a normal, healthy eating plan while at work.

My nightmare job was when I was a caseworker for child protection services and I was "on the street." I was doing home visits to all kinds of places, far-flung and inner city, places where you'd never stop and ask to use a toilet. I have a van and at that time I kept a children's port-a-potty in the back just in case (oh, no, I'm not revealing if it ever got used).

From: **Massachusetts**

IBS survivor
Regular Member

I have you all beat! I deliver the mail and I'm on the street five+ hours a day. Thank God I don't have IBS-D as bad as some of you. I rate mine about a 3 on a scale of 10. Sometimes it can be worse. Anyway, I have a bathroom when I'm at the station the first three hours of the day. After that, I'm on my own. I have several bathrooms on or close to my route, but if the need should arise, it would take five to ten minutes to get there.

Usually the first two hours of the day are the worst and those are spent at home. If I think it's going to be a "bad" day, I just stay home, because once you go to work, you're stuck! So far I've been lucky and have had no accidents, but I'm always thinking about it and what I would do if I got one of those knots in my gut. It's a scary thought! I just make sure that I take my meds everyday (Bentyl & Lomotil) and calcium which has helped my tremendously since I started taking it three weeks ago. Since I started the calcium, I have had no D and no urgency. The longer you go w/o those problems, the more confidence you get. I feel pretty good about myself right now.

Anyone who gets out there every day and works outside the home is a real trooper. Keep up the good work ....

From: **U.S.A.**

Pocahontas425
Regular Member

I commute to work for one hour on the subway to the city … I am a secretary and a full time student.

Honestly—sometimes, I don't know how I cope—but I do. I must admit that I am not as bad as many of the people on BB.

I eat a banana and oatmeal for breakfast, a "Campbell's Soup to Go" for lunch, and a bagel for dinner during the week.

I try to be as honest as possible with my supervisor and other colleagues. I am well known for my stomach problems. But I figure it this way—honesty is the best policy—if they know how serious this is, they will be a little more understanding and sympathetic to your situation. I have even been given a laptop to work from home on really bad days.

I consider myself thankful, and really lucky, that my colleagues, friends and family understand.

From: **New York**

Dkik
New Member

With IBS, you learn to survive … and find out where all the bathrooms are. I moved in to town to be closer to my job (no more 45 minute commute—without bathroom stops). I'm a photographer, and have become friendly with my clients so I can use the bathroom while shooting. I also take my phone with me—might as well get some work done, too. I was at a photo shoot one time, and had horrible cramps and D—couldn't concentrate. The end photos were not very good—and I ended up re-shooting on a "better" day. This IBS has really changed the way I live, but you cope. And you laugh. And you survive. What doesn't kill you only makes you stronger. My husband tells me that often. We try to laugh about it—it helps. When we are on long trips, he will look at every restroom and say "Well …?" But he knows when I say STOP, he needs to STOP RIGHT NOW! I hope that some day they will find CURE for this thing, not just a temporary Band-Aid.

We should all get together and have a telethon—"Help Stop Explosive D—Cure IBS"! Oh, well. Have a better day, all.

From: **Grand Rapids, MI**

WindyCityRich
Regular Member

I work in an office—I am the controller in my company. The bathrooms can be accessed pretty easily and discretely. I have let the management know that I have stomach and digestive problems.

(It's pretty easy for them to see that anyway as I never can eat the food that is sometimes brought in, or when I have to go to lunch with them.)

Being honest and upfront with them has really helped. I sometimes have to arrive late due to waiting for my IBS-D to subside. My bosses have told me to do what I have to do to take care of myself, allowing me some flexibility in work hours (coming in late some days if necessary, or leaving early if needed. I always make sure I make up the time). I work late whenever I can to make sure all my work gets done. My bosses understand that. As long as I get my work done, they're OK with my flexible hours. I know some companies and bosses may not be so accommodating. But if you let them know that you have certain digestive issues that won't jeopardize the quality of your work, they may be more accommodating than you would expect.

Those of you with jobs where you are on your feet most of the time—such as waiters or sales people—I really have to admire you; I don't think I could handle it too well.

Rich M

From: **Chicago, IL**

Styles
New Member

It is soooo interesting hearing everyone's replies .... I've always wondered how everyone else deals with this. Some days are great, others I think, "how am I gong to do this the rest of my life?? How did it get this far???" Arghh!! I'm a massage therapist, so if it's a BAD day I have to call in sick because I can't constantly excuse myself from treatments. However, everyone at my work knows and understands, my bosses are great ... I just feel guilty calling in sick when I have to ... plus I don't get paid sick days. This really sucks ... I've left a few other jobs and part of the reason was the bathroom situation ... isn't that nuts? Leaving a job because the bathroom is too out in the open or too many people sharing it, etc?! We've got several bathrooms where I'm at now ... thank God!!

From: **NS, Canada**

Mason_M
New Member

I'm an over-the-road truck driver with severe IBS-D. I have had it for 23 years and it seems to get worse every year that goes by. As you can imagine, bathrooms are often few and far between. I have learned to be pretty good at learning my particular "rhythms" and try to plan accordingly. I know that when I eat something at a truck stop I should not just jump in the truck and go, but wait around a few minutes because I know I will need to "go" within 10 minutes of eating.

There are those days when I have to make many, many stops on my way, and they are getting more and more often.

I fear that it won't be much longer until I can no longer do my job.

Mason

From: **Collinsville, VA, USA**

25CQ
New Member

I'm a med student and IBS creates huge problems for me. It is often just unaccept-able to leave in the middle of seeing a patient. I have had to leave the operating room before in the middle of a case. I basically try to eat almost nothing before I have to go to clinic. You would think it would be easy to explain this problem to other people in the medical field, but there is this weird understanding that med students and doctors don't get sick and don't let it interfere with their work. I am getting increasingly worried about what kind of work I'll be able to do (probably hard to work in the emergency room because you can't just leave whenever you want to). The times I've had trouble I have just had to leave and come back as quickly as possible. The worst part is that you don't want to go see a specialist for this because, who knows, a couple of months later you'll end up working with them!

From: **USA**

Akalways-Deb
New Member

I work in a legal office with five other women and two men. There are no facilities in our office, we must walk down the hall to the ladies room which is for the entire floor (fortunately there are four stalls). I have had several "accidents" but luckily no one knew it except me (which was bad enough, thank you very much!).

I am learning to better manage my IBS-D and hopefully, with new medications, my life will soon take form (deliberate "pun").

Deb

From: **New Orleans**

Discussion: Traveling with IBS-D

Having a body that makes urgent demands to get to a bathroom ASAP can make travel a nightmare. These posts offer lots of helpful advice to make traveling by trains, planes and automobiles a survivable experience.

Topic: Traveling with D

Shreyasf
New Member

Does anyone have any tips for handling long trips by car with D? I have to make a five-hour trip this weekend with relatives and am panicked!

From: **San Francisco**

FranC
New Member

Hi,

This past August I drove from NY to Disneyworld with my three kids. I basically didn't eat during the drive, which was kind of torturous when we stopped and everyone else was eating, but the thought of getting an attack of diarrhea on the road kind of suppressed my hunger. I also wore Serenity pads everyday (just in case I had an attack & couldn't make it to the bathroom in time). Throughout the trip, I only ate full meals when I was in or very close to my hotel room. I was away from home for 12 days (a record for me since I've been diagnosed w/IBS) & I am thrilled to say that I didn't have an attack. Go & enjoy yourself. Just take a couple of precautions and have fun!

FranC.

From: **Brooklyn, New York**

Shreyasf
New Member

Thanks. That info is encouraging. Did you drink water on the trip? Nibble on anything?

I think I can make it, but don't want to explain my problem to my family (in-laws!)

From: **San Francisco**

Homebound
Very Prolific Member

We went to Disneyland in July, which is a nine-hour drive for us. I took Imodium the day before we left, and I took some more an hour before we left. This may not be exactly good, but I didn't eat a THING while we were on the road. I'm one of those people who seem to start getting cramps as soon as I start chewing! So it was safer for me to eat once we got there.

I had a back-up outfit in the car, along with a wet rag and a dry towel for cleaning up (which I bring anyways since I have a 4-year-old who tends to get always get messy on car trips! LOL). I also put a Kotex back by my rear in case of an accident (which helps calm me about the whole accident problem).

I did drink soda actually, on the way down.

Once we were there, I did eat meals, mostly lunch and dinner (I would get toast while everyone else ate breakfast, morning are hard on my tummy). But our hotel was IN Disneyland and it gave me extra comfort knowing I was close enough to get back to the hotel quickly.

I do actually really well on trips, weird but better then when I'm home! But I know how you feel, our trip was also with ALL of my in-laws. All of which know about my IBS, but don't understand it worth beans. Once I did have to go back to the hotel room, but it was only a few pains, thankfully. I never did get any D.

But my best advice is to RELAX! You'll be fine, keep telling yourself that!

Have a great trip!

From: USA

Michele
Prolific Member

We have a nine-hour car trip to Kansas whenever we go to visit my parents. I take two Imodium the night before, then another two about two hours before we leave. I don't eat any meals while we're on the road, but I take some crackers to nibble on. I also know the location of almost every bathroom on the way! I do better when I'm the one driving, because I know that I can stop whenever I want to. Not that my husband wouldn't if I asked, but I guess it makes me feel better when I'm in control.

From: **Texas**

Redspruce
New Member

I understand your feelings. Things usually go in overdrive when I have to travel. I recently took my daughter back to university, a three-day trip. I used Imodium before leaving and after eating, avoided soda and milk products. Everything went well.

Relax and have a great trip.

From: **Brenton, NS, Canada**

Zappy
New Member

We do a lot of road traveling, which I really enjoyed until the IBS started, but I've learned if I take some crossword puzzles and some calming CD's to listen to, nibble on some crackers, and just try to relax and enjoy the trip, talk about the scenery with my husband, it helps. I also take a bucket with me, and keep trash bags in it, just in case, I've never had to use it, but I think the peace of mind that I can pull over, open the doors to the car, put the bucket down and have an instant potty is comforting in an odd way. I hope you have an enjoyable trip and just try to relax. Take some Imodium and calcium before you go.

From: **Mesa, AZ, USA**

Shreyasf
New Member

Wow! I was feeling so alone, frustrated and afraid, just dealing with my IBS. I felt so "different."

Now I feel I have found a group of friends who understand and encourage me to get out and about. Thanks to all of you.

I had even given up my volunteer work at hospice, which I love, but you have given me the courage to go back to it (but not on an early morning shift!).

Peace & Blessings to all of you
Shreya

From: **San Francisco**

Topic: Traveling Tips … Please

Tess McIntosh
Regular Member

Hi:

I have D and am getting ready to go on a long driving trip with my family. I am looking for any and all traveling tips! Any suggestions on how to make this trip better would be sooooo welcome.

I feel nervous about the trip but I will NOT let this darn IBS-D stop me from doing things. It restrains my life enough!

Thanks, Tess

From: **San Francisco, CA**

Kimba
Prolific Member

When I travel, it is usually to the city where there is a lot of stress for me. I have a hard time going there. Even though my Questran usually has everything under control, sometimes I panic and stuff. Here is what I do. Sometimes take some Xanax, sometimes some precautionary Imodium. Mostly though I make sure the people with me understand that when I say stop, I mean pull the D*** car over. I also travel with a bucket (five-gallon if you have the room), bags and TP. That way if I need to, I can have my own bathroom where ever I need to. I have not had to use it yet, but prior did leave little "presents" in many a farmer's field.

Good Luck,
Kimba

From: **Alberta, Canada**

Desirae
Regular Member

Imodium A-D!

From: **Dallas, TX**

HereIam
Prolific Member

Tess,

Good for you for not staying homebound!!

I, too, have found car rides nerve-wracking, especially if they involve city driving. Interstate driving doesn't bother me at all—there are lots of trees and woods along the way if necessary.

I have found that when a trip does involve city driving, if I do the driving I am in much better shape. This keeps my mind occupied on something other than my guts and also gives me a good sense of control, that if I need to stop I can. I also keep a bucket in the back of the van, just in case, and I've never had to use it.

Usually before a long car ride I take Lomotil to calm any spasms. I don't like Imodium, because for me it interrupts the natural schedule of a BM every morning and I'm so obsessed that if I don't go properly in the morning, I think about that missed one all day!!

Enjoy your trip.

From: **Massachusetts**

Michele
Prolific Member

I take Imodium at least two hours before we leave. If I take it later, we're going to have to stop so I can pee! I agree that being the driver helps me because I feel more in control. I also eat and drink as little as possible during the car trip. I know this isn't really good for me on a nine-hour car trip, but I do it anyway.

What I wouldn't do for an Interstate with trees and woods! There aren't a whole lot of those on I-35 from Texas through Oklahoma and Kansas, where my family lives. It's pretty much a whole lot of nothing for miles in every direction!

From: **Texas**

Glo
Regular Member

Tess:

Oh how I can understand, I do not like the city either, too much traffic and traffic jams.

When I have a trip I start three hours early, take two Imodium upon rising, two more an hour later, two more somewhere before leaving. Take SJW tincture and capsules during the three hours, and pack extra cloths. I also keep in the car lavender for smelling if I need to calm my nerves, crackers for calming my tummy, peppermint candies for tummy and I take a Pepsi with me too, this is also a calmer for me.

I have tissue and wipes in the car; you might take along a towel to put on your seat (especially if it is someone else's car) just in case. Also inform your driver of your problem (if they are not already aware), so they will know of your need. Perhaps make a list of conversation topics, I find if I am involved in a good conversation I don't have any problems. Keeps my mind on other things. Take a nap.

Sometimes I have to drive, too, but not all that often, anymore.

Hope this helps a little, have a great trip.

Glo

From: **USA**

Tess McIntosh
Regular Member

Thanks everyone for the traveling tips! I appreciate all the ideas. All of you totally understand what I go through … it is so nice to read your posts and hear the familiar feelings.

I'm looking forward to the trip. I will take a whole box of Imodium if necessary.

Thank goodness that the people I am going with understand (as much as they could without having IBS) and will stop. (Going with my husband, son and mom.)

Thanks again,

Tess

Oh, a tip I read somewhere else … thought I would share with the rest of you is to take along some Depends (adult diapers). I think this is a great idea. Just a little more safety.

From: **San Francisco, CA**

Topic: Airplane Travel

Adrianna1979
New Member

For the first time in my life I will be flying solo on a seven hour airplane trip. Needless to say, my nerves are already shot and I'm getting D every day due to the stress of just thinking about it. So I have some questions ...

1) Can you become immune to Imodium?

2) How long should I be fasting before I board the airplane?

3) Should I use a cleansing system the day before, like enemas or something to ensure I won't have incidents on the airplane?

Any help on this matter appreciated. Thanks!

From: **Canada**

HereIam
Prolific Member

Adrianna,

I sympathize with you on your nerves over flying, I experience the same thing every time I get on an airplane. Not only am I not fond of flying, I live in fear of messing my pants when that little seatbelt sign is lit.

To answer your questions—I don't think you can become immune to Imodium, it's not that kind of drug, I don't think a cleansing system the day before is a very good idea—it may irritate your bowel and cause more problems than it solves, and I also don't think fasting is a very good idea, either, as you'll feel lousy and weak.

Stick with a bland diet for a few days before the flight and don't overeat. If your doctor will prescribe you something like Valium or Ativan, that may help. If not, take two Dramamine pills, that will knock you down a bit and you'll be calm. Take a healthy dose of Imodium a few hours before the flight and even consider wearing an adult "diaper" for the seven hours. It will make you feel safer. Carry a change of clothes in your bag and remain calm if you can.

Try to focus on what you are afraid of and then take action: you are afraid of messing your pants. Okay, then deal with that—Imodium, adult briefs, something to calm your nerves and a change of clothes if all else fails.

Hope this helps and happy trails to you.

From: **Massachusetts**

Bushja1
Prolific Member

I travel quite a bit and know what you're feeling. Although I feel stupid doing it, I find wearing Depends helps me. More of a mental thing. I take Lomotil a couple hours before the flight and try to eat very little. Try to get up and walk around as much as you can. I find being cramped up that long bothers my intestines. Although I know it's not recommended, I have a drink at the bar before the flight and also on the plane. Luckily, I love to fly and find it very exciting. It's all the waiting on the ground that drives me nuts. Just reassure yourself that there are bathrooms on the plane and I've seen people use them even if the seatbelt sign is on.

From: **USA**

SirCrapsALot
New Member

Don't worry about that seat belt sign. I fly A LOT on business. Takeoff and landing are the times you can't be up. The rest is for your protection. I have always had a stern "I have no choice" work for me.

From: **TX**

WindyCityRich
Regular Member

Airplane travel is tough with IBS-D. I always take a Xanax before flying to calm me, so the anxiety doesn't create an even more severe problem. I have plenty of my anti-D medicine handy, and bring bottled water onto the plane so I can take pills if I need to. I usually take some anti-D medicine before I fly, even I don't currently have D, as a preventive measure, since I really don't want to deal with D on the flight!

Rich M

From: **Chicago, IL**

Zipman
Regular Member

I travel a lot as well and like Bushja1, Depends is the only way to get through it. Just remember nobody but you knows what you are wearing under your clothes.

From: **Home**

IBS survivor
Regular Member

You might also sit in an aisle seat at the back of the plane. That way you have an easy exit and not far to go!! I have a plane trip myself in a few weeks and I'm already dreading it because you just never know how you will feel on that day. Just sit back, relax, take a nap, and enjoy the flight … … …

From: **U.S.A.**

Jlady
New Member

Traveling can be a nightmare! I have severe IBS and wear the Attends briefs and that is the absolute best thing you can do if you even think that you might have an accident. Take it from somebody that has tried all the meds, and yes, some help, but NONE work 100%. Do yourself a favor and take the meds, and wear the protection … you won't regret it!

Good luck and God bless!

From: **So. Cal.**

Great_Beautician_in_the_Sky
New Member

Flying Munich to Toronto I was determined to fast the entire flight until I got the food … veggie lasagna … and I was so hungry I had to eat. Miraculously putting food into my body had the reverse effect as usual, and it stopped the D urges that kept pushing on my butt muscles and getting "caught" in the nick of time.

This was a once-in-a-lifetime thing for me. I fly about once a year and have all the same fears as you guys. I usually eat nothing but a few saltines when I get up in the morning, drink lots of hot tea, and carry a granola bar (I also tend to faint if I haven't eaten in a long time—I have to strike a balance).

I have never let myself have an IBS attack in the plane … those bathrooms don't look like they can handle it … with those tiny vacuuming holes. Plus I would be so embarrassed messing it up for the next person … I try my hardest to hold it in until I get out of the plane.

From: **Toronto, ON**

Topic: Travel = no eating

Sofia
New Member

Hi there

What do you guys do when you want to travel?

I always get SO worried when I go on a trip. I usually do not eat anything during the bus, car or plane ride even if it lasts hours and I am starving, and then I avoid eating anything if there is not a bathroom near. What a great way to enjoy a trip! I never taste delicious dishes in other cities or countries ...

How do you handle your guts when outside home?

I am going to the beach in two weeks and I am so worried I will get the attacks at some point.

Any advice? Thanks!

From: **Quito, Ecuador**

Kathleen M, Ph.D..
Very Prolific Member

Well the problem could be that sometimes not eating for extended periods of time can cause IBS symptoms due to eating any food at all much worse. It seems starving for a long time and then eating, sets off the post-eating reaction a lot more than just eating normally.

I would pack things that don't bother me and eat them on a regular schedule.

Basically you want to stick to whatever routine works for you as much as possible while on vacation. At restaurants order stuff you know usually doesn't bother you (like grilled chicken is good for many people) and then have just a taste of something more exotic from someone else's plate (or get it as an appetizer and split it).

K.

From: **Somewhere over the rainbow**

KCTony7
Regular Member

When I travel, I'm the same way; I don't eat all day or at least until late afternoon.

Usually when I fly I have to stop in Atlanta for my connecting flight, and at that point (when I'm on the flight to my final destination) I finally eat something (and usually a safe food like some saltines or pretzels).

I also take two to three doses of Imodium, a dose or two of Dicyclomine and, of course, a dose of Questran the night before.

The only good news I guess is I haven't had a blow-up traveling in over three years so it is working.

From: **Miami, FL**

Discussion: A Social Life with IBS-D

Living with IBS-D can sometimes make a person just want to stay home alone near a nice, clean bathroom. Such isolation, however, can quickly lead to feelings of despair and depression. The unpredictability of IBS-D can put a strain on relationships, leading to further feelings of loneliness. Learn how members have handled the topic of IBS with their spouses, dates and friends.

Topic: Does anyone's spouse (significant other) get angry at them when they're sick?

Mamamia
Prolific Member

Dear friends:

My hubby is usually pretty supportive. But sometimes he gets so angry. A couple of weeks ago I left work after having an accident (no one knew, thank God!) but of course I felt horrible, humiliated, etc. You know the drill.

Anyway, I came home from work three hours early and I'm laying on the couch, wishing for death, and my husband cops this huge attitude. We were having sandwiches that night for dinner, anyway. He says "Can't you even set the table???" (paper plates). And then he proceeded to be really icky the rest of the night, until I screamed bloody, blue murder that "I can't cope with this disease and your f—ing attitude!"

This is not the first time this has happened.

It's not that I don't try. I hardly EVER miss work or even family functions. I go sick or well, no one cares how I feel. Our home is always immaculate, I pay half the bills, and I just feel like the lowest life form when he does that.

I don't buy that, "he wants to fix it and can't" business. When I throw my back out, a problem HE ALSO has, he's all "sweetness and light."

Anybody else have this problem? Male or female?

Love and light to all,
Michele—

From: **New Jersey, USA**

LittleLisa
New Member

It's very hard for someone that doesn't have IBS to understand. Luckily my sister, aunt and mother all have it too, so when we all go out it's no big deal when someone is missing from the group in the bathroom. Or if my sister and I go shopping, I don't ever mind having to stop at the nearest, scummiest gas station if needed! We IBS sufferers are the ONLY ones that can understand our illness. When my hubby gets a stomach flu w/"D" it's like it's the end of the world for him. I say "sorry, no sympathy, welcome to my life just about EVERY DAY"!!! He is supportive like yours to a point, but he will never fully understand it. One time he was all proud of himself, scheduling a nice birthday dinner at a restaurant for us at an Italian place. I told him that I couldn't go there. It would kill my stomach, all the garlic, etc. He was so mad at me. I would rather of have soup and bread for my birthday because that way I wouldn't pay having terrible pains. Needless to say, he never understood. Hang in there and try to hang out with other IBS sufferers. It's a lot easier on your life!

From: **Pennsylvania**

KarenP
Prolific Member

Well, I certainly can relate. Sometimes my husband really gets mad at me when I don't want to eat out unless it's five minutes from home (and sometimes even that is tooooooo far). Most of the time he makes fun of me. I don't think he would find it too amusing to mess his pants. There isn't much restaurant food that I can eat and make it home safe (and clean). I'd much rather get something and take it home. I know what you mean about lying down after a bad bout. Sometimes it wipes you out so bad; you just need to lie down. If I'm wiped out when he gets home, he'll feed himself but not the three kids. They'll coming running up to the bathroom telling me how they're starving. You would think he'd feed them too! I think it's his way of punishing me ....

From: **Naperville, Illinois USA**

Luna
Very Prolific Member

Your hubby and mine are very similar, unfortunately.

Maybe that is part of the lack of sympathy ... he hasn't had any stomach problems for a while. When he does get a (ever-so-brief) bout with D, he is sooo much more sympathetic!!

I've really been having problems with energy levels and doing all the things I need to do, relaxing a little, and doing other stuff too. And he is being a real jerk lately about what I haven't done around the house. I'm doing the best I can. And I know he works more hours than me, but he COULD help out a little more. He has practically no commuting time, needs less sleep than I do and doesn't spend lots of time on the toilet or feeling poorly. So really I don't have all the free time he seems to think I have!

If you find a way to reduce or control the attitude popping out, I'd love to know! I'm still trying to find that switch on Mr. Luna that turns him from a nice guy to a jerk. There MUST be one somewhere!!

From: **Ohio, USA**

Honeybee
Regular Member

Boy do I know about this! I have two EX-husbands because of it. The last one pulled this trick: one day I was extremely sick all day at work, so I came home and immediately went to bed. At about 7:30 PM, he came up to my room, woke me up and said 'So are you coming down to make dinner or what?' My reply was 'not only am I not coming down to make dinner, I am not eating dinner, you are on your own'. Well, he didn't like this and went slamming out of my room, then proceeded to make dinner for himself, but not my kids. Luckily, my kids are old enough and have dealt with my illness long enough that they took care of themselves that night. After a few more of these episodes within the next couple weeks, he came home one day to find that his key didn't work on the locks! I have been sick all my life with this crap and I will not tolerate this type of behavior. If you can't be nice when someone is sick, you can't be around me! My sons' have learned to deal with it and are very supportive of me when I am sick. I think that someday they will be very loving to their women, so I think I am raising a new generation of boys in my house. Best of luck to you in dealing with your spouse, I personally choose not to deal with that type of behavior.

Honeybee (Melissa)

From: **Toledo, Ohio USA**

JB2
Prolific Member

To those of you that do not have supportive husbands or family, I think that LittleLisa hit the nail on the head. I don't believe that people who do not have IBS understand exactly what we go through.

This is not the first time that I have read posts such as this, unfortunately.

I told my wife and family exactly what my condition was like and said that if I was okay I would go out on trips or wherever, but if I didn't feel up to it then I would not be joining them and if they didn't like it, too bad. More polite than that but that was the message.

Fortunately, they are all very supportive, but I don't think they truly understand and probably never will.

All people are different, some supportive, some just downright pigs but it's good to have this BB where we can turn to people who DO understand, and although it doesn't solve anything, it is good to have a moan now and then, even if just to relieve the stress. You would think that our loved ones would be the first to support us and not to be selfish just thinking about themselves.

Maybe these selfish people will have an attitude change and be more sympathetic, although I doubt it.

I wonder how many men that have IBS have uncaring wives or family.

Peter

From: **England**

Momof4
Regular Member

Hi. I am married and have four kids. I have been dealing with IBS-D for most of my life (33 years) and especially since the birth of my first child 10 years ago. I can't believe what a downer it's been on my life. My husband of 11 years has recently been getting very upset with me when he wants to do things as a family. He says I'm using it as a control thing, making everybody else wait for me. He also says it's mostly "in my head" and that I should stop being so selfish and weak. I have explained IBS to him. I have humbled myself to tell him about all of the "close calls" with the bathroom and it seems that once I start crying, he backs off a little bit. The tears are not a sign of weakness, but signs of YEARS of frustration and embarrassment and worry about D and/or the urgency component. I don't think he will ever really believe me when I tell him that it's physiological and psychological. However, psycho or not, when it's time to go, it's time to go. I am a Christian. I pray about this every day. I ask God to rid this D from me so I can enjoy the life I've been given. It seems He answers me, but I'm always taken to "the edge" of comfort and confidence. I am in the habit of taking Imodium on a daily basis, as well as some good old Xanax for those trips away from home. I get sooo angry.

Reading other people's posting on this BB is like looking into a mirror. I just feel bad for all of us. I know it's not cancer or some other terminal disease but it's very life-limiting and emotionally draining. Today was a good day for me, though, and I feel great (although I didn't have to go anywhere, so does that count??) hee hee. There's always tomorrow and we'll be going to the graduation parties and being out-and-about and so I'll just load up on my meds and keep on praying. Take care, everybody.

From: **Wisconsin**

DDinSC
New Member

I have noticed my wife of 10 years is starting to get more impatient about it. I know she is not mad at me; it is the situation IBS causes that is getting to her. I can understand that. Imagine you are out to dinner for your tenth anniversary and being left at the table for 30 minutes or more. Of course, knowing she is out there alone and waiting only makes it worse for me. I would be willing to bet your spouses aren't mad at you, it is the IBS, but you just happen to be the object they can take it out on. I also believe the situation wasn't helped when we got a taste of a normal life when I was on Lotronex. Once you are normal you never want to go back.

From: **SC**

KarenP
Prolific Member

Sometimes my husband's attempts at humor aren't too funny. The other day I was starting to tell him something. I said, "Guess what I did today?"

He said, "You crapped in your pants?" I said, "No, not today." Isn't he just a riot?

From: **Naperville, Illinois USA**

Rocks
New Member

In the beginning, my husband was in la la land. Now by seeing me and what I go through, my husband over time has become pretty much 90% very supportive. The other 10%, I realize I have to look out for myself, where he would be absent-minded. I try to not fly off the handle when he wants to go for a two mile walk or other things I wish I could do, but can't, then I make a joke out of it. Joking about it does help. However, if hubby is stupid, try Ex-Lax on him, he may get the picture. Oh, be out and about when he's eaten it. No joke. It will shut him up fast.

From: **MIAMI**

Mamamia
Prolific Member

Dear friends:

So many of your stories are IDENTICAL to ones that I have experienced, even down to the conversation.

For example, I have been lying down on the bed, miserable and have been asked, "Are you getting up to make dinner?"

I DO realize that people who don't have IBS find it impossible to relate. I'm not asking them to relate, I am asking them to adjust.

Right now my hubby is having a terrible time at work, not his fault. I told him to go in and quit, we'll figure something out. I even told him I'd even increase my part-time hours (just what I need!) but he's my husband and you're supposed to do and care for one another.

To be made to feel like you are faking it, is the absolute worse!!! We have a picnic coming up way the heck out in PA, and I'm already rumbling. My dad has told me to tell my hubby that he is sick (my dad), he's almost 80, so that I'd have to care for him and not go to this picnic. I'm thinking about it.

Much love and light to you all, I need you guys so much, M—

From: **New Jersey, USA**

Rocks
New Member

Mamamia,

Be honest with hubby. Tell, him, "Hon., what should I do? I'm worried about the drive and facilities at the picnic." Put it on him to help you figure it out. It will make him a part of the choice. Sometimes, being a team will help you to come up with good strategies and ideas, i.e. put a bucket in the car/w TP. My mother suggested this; I thought it was gross (still do), however … it gave me more freedom to travel. Also, look for facilities and park yourself near there and enjoy the picnic. Don't let IBS cripple you, what you can improvise on go for it, and the stuff you can't work around, accept. Believe me; I have severe IBS, 12 times a day with 10-second warnings. You both may get very creative on your strategies.

From: **MIAMI**

Mamamia
Prolific Member

Dear Rocks:

I do like your suggestion about including him in on the decision. I just hope he doesn't shrug and say, "Don't think about it and you'll be okay."

I might be charged with homicide!!

(But I might try asking him anyway, thanx)

Love, M—

From: **New Jersey, USA**

Rocks
New Member

Mamamia,

Don't let him shrug it off with "don't think about it". If he say's anything like that, you need to take control of the conversation, NICELY. Say, "Hon, come on now, I really need you to be serious and help me figure this out. I need your help, I know you got some good ideas. (ego up)" Remind him NICELY, that you don't have the luxury to not think about it. Say "I wish I could, but I'm really worried here, so honey, help me think of something that can work so we both can have a good time".

I know spouses can be trying, but you need to get through to them that this IBS is no joke. My husband kept on putting the toilet seat cover down, which didn't help my 10 second dash. So I put a post-it note on the cover, "please leave the cover up". He laughed at the note and then stopped doing it. Trying, I know, but keep after them until they get it. It's wrong for these spouses not to understand and HELP YOU/US. This IBS is crippling.

From: **MIAMI**

Danaps
Prolific Member

I have had both experiences and I can say that my wonderful husband is so supportive of my IBS. He is the one who found Zofran when Lotronex was taken off the market, he is the one who encouraged me to see a therapist when I thought I would be stuck at home forever, he is the one who understands and stops whenever I say stop when I have a bout coming on. He lets me drive, he helped me tell his family so they understand and even though he get frustrated on occasion because I can't do something, it is not the most important thing, we just adjust the plans.

For example, this weekend we went on vacation with a lot of car riding (not the best thing) and he made an extra trip to take his son to a soccer game so that I would not have to be in the car for that period of time. I feel lucky and blessed to have found this wonderful man.

On the other side, my ex insisted that I had IBS to punish him, that I was making it all up, and all types of other not so nice things. He and I ended up driving everywhere in separate cars so that I would not bother him with my problem.

My son has seen both sides of the equation and he will be a supportive adult someday and I have my wonderful husband to thank for that.

So it can be good, it can be supportive and I have found that talking about it honestly (and sharing this BB with my DH) is the best thing to do.

From: **E. Windsor, NJ, USA**

Mamamia
Prolific Member

Dear Danaps:

Actually ALL of my family and friends are VERY supportive, it's just hubby who gets on my nerves when I think of it.

Even my granddaughter will say something like, "Hey Meema, don't have any of that ice cream cake we're having or you know what will happen" and she's only five!!!

Hubby is good in other ways, so I guess I'll have to keep him. If I had had this with my first hubby, he'd have made me feel like a complete idiot, I'm sure, and made fun of me mercilessly.

Love, M—

From: **New Jersey, USA**

OppOnn
Very Prolific Member

My husband, usually very supportive, drives me nuts every six months about a holiday to Mexico!

All I need! He says I can be careful what I eat.

Forget it, I kill the discussion dead, but he comes back again and again, because he's never been to Mexico and wants to go.

I think I'll send him on his own!!!!

O

From: **New York, USA**

Newlearner
Prolific Member

I adore every aspect of Mexico and would go there in the blink of an eye … I just take a lot of Imodium and I'm okay. Maybe your husband will take me! (Just kidding!)

From: **San Antonio TX, USA**

Topic: D, Dating, and Dignity

Turnoffmytummy
New Member

Hi All,

I recently found a great GI doctor who ruled out some things … which was good news. The bad news is: I just have frequent but seemingly random D (fantastic!). The hardest thing for me is dating. I have a boyfriend I love more than anything, and I know he loves me and is not judgmental. This is what I've been trying: acidophilus, high-fiber diet, fiber supplements, activated charcoal when I get gassy, and Imodium when my preventative measures don't work.

I'm going to visit him and his father next week, and I'm really seriously scared that I'll have that "explosive" D and totally embarrass myself. Regardless of their opinion, it is humiliating. I find that I try to be out of the house as much as possible when he visits, so that I can use public, anonymous bathrooms. Does anyone else do this? Feel anxious about being "trapped" at home where you can be heard/ smelled/whatever by a significant other? Advice and similar experiences would be hugely appreciated!

From: **PA**

Runningjude
New Member

Well, I'm so paranoid about the smell of diarrhea that I carry a very small air deodorizing spray in my bag—at all times. It's a habit, I feel better with it.

Jude

From: **Lancs, England**

Stillsuffering
New Member

I know what you mean about the dating thing. I eventually had to tell my boy-friend about it. I was running to the bathroom too many times without explana-tion. If he doesn't know, you're gonna have to tell him eventually. You can even make light of it by saying you have a sensitive stomach. When my extended family or people who don't know about it are over my house, I always feel uncomfort-able. Sometimes I used to take a shower or just run the shower to cover up the time I've been in the bathroom or to hide the smell.

I'll be thinking of you!

From: **USA**

Pat ...
Very Prolific Member

I always turn a tap on ... and carry a small spray of Neutradol ...!!!!

From: **England**

Lbcgeek21
New Member

I know how you feel. I have been dating my boyfriend for four years and he's probably been fully aware of my problem for about three and half years. We just don't discuss it in detail. Whenever I'm feeling sick and know that I'm going to have D, I always refer to it as "an upset stomach". In front of friends or people who are not familiar with my IBS, they aren't necessarily sure what I'm referring to.

My only tip would be this ... when I've ever had D at my boyfriend's parents' house, I do my best to use the upstairs bathroom. That way I don't have to worry about being so close to where all the people are sitting. I try to get my boyfriend to help me out with this ... like I'll whisper to him that I'm not feeling well, so let's go upstairs. That way, I can try to use the bathroom upstairs. Hope that helps some.

My boyfriend is pretty cool about it, it just frustrates him. When I'm not feeling well, he knows we're in for a night of just laying around. It's difficult to even put in a movie because we both know I'm going to be getting up three times in the middle of it to run to the bathroom. He's pretty good about it, but I've come to expect a disappointed sigh whenever I tell him my stomach is bothering me. He understands, but it's still frustrating for him.

From: **Naperville, IL**

Jes
New Member

About a year ago I decided it wasn't that embarrassing and I told myself to get over trying to hide it. I hate using public restrooms with many stalls in it. Like others here, I prefer my restroom at my house.

I don't really remember how I told my BF. I think the first time I got sick around him, I just told him "Oh I have a stomach problem. I get sick when I eat or whatnot." ... something like that.

Lucky me, his mom has IBS and he knows all about it.

We've been together a year and now live together and our bowel problems are something we openly chat about, hee hee.

I dunno why but I just feel so much better when people know I have IBS. It takes the stress of having to hide it off of me, and if I have to go to the bathroom a million times, everyone knows why.

From: **CA**

Topic: Traveling with friends

Sooz
Regular Member

This subject may have been discussed before, but how do you all cope with traveling in a car with another person and the IBS hits? The reason I am asking, is because I now have a boyfriend and he wants to take me out, but I am afraid of traveling in the car with him in case I get an attack.

Has anyone had this happen to them? If so, how did you cope? What did you do? He wants to take me out for dinner, but I think it is safer for me if I don't eat anything as sometimes it triggers IBS-D.

I would welcome any advice …

Sooz

From: **Perth, Australia**

Baby b
Very Prolific Member

Does your boyfriend know about your IBS? If not, tell him.

From: **Wisconsin**

Momof4
Regular Member

When my husband wants to take me out (of course he knows about my IBS-D) I make sure that it's somewhere close (within a 10 to 15 minute drive) and I load up on Imodium and my IBS meds and take a Xanax if I need it. (Sounds really romantic, doesn't it?) Any-hoo, most of the time, I ask if we can order in/carry out so I'm at home. That's more romantic anyway. hee hee. What's good about eating out at dinner is that you have the whole day to "clean out" and use the bathroom as much as you can and then take some Imodium. At the restaurant, eat light or half and take the rest home (you can always eat it later!). I avoid cola's to drink because that sets me off and I watch out for salads which also get me going. Good luck to you. I'm sure your boyfriend wants the best for you and will do what he needs to do to make sure you're comfortable. He probably doesn't want you to be embarrassed if the D starts a flowin'. You'll do great. Good luck and figure out the route to the restaurant so you can map out any bathrooms along the way. That really helps me, too. Geez, the things we IBS-D folks have to worry about …

From: **Wisconsin**

Sooz
Regular Member

Baby,

I haven't been with my boyfriend for very long, so I was worried about telling him about my IBS. I took your advice and told him … and guess what, he has IBS as well!

I was totally floored when he told me that. I couldn't believe it. He was afraid to tell me about it as well. (He is IBS-D)

Momo … I don't take any medication for it as I am a swinger—I either get the diarrhea or the constipation. Now that my boyfriend and I have discussed it all, it helps a lot.

Thank you to both of you for your help.

Sue

From: **Perth, Australia**

Forum IV: <u>IBS-Constipation (IBS-C)</u> <u>and Chronic Constipation</u>

"Use this forum to discuss any issues related to constipation-predominant IBS (IBS-C) and chronic idiopathic constipation."

The clinical description of the defining symptoms of IBS-C, e.g. abnormal stool frequency, hard or lumpy stools, and straining during a bowel movement, does not give a clear picture of the devastating impact that the disorder can have on a person's life. IBS-C sufferers can experience chronic severe pain, discomfort throughout the body, and the feared humiliation of leakage and gas. As with IBS-D, patients with constipation-predominant IBS often suffer in silence. The freedom to openly discuss embarrassing symptoms is what draws members with IBS-C to this forum.

<u>Discussion</u>: Dealing with Discomfort

Topic: Very Constipated—What to do for immediate relief?

Hma925
New Member

My constipation has been occurring more often and more severely recently (my stress level has been up.) I am increasing my water intake and fiber, but what can

I do for immediate relief? So far, I have unsuccessfully tried: a glycerin suppository, three Colace stool softeners, some prunes, a Fleets enema (an old fashioned water enema not mineral oil, or anything else), and just now another glycerin suppository and more Colace (out of enemas at home). I did have a miniscule bowel movement from first suppository.

I have trouble holding in enemas long enough to get much relief from them. I lie down in bed on my side to take them, start seeping a bit right away, and end up running to bathroom in fear I will have a BM on the floor on the way there if I wait any longer. (I am thinking of getting myself a bedpan. Then I could afford to wait longer and not worry about "messing". I could use the bedpan if I couldn't make it to bathroom.) I usually get to the toilet and expel the water from the enema about three minutes after giving it, with just little flecks of stool. And that is what happened last night. I still feel "full" for lack of a better way to state it. And last night I didn't eat much because I am constipated but ended up with headache, in part from not eating much, I am sure. Any suggestions would be very welcome. I will have to call my doctor (PCP) later today if nothing else works.

From: **PA**

Alexandragirl
Regular Member

I am sorry to hear about your tough time. We have all been there. I highly recommend Fleets phospho soda at this point. It doesn't taste good, but it works and will clean you out. I would take it on a very empty stomach and it should work pretty quickly, about 30 minutes to two hours. I like to take a walk after I drink it to get it working faster. Good luck.

From: **Texas**

Miranda Fox
Regular Member

Maybe try one or two Dulcolax? You will probably have a lot of cramping, but you also might be willing to deal with that instead of being overly 'full'. Afterwards, have a bowl of oatmeal for your next meal, and try to have some every day for a couple days until your system settles down. The oatmeal is a soluble fiber—good for those of us with C.

Also, you could drink Ensure—all the vitamins and stuff you need, but your system has a chance to rest. Ensure is also lactose-free, as opposed to some of the 'diet' drinks.

Good luck—I know how miserable being extremely C can be!

From: **Florida**

I'll B Snookered
Prolific Member

Try magnesium (500mg or so) and vitamin C (3000mg or so) at bedtime. Also, keep up with the prunes, and eat some fruit at every meal. The "p" fruits seem to be good—pineapple, pears, prunes, peaches, papaya. Also, you should look into Digest Gold digestive enzymes and papaya enzymes. I take them before and after every meal, and they help. Finally, take some sort of probiotics. I've done all this, and now I still have the incomplete evacuation, but once I have my last bowel movement (diarrhea-like), I am much better (not good or even okay, but better).

I forgot to mention that I also take Zelnorm, Zoloft, 1 Colace, Miralax, and Metamucil—the last three an hour or two before bedtime. It seems that the more time I give the stuff to work, the better. Oh, and I also drink licorice tea and ginger tea in the morning along with eating some fruit and possibly taking some caffeine to get me going … My word, I do a lot of stuff (and spend a lot of money) on this crap.

AAAAAAAAAAAAARRRRRRRRRRRRRGGGGGGGGGGGGHHHH!!!

From: **SF Bay Area, CA**

4WillieC
New Member

For a quick, gentle solution, try a glycerin suppository … that should help.

From: **USA**

Loveholli
New Member

I do hope you found some relief by now. However, I found strong stimulant laxatives do the trick ... I take three before bed and the next day my system is cleaned out. It's crampy and very inconvenient, but it works. Just don't abuse stimulant laxatives. I'm not sure how often is safe. But I do not do that more than once a month.

From: **Indiana**

Topic: Feel constipated after I go to the bathroom?

Patm34
New Member

I have been going on a period of about a little over two weeks, I will go to the bathroom a little bit, but its not very much, and I still feel constipated like I still have stuff to poop out but it doesn't want to come out. I'm starting to get worried. I take fiber every night and I'm on a low dose of anti-depressant to calm my stomach? Can anyone help?

From: **MN**

Type 0
Prolific Member

Hi Pam—The first thing an anti-depressant will do for me is totally deaden my intestines or colon, so that I can't feel anything happening in there at all. Feels dead. Pam, did this constipation problem start when you started the medication? Drink lots of water if you are taking any fiber. I have been helped with magnesium oxide and fiber. I also take MSM for my joints and I think that also helps things move along. Not sure though. But I still have the incomplete bowel movements most days. It's a rare day that I can totally clean myself out.

Keep us posted, okay?

From: **Canada**

Bewitched-Bothered and Bewildered
Prolific Member

Same problem here ... I could go eight times a day and still feel like I have to go! It's so frustrating! I do a warm water enema every morning and that seems to help a little. I use about eight ounces of water. That's not a whole lot, but it gets rid of anything in my lower colon—I wish I had some better advice—Wendi—

From: **Arlington Heights, Illinois**

NancyCat
Very Prolific Member

Same here, its awful that I can feel C after just one day of not going. If it is incomplete evacuations, I can't imagine how much poop would be there (sorry, gross) if they were complete. Some days I go so much I can't imagine where it all comes from. It's the worst part of IBS for me and is very frustrating.

Nancy

From: **Massachusetts**

Modgy
Prolific Member

Yes I feel the same. When I used to smoke, the morning cigarette sometimes gave me a BM that felt like it "cleaned me out", but since I quit, this incomplete evacuations business has become a permanent nightmare.

From: **Sydney, Australia**

Lorilou
Regular Member

I have the same problem. It is so frustrating to go and not really "go good". I take Bentyl, Reglan, Zelnorm and mega-doses of fiber every night. Wish I had an answer.

From: **VA**

Cicelyak
New Member

Has anyone been checked for anismus by a colorectal surgeon?

Has anyone tried low doses of Valium to relax the anal sphincter?

From: **Long Island, New York**

NancyCat
Very Prolific Member

What is anismus? Valium never helped me with relaxing abdominal muscles.

Nancy

From: **Massachusetts**

Cicelyak
New Member

Anismus is the term used to describe an anal sphincter that contracts paradoxically instead of relaxing when one tries to move their bowels.

Valium relaxes smooth muscle, which is what the external anal sphincter is comprised of, and has helped me in the past.

From: **Long Island, New York**

Ira
Regular Member

Hello:

This sense of feeling constipated after bowel movements, or even after many bowel movements, is essentially how IBS manifests itself in my own case.

Along with this, I feel a high degree of pressure or tightness in the area of the rectum anal sphincter. This builds up to pain and finally leads into urinary symptoms as well.

As far as relaxing the sphincter and rectal muscles, has anyone here had much luck with "Kegels" and is there an optimal way of doing these?

My MD suggested that I try this recently, but I would like more specificity as to different ways of doing these and which are likely the best for this type of condition.

—Ira

From: **USA**

Cicelyak
New Member

Ira,

I have exactly the same symptoms, which the colorectal surgeon diagnosed as "non-relaxing puborectalis syndrome". The anal sphincter contracts instead of relaxing. I get urinary urgency and frequency if stool is not expelled completely.

Valium at low dosage helps.

All symptoms started for me after 10 days of the antibiotic Biaxin about two months ago.

Kegels only worsened my pain.

From: **Long Island, New York**

NancyCat
Very Prolific Member

Cicelyak—Biaxin absolutely ruined me. It took me many months to get back to normal (for me) and I was especially sensitive to foods that normally didn't bother me. I will NEVER take it again unless they tell me I will die if I don't.

From: **Massachusetts**

Poo Pea
Prolific Member

I have the same problem. I have found if I eat a lot less, and the meals are a lot smaller, then I don't feel so bad. Also, I try and avoid eating after 7:00 PM.

It's a horrid feeling, but it is one you learn to deal with. It's been 17 odd years for me and it is only in the last year that I'm coping better.

From: **Planet Earth**

Spml
New Member

I have anismus, which was determined by the anorectal manometry test. Following that test, I had ano-biofeedback training, which teaches you to relax the external anal sphincter. This helped me greatly for several months, and then failed. But biofeedback does help some people, so, as I've suggested in other posts, I think it's worth asking your MD if you might have PFD—pelvic floor dysfunction. (Anismus is a type of PFD)

Valium did not work for me.

From: **Millis, MA**

Suev
Prolific Member

You folks are SO lucky—at least your doctors take you seriously. I've had IBS-C for about seven or eight years and I have never heard of ANY of these things. The best help I've had is from an allergy specialist who was absolute bliss, and with good dietary management I can just about keep the old bowels moving, though still suffer with a helluvalot of gas and bloating, particularly around my period. I have had the basic tests, though nobody has offered to look at my bowels. I've never heard of all these tests on the boards, still I reckon it can't be anything too drastic as I've had these symptoms for this long and I'm not dead yet!! Good luck with you all.

Sue, Manchester UK

From: **Cheshire.UK**

Rosmaria
New Member

I can't believe I am not alone with this horrible problem. IBS with C is SO much worse than IBS with loose movements. It is awful to feel bound up all the time. I have Graves Disease as well, which usually produces loose movements, but my IBS is so bad that I don't get them at all. In fact, just the opposite. The only time I have felt totally cleaned out is after a Fleet's enema. It is awful!!

Does anyone else have a bloating problem primarily in lower abdomen as well? I exercise like crazy, but can't get my stomach flat the way it used to be before this IBS set in. It is so frustrating. I am taking fiber and drinking water. I don't know what else to do about the bloating, gas and C.

HELP!!

Rosmaria

From: **Long Island, NY**

Legseleven
New Member

Hi Patma34.

I am so sorry and yet relieved to hear someone else has incomplete evacuations like me.

I was beginning to feel I was the only one having this miserable complaint. The MUCUS after, I hate. Any suggestions anybody? I take lots of fiber, doesn't help the mucus at all.

From: **Ontario**

Stillstanding
New Member

I feel like I have mucus coming out when I don't have to have a BM, especially on days where I feel really bad from incomplete evacuation. I don't know what to do, but can relate to all of your guys symptoms. Worse one is the wetness I always have from not getting "it" all out. I hate it. Tried fiber, no luck, of course. Just want to beat this damn disease so I can get on with my life. 20-years-old and confining myself to my dorm room isn't a life I want to live. I take Xanax to help with the anxiety from it ... but it doesn't help the base of the problem.

From: **Vermont**

Lilscar2003
New Member

Just a suggestion. Sometimes if I feel like I still have to go after having a BM. I take a glycerin suppository. It works for me. I tried the Fleet enema, but it causes my bowels to go into painful spasms.

From: **New Jersey, USA**

Topic: Is this question unanswerable?

Rob Marks
New Member

For years I have sought the answer to this question without success:

Exactly what causes a part of my stool—the first to come out during a bowel movement—to turn to clay?

I've read everything, seen my gastro, taken everything and still ... still the first third of every bowel movement is torture. The remaining two-thirds are easy and soft. But, that first part is hard, hard, hard. Just like clay. And no one can tell me why. Without knowing the answer, there's little more I can do to alleviate the problem. Only suffer.

Thanks for any help.

From: **Tucson, Arizona**

Italianpet
New Member

Rob, I know what you mean. When I have to go and it feels like I need to go right away, I have such the hardest time going. I feel that this big, fat something is going to come out and it turns out to be something so small. But, when that first piece is out, I have such an easy flow after that. I just don't understand it ... ... Sorry, I can't help you but will read if someone else can. I need the help too!

From: **Brooklyn, New York**

Jolan
New Member

I always figured that that first portion was the 'front' of the engine and sat there a lot longer—thus drying out more—the rest seemed to go at a pace behind the 'engine' once it decided to start moving. I find once the 'engine' (often a painful process) makes it through—the softer cabooses follow.

From: **Saskatoon, Saskatchewan, Canada**

Ghitta
Prolific Member

Jolan is right. Those hard stools that are hard to pass are, in fact, the definition of constipation. Most people think that C is not having stools, but in fact it is hard to pass, dry stool that defines C. A primary cause of this is not going to the bathroom when the urge arises because of psychological discomfort: example, not wanting to use a public restroom, or go at work, or rushing the morning clock and not going, or not going at another's house, etc., etc. Another cause, of course, is not enough water and/or lubricant in the bowel: this can be dealt with by drinking more water, consuming more olive oil or other "good" fats. There are, of course, foods that help with this (cooked greens, artichokes, prunes and figs, pears, etc) and for many of us, magnesium supplements, taken with meals helps to draw water into the bowel, hence softening the stool. I basically have gone from C to practically D (which I prefer) using magnesium over the past two years.

From: **Florida**

Topic: Has anybody had a problem with poop leakage?

Poopgirl
New Member

I have a problem with constipation. I will go five days or longer without a BM. Sometimes (quite frequently) I will feel like I need to go and will try, but can't go. Then I will go shopping or something where I do a good bit of walking. When I get home (sometimes before I get home) I will smell poop and will go to the bathroom to find I have pooped and didn't even know it. I'm not talking about runny poop. I'm talking solid poop. But I still can't get any to come out on its own. I guess I get so backed up that some just leaks out. Oh, I don't have to necessarily walk for some to leak out. It is just more when I have been walking. I don't ever know that I have done it until I either smell it or notice that my undies are stuck to my butt. Please tell me that there are other people out there that have this same problem. This problem is so embarrassing! Please let me know if any of you have this same problem or have experienced something at least similar. Thanks!

From: **Georgia**

I'll B Snookered
Prolific Member

You should have some anorectal manometry done, because it seems as though you have fecal incontinence to some degree. I believe I have very minor incontinence, thus inducing "gas" issues. Kegels might be beneficial for you (or possibly sphincter surgery). See a doctor.

From: **SF Bay Area, CA**

Bkitepilot
Prolific Member

Poopgirl, I have a problem with leakage when I'm full of 'it' (and sometimes when I'm not). Mostly mucus leaks out, but occasionally enough stool to soil my panties and put me in a panic. Sometimes I feel it happen, but most times I don't. I have some internal hemorrhoids and wonder if it sneaks by them. If I have D … OMG it's protection in the panties, because I don't trust that faulty sphincter.

I'm going to do more studies on the Kegel exercises, like many here are talking about, for leaky gas.

Belinda

From: **North Georgia**

Feisty
Very Prolific Member

Kegels can help strengthen the pelvic floor to a certain degree, but if you have a weak or damaged sphincter muscle, it won't help. Snookered is right, an anorectal manometry would be a good test to have done.

I have the same problems. I had to have major pelvic floor reconstruction surgery (two phases) to repair as much as possible. It was found that I only have 1/2 inch of good sphincter muscle, which gives me very little control. It was tightened during Phase Two of the surgery, and it will buy me a few years of somewhat better control, but it will by no means hold forever.

The colon/rectal surgeon specialist said most of the damage to the sphincter muscle and pelvic floor was due to childbirth (very fast deliveries), a bad episiotomy and a botched hemorrhoidectomy.

Because of a lot of nerve damage, I have little to no feeling, so I can understand your embarrassment. It really gets me down at times, but there is nothing I can do about it. I plan everything around "where's a bathroom" and I deal with more "C" than "D" also.

From: **USA**

Bkitepilot
Prolific Member

Thanks Fiesty, for the eye-opening info. I had a 4th degree tear giving birth to my daughter almost 20 years ago requiring hours of repairing—and a major epesiotomy with my son six years later … hmmm, I'll bet that has something to do with it. (that hadn't even crossed my mind).

Don't know how bad I'd want to go through surgery again … ugh! Too much cutting already all over this body. I surely will ask to do the manometry test.

Good grief, I feel like my geriatric patients with incontinence creeping up on me. NOT COOL!

Me and my stinky butt, locked in a love-hate relationship forever!

From: **North Georgia**

Topic: Does anyone have to push on the rectal area to help poop come out

LK38
Regular Member

I know this sounds gross, but I saw this question on the chronic constipation poll. I have been doing this a very long time. I really didn't think too much of it until I read it on the poll. What does this mean? Is this really bad? Obviously when I am in the constipation phase, this happens. Now I am scared. I have never even mentioned it to the doctor before. Can it be related to a weak pelvic floor?

From: **Long Island, NY**

Kathleen M, Ph.D..
Very Prolific Member

As far as I know it isn't harmful, just one of the ways people cope.

I generally don't have much constipation and so I only do this once in awhile, and I think my Pelvic Floor function is quite normal (don't have any of the symptoms people with this issue have).

Now, if you cannot go unless you do this, it might be a sign that you need to have things checked out, but if it is just a way to avoid having to strain more, I think it is just a harmless coping mechanism—a way to make things better faster.

K.

From: **Somewhere over the rainbow**

LK38
Regular Member

OK, thanks for the replies. I will have to take note if I do this with every constipated BM or not. Like I said I never gave it much thought until I read that questionnaire. I have to stop reading—it gives me even more agita. I know I do have a weakened pelvic floor because I pee in my pants sometimes when I cough or sneeze. Doc recommends Kegel exercises, but I honestly never know if I am doing them right.

From: **Long Island, NY**

Glenda
Prolific Member

When I've gone as much as I can, but still need to go, I use a water enema to insure the rest of the bowel movement comes out. It works well for me!

From: **Washington**

Spml
New Member

LK38,

You may have a form of pelvic floor dysfunction in which the anal sphincter contracts (closes) when it should be relaxing (opening) to let the stool out. If so, ano-biofeedback training might help you. The problem is detected by a test called anorectal manometry. I would raise this issue with your doctor.

From: **Millis, MA**

LK38
Regular Member

How do they treat a dysfunctional sphincter? Sounds creepy to me. My husband was told by his colorectal surgeon that his sphincter is too relaxed. He leaks. So typical that I might have the exact opposite problem as my husband.

From: **Long Island, NY**

Fourstars
New Member

I may not want to know this—ha ha! But what is an anorectal manometry?

Thanks in advance.

Pam

From: **DFW Texas**

G2004
Regular Member

Glenda: What is a water enema? How does it work?
        (Sorry if a stupid question)

Thanks.

From: **New Jersey**

Spml
New Member

In the anorectal manometry test, they stick sensors into the rectum and perform some measurements. One is to test the strength of the external anal sphincter. For that, they ask you to squeeze (tighten) the sphincter. They also measure sphincter pressure in the relaxed state. Then they insert a balloon. As they fill the balloon, they measure at what point (balloon volume) you first feel pressure, and at what point you feel the urge to go. Sometimes they continue to fill the balloon to the point where you first feel pain, but I don't believe that measurement is necessary.

Finally, they ask you to try to expel the balloon. If you fail to expel the balloon (as I did), they will probably schedule anobiofeedback training. There they train you to keep the anal sphincter relaxed (open) while at the same time pushing to expel what would be the stool. Pushing is actually accomplished by inhaling, which is the opposite of what I'd expect. You inhale through the abdomen, rather than the chest. For a lot of people with pelvic floor dysfunction, learning this technique helps a lot.

At first I didn't want to do the test, but actually it's completely painless, except if they fill the balloon to the point where you feel pain, but again, I don't think that's necessary.

From: **Millis, MA**

Pottymouth
New Member

This has to be one of the funniest posts … LK38 I am SO sympathetic! I have had IBS-C for about five years, and after I had twins my minor hemorrhoids turned MAJOR and NOTHING would come out and yes, I had to do that thing you mentioned. How come no IBS-Cers ever talk about 'roids? It seems to go hand in hand with mine. LK, I don't know if it would help, but I use Prep H suppositories OFTEN. (nighttime only) Makes things come out easier, so to speak. When I had the major problem post pregnancy, I took stool softeners and glycerin suppositories. I keep meaning to ask my doc about better 'roid meds. And my pelvic floor … well don't tell me jokes if I have any fair amount of urine in my bladder. And if I sneeze … I go change. I bet you have kids if your PF is shot like mine. I really don't think it relates to the constipation/straining thing. It is just something else FUN you get to deal with! Good luck!

From: **Richmond, VA USA**

Walkinglady
Regular Member

Glenda, a water enema can be done in several ways. I use mineral oil enemas occasionally, which I purchase at the drugstore for about two dollars. I clean the little plastic bottle they come in carefully with soap and water and reuse them with water, also occasionally. They are good for getting out the bits and pieces that remain in the rectum sometimes and can get against a nerve and set up a "howl".

Or you can use an enema bag. Ordinary hot water bottles usually come with the enema closure as well as the regular stopper and also the hose and syringe. You put anywhere from a pint to a quart of water in the bag, warm, but not hot. My mother used to use soapsuds in the water when I was a child. I just use water, but rinse the bag out with soapy water afterwards. I haven't done one of those for a long time. You have to hang the bag from a hook or something that is higher than your abdomen. Then you put Vaseline on the syringe, place it in your rectum and release the little gadget that keeps the water from coming out before you are ready. The water flows in. When you feel you have had enough you close the gadget, hold the water for awhile if you can. This usually produces results, though not always. It is a messy, uncomfortable procedure to say the least.

The little "disposable" enemas are much easier. I am beginning to wonder some about reusing the bottles since people have begun to say that one should not reuse bottles from store-bought drinking water. That's probably more information than you wanted!

Strack2004

From: **Gibbon, MN**

Topic: Major laxative problem help!!! Anyone else with this problem???

T7d3dek0fsk1
New Member

I have irritable bowel with constipation. I'm pretty sure I've abused laxatives and my bowel has become lazy. Is there anything I can do to bring it back? It's so bad that I'll lose my voice. I've tried Lactulose but that didn't do anything. Miralax didn't move anything either, but maybe it takes a number of days. I've tried everything. Right now I've been trying Epsom salts. I'm panicking because I don't know what to do. I'm on disability for now for depression. I'm on an antidepressant. I had this problem before taking the antidepressant. Is there anybody out there that has had this happened? I just don't know what to do. I even lose my voice because of this, because it backs up so bad. I can't even go on my own. I've tried Citrucel, Metamucil, Zelnorm, which stopped working after a few weeks, Senna, and Milk of Magnesia. I don't see the gastro doctor until July 1st. I know I must not be alone.

Thanks!!!

From: **Davenport, FL**

T7d3dek0fsk1
New Member

I don't know what else to do. The Epsom salts work a little bit. How do you survive on disability? I'm in constant pain. My name is Tim and I'm 30 years old. Please help!!!!

From: **Davenport, FL**

Bewitched-Bothered and Bewildered
Prolific Member

I had to fight for two years to get disability. My boyfriend helped a little financially, but mostly I lived off of money that I had in savings. I had to get a lawyer and several letters from my doctors explaining my condition. Finally I had a court hearing with my doctor and the judge approved my case. I still have not gotten money yet, because it can take months to see any money after you win your case. It's definitely a last alternative.

Have you tried magnesium? They say it works better taken with vitamin C. I'm trying this therapy now, so I still don't know yet how it will work out. It really does take some patience. I know that it's not easy.

Oh …., I almost forgot, I take stool softeners too. It's called Colace, not Peri-Colace, because that has a laxative in it. I just take a generic brand of Colace from Walgreen's or Wal-Mart since it's the same thing, only cheaper.

From: **Arlington Heights, Illinois**

Sean
Regular Member

Tim, it sounds as if we could be twins. I have tried all of the things you have for years, and still have severe, chronic constipation. When the Zelnorm and Miralax stops working and it has been three days since my last BM, my doctor has me give myself a warm water enema. Believe me, it works. Have you tried that? It sounds as though you may have little choice at this point.

From: **Houston, Texas USA**

Bewitched-Bothered and Bewildered
Prolific Member

I also have tried all the things you listed and more. There is just no easy solution. Sean, I also use warm water enemas. I use them everyday before I get into the shower. It does offer some relief. Tim, you should try that. I get into this really strange position when I do an enema. On my hands and knees, then I lay my left arm across, stretching to my right shoulder. Kind of balancing on my left shoulder with my butt on the air. It must look crazy, but it helps the water get further down.

From: **Arlington Heights, Illinois**

NancyCat
Very Prolific Member

Tim, you are not alone. I am IBS-C and D (leaning more to C), and haven't gone at all for three days and I am freaking out. I get so panicked that I feel like I will never go again, which is only making it worse. What antidepressant are you on? I am on Elavil, which has a slight constipating effect that I can usually deal with. I'm not in so much pain and discomfort but rather am very anxious because I want to go and need to go very badly. It seems like all I do is try and go, till I can't stop sometimes, but no matter what I do, I am so mad!!!! This totally sucks!!!! I'm probably not helping you much by my venting, but please know that you are certainly NOT alone. I'm seeing my GI the last week in June but I'm not a candidate for Zelnorm (I have adhesions from a C-section and another abdominal surgery, gallstones and a history of D which are all contraindications for it). I'm thinking about asking my GI for the name of a therapist who works with IBS patients. I hope you can get some relief, I do know what this is like, especially the anxious, panicky feeling. Hope this helps.

From: **Massachusetts**

Hootmouse
New Member

Hi,

Have you tried the liquid Magnesium Citrate? It will get things going quick. I do not know of anything that will help with the lazy bowel though. I suppose I have the same problem, I have had to use laxatives for years. It makes no sense to tell people not to use them except for short periods of time. To me, when your bowels do not function properly, it is the same as when someone's heart does not function properly. They would not tell someone with a heart condition to use the medication for a short period of time because their heart may become dependent on it, would they? I just do not think doctors take constipation very seriously. To me, it is a very serious problem.

Good luck!

From: **Colorado**

Type 0
Prolific Member

It's hard to see so many people with this problem also. I've abused laxatives (herbal). Zelnorm didn't really work well for me and made my back sore for some reason. It got so that the laxatives worked too well and gave me spasms that were just awful, just a vicious cycle. Seems things worked for a while and then stopped. I am right now drinking Noni juice and it is working—I am keeping my fingers crossed that it will keep working and not stop in a month or so, because I don't know what I'll do then. My bloating has gone way down—my daughter asked me if I had lost weight on my stomach area!!! It's so hard, Noni juice is expensive, but I'm thinking if I can throw away all the other stuff that I was taking, it'll be cheaper in the long run. Zelnorm was terribly expensive. Hope you can find something that works soon.

From: **Canada**

CJSJ
New Member

Noni juice, like many other herbal laxatives, has a mixture of anthraquinones as the active agent. Anthraquinones are responsible for the laxative effect of Senna.

This is not to say that you shouldn't use the Noni Juice, but rather that you may have trouble with long-term usage. Some of the other treatments that you will find in the posts to this board, such as Magnesium Oxide, may cause less long-term problems.

From: **Clearwater. FL**

Type 0
Prolific Member

Hi, thanks for your info and you are right, but noni juice isn't just sold as an herbal laxative. It will also help diarrhea, so I'm told by the guy I bought it from. It makes me feel normal, go normal and be normal, nothing else has made me that way, including magnesium. Believe me I've tried it all. I am wondering just what kinds of roots the people of Africa are eating when we're told they never have digestion problems, probably roots containing anthraquinones? Maybe turkey rhubarb root, who knows? I'm drinking a fruit juice, a crappy tasting one, but it's not like Senna on my system and doesn't cramp me up. Like I said it just makes me normal and it's so good to feel normal with this problem. I am to the point where, what's worse, not ever going on my own or trying to find something that works and is not hard on my body? Triphala also has these anthraquinone properties in it, but is said to be great for the digestive system. Who knows about all this stuff, I am tired of trying to figure it all out. I have been coping with IBS for 30 years now and yes, I'm tired of trying this, trying that. Don't mean to sound fed up, but some days I am. Take care.

From: **Canada**

Topic: Too many enemas make sigmoid lazy?

Joan Gregg
Prolific Member

For the past two weeks, not only can't I empty the rectum, I can't empty the sigmoid. Too many water bag enemas? Please respond. Can I re-train? I still have that transit disorder that affects my WHOLE gastrointestinal system, according to a Pennsylvania hospital doctor.

From: **Philadelphia, PA**

NancyCat
Very Prolific Member

JG—You need to set a time each day to sit on the potty and "try" to go, even if you can't. Hopefully you can train your body to get the proper urge and to go after a while. It can't hurt and may help. Hope this helps.

Nancy

From: **Massachusetts**

Ghitta
Prolific Member

Joan, sorry to have to tell you this, but enemas are addictive just like stimulatory laxatives. And just like stimulatory laxatives, once in a while is fine, but on a regular continuing basis, they will mess you up permanently (Mae West was a known enema addict and ended up incontinent in her old age). If you can find other solutions, that would be better (same old, same old: diet, exercise, mental health, relaxation techniques, supplements, things that are fast to digest if you have slow transit: fruit, green vegetables, etc.), but try to stay away from enemas on a regular basis.

From: **Florida**

Paula J.
Very Prolific Member

I'd call the doctor's office, and ask what you can do for this problem.

I'm more screwed up when I don't use something then when I do, but I'm screwed either way. I've eaten plenty of bran and it's gassy but it does help, and I still need assistance going. I've gone four to five days without going, and I just will not do that anymore. When I have incomplete evacuation, I use an enema. I mean you have to use something, or sit with that discomfort all day. It's one thing or another to me.

I have read various opinions, but there are some gastroenterologists who don't believe you can get addicted to laxatives. I think you can retrain quite easily if you want to go through not going for a while. Eventually you'll go if you are eating fiber and fruit. I took some cascara segrada, an herb just to see if it would help me go last week and it did nothing. I've taken laxatives and nothing or very little. Suppositories cause me to go, and an enema to top it off if necessary. Works like a charm. I feel moving the bowels is important and really we should go a couple times a day. I never did, but it would be better if you did. Doctors say it's however your body goes, but they don't have to live with that sluggish feeling till they go.

I think diet has a lot to do with it also. Too much dry food is no good. Bread, chips and nachos have no water in them. Eat foods with water and drink water and other liquids. Eating more soup. Soup should be a staple.

My grandpa used to drink Fernet every morning, and he went like a charm. This is a liquor, and you might have to order over the internet because liquor stores don't readily have it. I got some Angostura bitters, but they didn't work. Not going runs in my family way back to my great-grandmother, but I have no clue what they did, except for my grandpa. The Fernet is hard to take because my grandpa made a big scrunched up face when he took a shot, and the bitters are bitter.

I wish I could help, but I have no clue. I just do what I do, and I'm quite gassy, but at least I can go. I'm gassy either way because I've tried everything.

From: **Tennessee**

Topic: IBS-D turned to IBS-C?

Starcrossedlvr
New Member

Hi everyone … I'm new here, I was diagnosed with IBS-C about two years ago, even though I have had it for about three or four years. I am currently 23 and the IBS-C started when I was about 19. The thing is between the ages of 12 and 18, I was the opposite. I had constant D. I always had to watch what I ate because I got sick easily. Ironically, now that I am a more healthy vegetarian (going on two-and-a-half years), I flipped to IBS-C. Has anyone experienced such a dramatic flip? Could it be a change in lifestyle that did it? Any ideas?

From: **New Paltz, NY**

Leanned
New Member

Yes … I was initially IBS-D for about the first one-and-a-half years after I was diagnosed … I have been IBS-C for the last seven or eight years now. I can't say that I noticed any reason or cause for the change … I would say I preferred

IBS-D to my current state, but then again I always say anything is better than this ... funny how time makes you forget. Good luck.

From: **Atlanta**

AussieGirl37
New Member

Hi, yes, I used to be IBS-D for about 10 years and now IBS-C for about one year. I think it's because I adopted such a low fiber diet and eliminated all fruits, as I may be fructose intolerant (not sure), so now I get constipated instead! Can't win, hey! Now I take psyllium to help keep motions bulky and moving and that seems to be helping at the moment. But, as you know, it is so different for all. I did get a colonoscopy done though, as my stool shape changed, so wanted to be sure there were no blockages. Plus, they told me to get more exercise, as this helps to keep your system moving.

Good luck.

From: **Australia**

Legseleven
New Member

I too have changed from D to C. Don't know which is worst. I also take psyllium [Prodium]. It is very good, take small amounts at first, until you get used to it. Can be a problem if you take too much, and drink lots of water.

My problem is mucus afterwards, has anyone else experienced that?

From: **Ontario**

NancyCat
Very Prolific Member

Happens to me like that too. The doctor told me you can alternate at different intervals, days, weeks, months and even years. I was IBS-D for the four years when I was pregnant and for the next three years. Then I wasn't C, but I'd go a lot, which I think is actually a subset of being D, cause the poops happen abnormally often (like eight nine times a day but not D). I'm not terribly clear on that, but I think D is defined as frequent or loose or watery stools, or all three. Anyway I'd rather be C, but both are MISERABLE.

Nancy

From: **Massachusetts**

RT
Regular Member

My IBS-D just turned into IBS-C in the last two days. I wonder if it is because my diet changes helped with the D, but not the C. It's a fine balancing act and I'll let you know if I find a formula! I do take a dose of Citrucel before each dinner (mainly because that is the one meal where I sometimes cheat and splurge on an item I normally have eliminated from my diet).

R.T.

From: **Portland, Oregon**

Starcrossedlvr
New Member

Thanks for the replies everyone!! I don't know what it is ... my IBS-C has been horrible the past couple months ... I think my D may have turned to C because of college (it is mental I believe), b/c that is when it changed ... but I don't know, b/c when I took time off from school it got better, but then acted up again later ... I do think its linked to a different kind of stress or depression then the kind I had when I had D as a teenager. Well ... maybe when I graduate things will improve or change! I think I'm gonna try the whole Vitamin C and magnesium supplement thing I've been reading about ... ciao

From: **New Paltz, NY**

Topic: Desperate for Hemorrhoid Relief. HELP!

IBSinAZ
Regular Member

I have nasty internal hemmies and some days they just bleed out in the toilet and shower. The loss of blood is incredible. I have an appt. with a surgeon on Tuesday, but have heard from EVERYONE that surgery is worse. Have any of you dealt with vicious ones and have healed yourself without surgery? Please, I am begging any of you to help me out. I am at the point of giving up on life. I just can't go on living my life with this problem. I am only 26! I take three stool softeners a night and drink water all day long. Please help a desperate person out! Thanks!!

Matt

From: **Arizona**

LifeLostW/IBS
New Member

I had surgery in July to remove my hemorrhoids. It was not fun, the pain was horrible, and there is no worse feeling in the world when you have a BM. But to look back, it was the best thing I have ever done. To suffer years of the pain from them, it was well worth the initial pain to now be pain-free. My only regret is that I did not take the pain meds until it got really bad. I was worried about constipation and terrified to have a BM. I called the Doctor and told him this. He said "take the pain pills and stay on top of the pain" and prescribed a stool softener which did wonders. It was not so bad to have a BM. I had a Sitz bath waiting for me for when I was done. What relief I would get and it helped to speed up the healing process. I still suffer from the dreaded C word, but no hemorrhoids. It was so worth it.

From: **PA**

Lalarainbow
New Member

Hi,

I sure can sympathize with you. Been having problems with 'outies', sheesh! It is usually from diarrhea, but then a med I take for IC causes constipation. I take Metamucil trying to keep things normal. I use Prep H and soak, but this sure is painful. Surgery would be my last resort, but if they could promise no more pain after that, I would go for it ...

This is the pits!!

Hope you feel better real soon.

~~Pam~~

From: **Nova Scotia, Canada**

Ghitta
Prolific Member

The thing is, if your 'roids have thrombosed and hardened up, the only real solution is the scalpel and DON'T LET THE SURGEON DO IT BY LASER! It is an amazement to me that they use laser surgery in America for 'roids as opposed to the old-fashioned knife. I had a hemorrhoidectomy in '99 and although it was vile at the time, it was the best thing I could have done—however—I retrained my bowel and everything else afterwards, so I would not suffer C too much again. In the meantime, the important thing is to keep your stools SOFT AND LOOSE: water, softeners, magnesium supplements, tons of cooked greens and other vegetables, prunes and prune juice, olive oil, etc. etc. Another thing is to address the circulatory issue of 'roids: exercise and there are supplements found in health food stores that boost your blood circulation. Good luck!

From: **Florida**

Topic: Constipation and Headaches

Gary
New Member

I have a moderate level of chronic constipation, that's mostly kept in check with Miralax and fiber. However, when I do get constipated, I tend to get headaches. Not excruciating ones, but dull, throbbing, headaches, usually on one side of the head. The usual over-the-counter medicines don't do much. Headache frequently is relieved by a BM.

Does anyone share this symptom, and what do you do about it?

From: **USA**

NicoleG
Prolific Member

I get this as well. It is unbearable. Mine are right above my right or left eye. Just last week I found something that helps, finally, after almost 10 years.

I take a cayenne capsule before I go to sleep. Cayenne somehow reduces substance P, a chemical that sends pain from peripheral nerves to your brain. I am assuming that this is why it is helping me. All I can tell you is that it helps me a ton with the headaches and I am very glad to have found this out.

From: **Wharton, NJ USA**

Suev
Prolific Member

Gary—sounds stupid—but how much fluid do you drink? I'm IBS-C and am terrible about not drinking the requisite amount of dreaded water (hate the stuff), but you might be headachy because you are dehydrated. I now try to have a glass of water first thing in the morning, which seems to make me feel more awake if nothing else. See if that helps—dead obvious I know!!

All the best anyway.

Sue, Manchester

From: **Cheshire.UK**

Gary
New Member

Thanks for the info.

I think I'm good about drinking enough water, but now I'll be more conscious of the issue, and at least have a sense of whether I'm getting the headaches when I've been drinking less than usual.

Nicole, it sounds as if you're getting the headaches a lot more frequently than I am. Mine are maybe twice a month, so if I'd gone a week without one, I wouldn't be convinced that I'd found a remedy. I hope it continues to work for you!

Has anyone heard of constipation being a trigger for migraines? Is it possible that a migraine is somehow being triggered by the same thing that triggers the constipation?

From: **USA**

NicoleG
Prolific Member

This is how it works for me. When I have to go to the bathroom, I get a pain over my eye, usually my right eye. My left eye will also twitch. I have virtually no sensation down there when I have to go to the bathroom. Instead of feeling like I have to go, I get the head pain and eye-twitching. It is very odd. The pain is excruciating. Then, when I go to the bathroom, the head pain IMMEDIATELY goes away. This leads me to believe that the stool must be pressing on a nerve that is signaling my brain to produce this head pain. No doctor has been able to find a reason for this. I know it is real though, I have been dealing with it for almost 10 years now. Every day. But, the cayenne does help dull the pain.

From: **Wharton, NJ USA**

GNW12
New Member

Gary,

I have had hormonal migraines for years. My GI says that my migraines and IBS-C are definitely connected. I assume it's because of the serotonin. I'm going to ask him more about it when I see him next. I understand that 95% of the serotonin in the body is in the gut, & I understand that the brain has serotonin. I know that Zelnorm is supposed to target the No. 4 receptor site for serotonin in the gut, although it didn't do anything for me.

From: **Louisville, KY**

Ira
Regular Member

Gary:

Yes, IBS-related constipation is often linked with headaches in my own case. They are similar in location to what Nicole describes. Sometimes I can't even tell if the pain is coming from above my eye or from the gut. Kinda feels like rapid oscillation.

I have had quite a degree of relief from these by reducing caffeine intake by half. At first, I got some caffeine withdrawal headaches. But after a while the C-related headaches lessened in intensity.

—Ira

From: **USA**

Discussion: Things that Help

Many individuals with IBS-C are frustrated by the lack of help that they receive from the medical profession. Often, there is no "magic pill" to make it all better. Luckily, members in this forum are generous with their advice. As you read the following posts, you will see that there are lots of things that you can try. Dealing with IBS-C requires a multi-prong approach, with a great deal of trial-and-error, to get things moving in a manageable way.

Topic: Bowel Retraining?

MicheleL
Regular Member

Hi,

Anyone with IBS-C and spasms ever have luck with bowel retraining? I read that you should sit on toilet 30 minutes after eating, for 10 to15 minutes, and do it consistently.

From: **United States**

NancyCat
Very Prolific Member

Yes. It has worked for me, even though it can be discouraging at times. I am IBS-A, and even when I'm not C, it can be difficult to get things going, so to speak. I go, or don't but feel like I have to, in the morning. Whatever happens, or doesn't, its easier to get it all done at once, when I'm at my "best". I usually drink a cup of coffee rather than eat.

In my experience, it takes a really long time (months) and you do have to be consistent. If you flare up (I go both ways, D flares or C flares) it can mess things up.

But I think the key to it is to get into a regular routine. I also need to get enough uninterrupted sleep, because when I wake up, my bowel does too, and often the contractions start shortly after.

When my son was a baby, things were especially problematic because I was up all the time. When you eat, it often stimulates bowel contractions (I think its actually considered normal), so it's probably easier to poop then. It's worth a shot trying to do this, it's easy and non-invasive. Hope this helps.

Nancy

From: **Massachusetts**

Ghitta
Prolific Member

Here's how I did it, years ago, and it still works for me—

I arranged my work life so as to no longer rush a morning clock. I changed my bedtime to go to bed earlier and I began to rise at dawn. I began to drink hot tea and/or coffee or hot water with lemon, first thing in the morning. I would take, and sometimes still do, a tablespoon of olive oil mixed with fresh lemon juice on an empty stomach, followed by a glass of bottled water, followed by my hot drinks. I did NOT give up smoking. I allowed myself at least three hours before leaving the house and I did NOT eat breakfast until I had eliminated one way or another. I added magnesium supplements to my dinner, along with a flax oil pill. I made sure I moved my body enough during the day and drank a lot of water, never tap, never carbonated. I walked instead of drove, if possible, used the bike if possible, added tons more cooked leafy greens, artichoke hearts, cooked fruits and vegetables to my diet, stayed away from wheat, dairy and corn as much as possible, and so far …. IT MOSTLY WORKS. I did all this over a period of four to six months, back in 1999 and I still do it … … and it works for me.

From: **Florida**

Midwinter madness
Prolific Member

But is there anyway of doing this without having to get up at the crack of dawn? That is the way I manage it at the moment and I hate it—spending the first few hours of the day on the toilet with cigs and hot drinks—it makes me feel so abnormal and is making me very scared about how I'll cope when I stay with friends over the New Year. I used to say "no" to these kinds of invitations because of my gut, but I'm determined to go this time. I'm tired of missing out because of it. I guess maybe I just need to keep persevering with the suggestions I was given.

Take care MW

From: **London**

Jo-Jo
Very Prolific Member

I think (like Ghitta said) giving yourself enough time in the morning is the key. I'm up at 4:30 AM weekdays to give myself enough time. Sick time to get up, I know. My mornings are crucial. You get used to it after a while. I don't sleep over anywhere unless I can be totally undisturbed; friends and family are out of the question.

My gastro doc tells me to sit on the toilet each day for 15 minutes after each meal. Tried it and it didn't work for me. I do the glycerin supplements and that has been the only thing that has kept me "pain free" for most of the time. I don't think I could be able to work without them. The pain would be excruciating. Food-wise, I try to eat a lot of vegetables—peppers, squash, cooked spinach, and pears work great. I don't take any fiber supplements anymore (Metamucil), I was in more pain with them. I take 425mg of magnesium oxide after supper each day, which helps a lot.

I have never been a regular person. I remember taking castor oil everyday when I was little because I was always constipated. I will never forget that nasty taste.

From: **Oh Canada!**

Ghitta
Prolific Member

There is a whole school of thought that if one has chronic C with a probable tendency to hemorrhoids, the last thing you want to do is sit on the loo, unless you really feel the need to "go" ... ... this business about sitting on the loo after every meal is the most ridiculous thing I've ever heard of and I've never known anyone it's ever worked for; on the contrary, sitting there without going and probably straining will bring those 'roids faster than a New York minute!

From: **Florida**

Topic: Insoluble vs. Soluble Fiber?

Baltezaar
New Member

I know there are two kinds of fiber, soluble and insoluble. I know the difference (one dissolves and one doesn't!)

However, is one overall better for C? Right now my main sources of fiber are wheat bran on my oatmeal, and Metamucil wafers. I've read a lot of folks here take Citrucel, which is mainly soluble fiber.

A friend who sells Shaklee says I should be taking their fiber pills which are mostly insoluble fiber. She also recommends acidophilus.

Is one kind of fiber better than the other? Can I "mix" them (i.e., wheat bran and Citrucel)? Does it mostly just depend on the individual's body and reactions?

From: **Ohio**

Austin
Prolific Member

I really don't know the answers to your questions, but wanted to say that I tried Benefiber yesterday (I was feeling quite unwell) and it seems to have been just the thing to get me back on track (along with prayer, visualization, Zelnorm, and a few other things). Anyway, I was also wondering about fibers and if others have had positive experience with Benefiber, and is it insoluble or soluble (I'm guessing soluble)?

Another thing I wanted to say about the Benefiber is that it is made from gar gum only, and this seems to be a substance that I do not have an intolerance to. What frightens me about most of these products is that I'm not sure what's in them and how I will react to the ingredients, but on the web site I learned that there are no additives to the main and only ingredient. So I felt safe trying it. I also use flax seed, grind them myself so I'll know exactly what I'm getting. I'm thinking with the addition of the Benefiber, I've got a workable combo.

Jimmye

From: **Austin, TX**

Isis1
Prolific Member

The traditional school of thought seems to be that insoluble fiber is better. That's what my original meal plan was based on, given to me by the nutritionist my first GI doc sent me to. At that time Citrucel 3x/day was also part of my treatment.

What I've heard over and over is soluble fiber softens the stool, making it easier to pass, while insoluble fiber bulks it up. What has been confusing to me is that I've seen posts from many people here with IBS-C who say soluble fiber has been bad for them, that the insoluble type is much better. You're right; it's a very individual thing.

Personally I need both, but far less of the insoluble type. I try to eat foods all day that are high in soluble fiber, including a bowl of oat bran cereal every morning. I mix a couple of tablespoons of flaxseed meal into the cooked cereal and it works really well. When I checked the label I saw that flaxseed meal is almost 50/50 soluble/insoluble fiber. The rest of my diet has small amounts of insoluble fiber in it as well.

So for me, it's a matter of degree, keeping this ratio of roughly 80/20 between the two. I hope this helps ...

From: **Boston**

Tiss
Very Prolific Member

I seem to need both types of fiber. I use Benefiber (LOVE that stuff!), Citrucel (4 tablets/day), psyllium, and pectin in a capsule.

Tiss

From: **Mid USA**

Baltezaar
New Member

Thanks to everyone for their replies. I also looked at Benefiber, which is soluble.

Just tired of feeling overwhelmed by both the amount of things I **don't** know and the dizzying array of methods used by posters here. It's hard to know where to begin.

From: **Ohio**

Isis1
Prolific Member

Baltezaar,

I know what you mean about the overwhelm! It was daunting to me at first. It helped me a lot to do/learn these things:

1) Keep weighing my options according to what these things do:
   Stool softeners (Colace)
   Fiber supplements (Metamucil, Citrucel etc.)
   Osmotic laxatives (Milk of Magnesia)
   Antispasmodics
   Lubricants (Mineral oil, etc.)
   Suppositories (Glycerin)
   Stimulant laxatives (Senna, aloe, cascara etc.)
   SSRIs
   Zelnorm

2) Distinguish between things that are safe on a daily basis (the first two things), things that are safe for a limited period of time (the last three things), and get familiar with what falls between. I will often check in with the doctor about those in-between things, as I need to.

3) Be aware that there's a lot of snake oil being sold out there. If I can't find a clear direct description of how and why something is supposed to work, and I can't find valid info about it on sites like PubMed, Medline, or other reputable sources, then I'm suspicious.

4) Know that while there are some general things that work for most of us, we're all different in terms of specifically what works for each us.

5) Anything that works could just stop working at any time. It helps me to be ready with another alternative as soon as I notice that's happening. If I catch it like that, I can actually stop a flare-up from happening. There's no guarantee that something new will work, but it's not a shot in the dark anymore. That's where this site has been invaluable. I do have more control than I used to.

I didn't think there was much I could do before, now I know there are many options and combinations of things to try the next time I'm in trouble. I'm also much more comfortable now on a daily basis, with fewer flare-ups than before I found this site. This is a very valuable resource. Just keep coming back!

I hope this was helpful to you …

From: **Boston**

Baltezaar
New Member

Isis, that post was INCREDIBLY helpful. Thanks for presenting the information in an organized, logical way.

While I have read a lot of helpful ideas here (NEVER would have imagined that flax seed would be good for C!), most of the posters seem to write as if everyone already knows what stuff is, what it does and where to get it.

I'm also dealing with mild C, though it seems to have switched on me lately. Used to be better and regular about going at work and not so much at home; now home is more "productive" than work. Makes the working day a lot more uncomfortable.

From: **Ohio**

Ganas
Prolific Member

For me insoluble fiber most often seems to be my trigger. I am of the opinion of the 80 soluble/20 insoluble, making sure to eat soluble first. Just have to find what works best for you. It will depend a lot on if you are predominately C or D.

From: **Michigan**

Ghitta
Prolific Member

I can't do any of those bulk-forming fiber supplements and I hate measuring out what I eat in the 80/20% thing. I figure that 99% of the planet's population doesn't worry about this stuff and it's because we eat such a refined diet in North America that we have to seek out solutions in hay and straw (which is what pysllium and flax seeds taste like to me ....) In order to bulk up and soften my stool I use food and magnesium supplements. I've said this before but I'm going to post it yet again: try eating a plate of cooked fresh spinach smothered in olive oil topped with half a dozen canned and rinsed artichoke hearts with perhaps a little brown rice or millet on the side followed by a dish of stewed prunes and see if you don't go to the bathroom first thing in the morning!

This is a non-exhaustive list of foods I use as fiber instead of fiber supplements: cooked apples and pears, mangos and pineapple, oranges and grapefruits (the fruit, not the juice,) well-cooked broccoli, cooked carrots, cooked greens of all types, cooked onions and garlic, cooked celery, potatoes of all types WITH SKINS ON (hence, organic only), brown rice, white rice, rice crackers and rice pastas, white beans and pinto beans, polenta (corn meal,) and most importantly: those arti-choke hearts!—if one sticks to a diet of frozen microwave foods, those hideous weight-watcher-type, low-calorie frozen meals, processed junk, it is no wonder one is C-ed up. So you get a little gas from eating beans and rice, you might be farty but you sure as heck will be pooping … … g—

From: **Florida**

Believer
New Member

Ghitta—

Thanks for the info in your post. I haven't had much success with fiber supple-ments, either. In reading through some of your previous posts, I realized I have become a little lax on the amount of fiber I'm consuming from "real food." I have been trying to incorporate some of your ideas and it has made a difference. Thanks for sharing your insight.

From: **Dallas, TX**

DavidLA
Prolific Member

Ghitta—Great post!

I personally avoid all PRODUCTS that boast to help constipation. I sincerely believe that foods are the BEST medicine. I believe basically that the S.A.D. (Standard American Diet) = Digestive Problems. I was taught (later in life) to always shop on the outskirts of the Market ... Produce sections first. Thanks again!!!

From: **Sherman Oaks, CA, USA**

Cordelia
Prolific Member

Last night I had six artichoke hearts and five prunes (stewed), among other things, and today I went wonderfully well! Yippee, yeah, Ghitta, thanks!

From: **United States**

Ghitta
Prolific Member

Ain't nothin' like dem artichoke hearts, I swear! Glad to hear it worked for ya, Cordelia. Here's another recipe tip: sautéed onions and garlic in olive oil in a pot, add chopped tomatoes WITH SKINS ON and seeds, throw in a handful of spinach, fresh or frozen, throw in a dozen artichoke hearts cut in half or quarters, throw in a can of cannellini beans, cover with organic chicken broth or just plain water, bring to a boil, then simmer for an hour and voila! Easy healthy fiber soup. Eat for dinner with bread of your choice or rice crackers and soy cheese slices. G—

From: **Florida**

Topic: Frustrated with Fiber

Spongebob_mom
New Member

I posted this on a different message board and haven't gotten any responses. Hopefully, there will be more help here.

I have had IBS C & D since I was a teenager (I'm 32). However, lately, it's the C that's been acting up. My problem is that Citrucel and Metamucil make my constipation WORSE. I know that they "bulk" your stool and I have found they just do not help me. However, other types of fiber do help. I was hoping that I'm not the only one that has worsening C with fiber supplements. Also, if so, what types of fiber-rich foods DO help your C?

By the way, I am a very big advocate of Miralax, but I would like to find natural ways, such as diet, to help my IBS as well.

Thank you in advance,

Jane

From: **Michigan**

Michele Brake
Prolific Member

Hi, I have had IBS since I was about 15, now 33. I have IBS-C and am currently working my way off Miralax after more than three years! I am planning on trying to get pregnant this spring and want to reduce the chemicals I am putting in my body. I am only able to do this by adding acacia to my diet. Acacia is a soluble fiber powder. When I first started it made me REALLY gassy for a couple weeks. I was told I started at too high a dose. Over the past four to six weeks I've increased the acacia and decreased the Miralax. I am currently taking three teaspoons of acacia in the AM and PM and only taking half a dose of Miralax every other day! Before the Miralax, I was dependant on over-the-counter laxatives.

A lot of people who try fiber supplements are not taking enough! And in order for them to work you need a TON of water. I drink 10 to 12 glasses of water a day! I also find exercise to be very important—keeps things moving!

I find nothing cleans me out like a nice big salad! Raisin bran also speeds things up. Sometimes they do cause a little D! What kind of diet are you eating and how much fiber supplement are you taking?? Also, the different brands seem to make in difference in different people.

From: **Detroit**

LK
Prolific Member

Hey Spongebob_mom,

You are definitely not the only one who gets worse with fiber supplements, although there seems to be only a few of us on this board. I spent two bloated, gassy years trying to get them to work for me; and they did to some extent, but only if I drank water constantly through the day.

There are two types of fiber: soluble and insoluble. Soluble fiber is the main ingredient in most fiber supplements. It is also typically the fiber that is found in fruit and legumes. Insoluble fiber is typically found in veggies.

Soluble fiber works by forming a gel-like substance, which is supposed to help things along. However, if you are not getting enough water into your colon (which is often the case with us constipated folk) then instead of a gel, it just becomes a sticky glue, hence making things way worse.

Insoluble fiber on the other hand, just holds water in the fibrous material.

After a recommendation from someone on this board, I tried taking magnesium supplements instead and eventually went cold turkey on the fiber supplements; this has worked wonders for me.

As for soluble, I now avoid it at all costs, which includes really watching what I eat. I find whenever I eat something with high soluble fiber, I get backed up again and very gassy. In addition to fruits and beans, this includes a lot of processed foods, as a common food additive is gum, i.e. guar gum, carob bean gum, etc., which are all soluble fibers. They are most often found in dairy products and sauces, as they are used as thickeners to keep products from separating.

Anyhow, I recommend you try laying off the fiber supplements if they are not working for you. Try eating more insoluble fibers and give the magnesium supplements a shot.

Good Luck.

Linda

From: **Canada**

Ghitta
Prolific Member

I've posted this a gazillion times and I'm gonna post yet one more time: cooked leafy (fresh) greens like spinach, kale, chard, etc, canned artichoke hearts, white canella beans, pinto beans, black-eyed peas, (cooked, never raw), broccoli, carrots, green beans, asparagus, white potatoes with skin on (organic only), yams and sweet potatoes, white bread, rice crackers, rice cereals or diverse grains such as millet, amaranth, couscous, spelt; cooked fruits: apples, pears, raw fruit: tropical only—pineapple, mango, papaya, cherries.—raw lettuce OK, but not iceberg because boring and tasteless without nutrients.—goat/sheep's yoghurt, organic kefir, cranberry juice, tomatoes with skins on, cucumbers, sprouts. Now, try this foolproof recipe: a plate of rinsed canned artichoke hearts mixed with garbanzo beans and cooked spinach, and some tuna if you want. Eat it at night and take a magnesium supplement with dinner as well. Drink water or herb tea only from dinnertime to bedtime; see what happens in the morning! G—

From: **Florida**

H8_IBS
Prolific Member

I am right there with you. Those fiber supplements are miserable. I will NEVER, and I mean never, take them again as long as I have IBS.

What helps me with C and doesn't cause me pain or bloating like Metamucil can:

Benefiber is the only fiber I would recommend as far as those fibers go …

Slippery Elm supplements as directed on bottle, on an empty stomach between meals

Sunflower Seed Kernels

Almonds

The soymilk I drink has four grams of fiber per serving

Cooked/over-cooked veggies

From: **NJ**

Topic: I eat 8 prunes a day just to go ...

Beach
Prolific Member

If I didn't have my prunes with me, I don't think I would go. I have five in the morning with breakfast, and three when I come home ... in order to go. Thank goodness for prunes!!

From: **NY**

AMC
Very Prolific Member

Wow ... . I've never tried prunes, but I'm willing to try just about anything some days, LOL!! I don't know if I've ever even HAD prunes?? Do they taste alright?? Or is it one of those things you just sort of have to pinch your nose and swallow real quick so you don't taste it??

From: **United States**

Beach
Prolific Member

I actually really like the taste. Nice and sweet, like raisins.

From: **NY**

Gottogo
Prolific Member

When I turned 40, a few friends all got me a bottle of prune juice as a joke. Well being an IBS-CG person, I decided to try it. Oh, it was the worst stuff I ever drank. I gagged. Then I dumped it down the drain. Never again will I drink prune juice. Hopefully the prunes have a better flavor.

From: **Ohio**

Tiss
Very Prolific Member

I eat six every day and I think they help a lot.

From: **Mid USA**

Chmiel0613
New Member

I have never tried prunes or prune juice either. Everything in the world consti-
pates me. I would love to try something natural that would help me completely
go. So, prunes are better tasting than prune juice?

From: **NY**

I'll B Snookered
Prolific Member

Prunes are good. I eat six to eight per day at about 8:00 PM. If nothing else,
they've got some good antioxidant properties.

From: **SF Bay Area, CA**

Ghitta
Prolific Member

Stewed prunes are great. Organically-grown prunes are even better, because they
don't have all the hideous sulfites and nitrates and all matter of crap that you find
in regular prunes (like Sunsweet's). If you want good-tasting prune juice, just soak
your dried prunes overnight in the fridge in water and in the morning drink the
water. You can also add a little good maple syrup (also good for C). Try stewed
prunes over vanilla ice cream (if you do dairy) or soy/rice ice cream if you don't
(do dairy, that is,) for dessert at night.

Here's another anti C recipe:

Take as many dried prunes as you wish, throw them into a small pot with a handful of raisins, some tapioca, a little vanilla extract, and some cinnamon; cover with water, bring to a boil, lower to a simmer; eat like soup at nighttime or first thing in the morning. By the way, figs are even higher in fiber than prunes—if you can get your hands on fresh figs (not easy in America) pig out on them. Immediate relief from C with no digestive upset. Prunes can cause gas in some people sensitive to fructose, etc. A little note to those not familiar with prunes: they are what plums become when dried.

From: **Florida**

Brook0114
New Member

I've tried drinking warm prune juice. It helps, but it tastes very gross.

From: **Louisiana**

Ghitta
Prolific Member

Try mixing prune juice with pear or apple juice, and by all means, drink it cold!

From: **Florida**

Topic: Flaxseed

Gonowoften
Prolific Member

Well, as of three weeks ago, I began using ground flaxseed, and the change from the prune juice is mind-boggling. I'm having regular movements, several times a day (average of five or so) and, for the first time in nearly a year, I'm feeling "clean", like I don't have waste within me. I don't have the urgent feeling that prune juice would induce and I just feel "normal" again. It's great. It only took half a day for the flaxseed to take effect for me. I've purchased golden organic flaxseed and a coffee grinder. Every day, I take two ground tablespoons in the morning with some cranberry juice for a mini-breakfast, and then three more tablespoons at night, a bit before bed.

From: **Melbourne, Australia**

Tiss
Very Prolific Member

Hi, I use whole flaxseeds (my doc says it's great to eat ground or whole—I prefer it whole). It definitely helps. I use it in my oatmeal everyday and I love the taste!

Tiss

From: **Mid USA**

Byte
Regular Member

Is there any difference if you took it as the flaxseed itself or if you took the flaxseed oil supplement??

From: **Melbourne**

Tiss
Very Prolific Member

Flaxseed, ground or whole, acts like psyllium in that it absorbs fluid and makes a BM softer and easier to pass.

I put them in my oatmeal (whole flaxseeds) and then microwave it all together. I love the crunch and the taste of the flaxseeds. It is better for my C than ground. Don't know why.

Tiss

From: **Mid USA**

Laylo
Regular Member

Byte,

It's the fiber in whole or ground flaxseeds that alleviates constipation. Flaxseed oil and pills do not have fiber.

Also, whole and ground flaxseeds have a mucilaginous quality that soothes and heals the gut lining. Try soaking a few tablespoons of whole flax seeds in 8 oz. of water overnight, and you'll see what I mean by mucus. It's actually not too bad. You can drink the whole thing down. I don't know if this would be as helpful as ground flax, though, for constipation relief.

L

From: **Santa Cruz, California**

GSNAILS
New Member

Can you tell me why grind them? I also have constipation, and have bought some flax seeds but now I do not know whether to eat them whole or grind them. I feel hopeless.

R.

From: **GEORGIA**

Kathleen M, Ph.D..
Very Prolific Member

I think people grind them because that gets the fiber out of the hard shell of the seed to where it might do you some good.

Otherwise you just pass the hard seeds whole, and that probably won't be all that helpful.

K

From: **Somewhere over the rainbow**

SpaceNeedle
Regular Member

Flax oil has been a big help for me. I've got diverticulitus, so eating small seeds is a no-no. I buy the pre-liquefied brand, the type that's in the cooler section of your local health food store. Flax oil puts tons more moisture into your GI than Miralax. Also, peppermint pills have been a huge help.

I take two peppermint pills in the morning, four to six tablespoons of flax oil, one or two peppermint pills before lunch, then four to six tablespoons of flax before dinner.

From: **Bellevue, WA**

Gonowoften
Prolific Member

I prefer not to use the whole flaxseeds because I have been told by professionals that the shells have a very sharp point that can irritate an inflamed bowel and lodge in any diverticular pouches that may exist, thereby causing further discomfort.

I believe the perfect way to take flaxseed is to follow Dr Budwig's suggestion, which also allows us the perfect daily allowance of Omega-3 & Omega-6.

One dessert-spoonful of oil mixed with equal amount of plain cottage cheese or yoghurt.

It is important to buy cold pressed flax oil in glass bottles from a store where it is kept in a refrigerator and in a light-proof container (usually a cardboard cylinder capped top & bottom.) This ensures you are getting the very best.

If any of you are familiar with oil painting you will know all too well the smell of linseed oil as it is used in the medium & mixed with turpentine. This is nothing less than rancid flax oil, so you need to be diligent when making your purchase!!

From: **Melbourne, Australia**

Tiss
Very Prolific Member

I just don't think I could take the oil alone or in something. I use Barlean's cold pressed high lignan flaxseed oil in capsules that are kept in a fridge. I use two in the AM and one at night. Lots of Omega-3.

Tiss

From: **Mid USA**

Gonowoften
Prolific Member

Tiss,

The fresh cold-pressed oil has a bland nutty taste, not at all like when it is rancid and doesn't smell unpleasant either. You could even add it to salads, etc.

From: **Melbourne, Australia**

Modgy
Prolific Member

Are people finding flax oil helps C much??

I'm using it because unlike just about everything else I could take for C, including any kind of fiber supplement, it doesn't leave me in agony.

Although I can't really tell if it's helping or not …

From: **Sydney, Australia**

Gonowoften
Prolific Member

If it doesn't leave you in agony it must be soothing your gut. Stick with it & you might like to try Slippery Elm also!

From: **Melbourne, Australia**

Modgy
Prolific Member

Hey Gonowoften,

Does slippery elm swell in size in your gut?? If it does, it would be a no no for me. I am finding "oiling" my diet up is helping more than any fiber supplement. I don't tolerate any kind of "distending" substances.

I am sticking with the flax oil, and upping my dose, in fact.

From: **Sydney, Australia**

Gonowoften
Prolific Member

Modgy,

Slippery elm does not swell up in the gut. It is a highly nutritious food that American native Indians have proved you can practically survive on. It is available in either tablets or powder, & when mixed with a little milk or soy to a paste, then hot water added, can make a huge difference to your condition.

Slippery Elm when mixed with liquids changes into a form of mucilage that soothes the whole of the G.I tract for at least 36 hours.

It is a Godsend for those unable to keep other foods down.

From: **Melbourne, Australia**

Topic: Flaxseed

Rose
Very Prolific Member

I have diverticulosis and absolutely cannot eat any kind of seeds. Does anybody know if the flaxseeds are ground into powder, is there a possibility some parts of the seeds could be in the powder?

From: **Massachusetts**

Kathleen M, Ph.D..
Very Prolific Member

I think it depends on the grind. If ground as fine as most psyllium husk powders are, I would think it would be OK ...

I mean Metamucil is OK, and it is psyllium husk (which whole I think would be a no-no) and that is often used for people with diverticular issues ... I think.

K.

From: **Somewhere over the rainbow**

Better Life
New Member

I used ground flaxseed for the first time this morning with my oatmeal, two table-spoons. Metamucil or Citracel does not work on me. I know that flaxseed swells in size in your intestine, but I feel full and a bit uncomfortable. And it's making me less hungry. When I feel this way, I tend to want to eat more. Is this normal? If this is how it feels all the time, I don't know if I want to take it. I've been a sufferer of constipation, bloating and gas for 10 years. I have yet to find a good remedy. Please help.

P.S. I do not believe in prescriptive drugs.

From: **California**

Ghitta
Prolific Member

Very well ground flax seeds (in a coffee grinder, for example) should not trouble those bothered with diverticulosis, but they can bloat, ground or not. To Better Life I suggest lots of fennel, artichokes, parsley both in vegetable form, well cooked, and in tea form. I find fennel tea with a bit of honey and/or lemon really helps when I'm gassy and contributing to the hole in the ozone layer!

From: **Florida**

Suev
Prolific Member

I've had IBS for about seven/eight years and I have just tried to be a little more proactive about managing my condition. The local health food shop is brilliant (and the lady in there, spoke the most sense of all the folk I've seen in my dealings with IBS) and I am now on a probiotic and linseed. I have a problem with gluten and therefore was eating a very fiber-poor diet which was making my constipation and sluggish bowels even worse. I'm not saying I'm cured (as I don't believe there is one) but I will say that for the two weeks (which I know is only a very short while), I have had better bowel movements (something we are all aiming for—right!) and much less rumbling and wind than for many a long year, so this might be worth a try.

All the best

Sue, near Manchester UK

From: **Cheshire.UK**

MrTIBS
New Member

I don't think I saw this mentioned yet, but many people were wondering. Whole flaxseed provides only one thing—insoluble fiber. The seed is too tough to break down or digest, so you don't get any of the oil benefits. Ground seed provides a (supposedly perfect) balance of insoluble and soluble fiber, plus you get the oil benefits. "High Lignan" oil is oil that contains ground seed bits—they actually add it back into the oil once it's been pressed (in much lower quantity than just using ground seed). I think you have to look at the brand for "particulate matter content" or something like that.

I've tried ground flaxseed on and off, with inconclusive results. I keep meaning to try it again sometime, but I've found success with Prodiem (the Citrucel-style). If you're sensitive at all to insoluble fiber, then be careful with flaxseed, whether it's ground or not. I don't think grinding to a fine powder eliminates the insoluble fiber (it comes from the outer shell and it will still be there, fine powder or not). I did try the Omega Nutrition flaxseed powder, but I found that grinding it myself was easy and it tasted/smelled much better. It goes rancid easily and the place where I bought the powder kept it on a shelf, not in the fridge.

I've been using flax oil for probably over two years now—at first it made a BIG difference (I believe it worked within a few days). Supposedly the oil helps constipation because it lubes the plumbing. The good effects slowly wore off, though. But I still take it, because I've cut out most other fat from my diet, and it's all unsaturated fat. I take about 1 to 1 1/2 tablespoons a day, depending on what other fats I eat that day.

Someone asked about fish vs. flax oil. I haven't tried fish oil, but I've read that it's better for you because it has a better balance of natural oils. Flax only contains omega-3 fatty acids. Also I've wondered about the "purity" of fish oils, given all the controversy over pollutants in fish (I'm not making any claims one way or the other; I haven't researched the subject).

I don't think there's any difference between fresh bottled oil and oil capsules. Just keep in mind that to get 1 tbsp. of oil, you need a lot of capsules! The capsules are much more portable, though.

If you want a good read about oils, try "Fats that Heal Fats that Kill" by Udo Erasmus. I found it enlightening, and he talks about how much oil to take, and how to balance it properly with other oils (omega-6,-9, and-12) which is important too. A diet too high in omega-3 oils can lead to other problems. I don't currently use his oil—I tried it and it did taste good, but I didn't want all the stuff he mixes into it. I just use a mix of sunflower and flax oils, and cook/bake with canola.

If you use the oil or ground seeds, make sure they're fresh and stored cold (you can even freeze the oil to prolong its shelf life). Don't cook or bake with flax oil. Don't reheat something that has flax oil or ground flaxseed in it. Heating the oil creates—something, I forget what, but I think it's related to free radicals and all that. Bad stuff. I've read that you can bake with ground flaxseed, and it's great to add fiber to quick breads, muffins, etc. You can even use it as an egg replacement.

Oh, an important point that I don't think anyone mentioned is that if you do take flaxseed—ground or whole—drink lots of water. Something like a cup or more of water per tablespoon flax. And start out slowly.

Start gradually, as with any fiber supplement! Maybe start with a teaspoon and work your way up. Any fiber supplement will help make you feel full. That's what some diet supplements are—the theory being the more full you feel the less you eat.

I never found a guide for how much seed to take, probably because everyone's different. You might have to figure out what other fiber sources you have, and aim for that 35+ grams of fiber per day. Of course, that doesn't take IBS into account. Be aware, though, I think I heard that over 50 grams per day could start causing problems, such as nutrient loss.

From: **Canada**

Hope
New Member

Flaxseed can be made into a tea rather like porridge. You can grind it in a blender, once ground, it will last a while—even longer in the freezer. Yes, it can be purchased at health food stores already ground—look in the sections that have gluten-free items and unusual pre-packaged flour—but grinding it in a blender will work just fine.

I have used it for years for stomachaches as a tea: put a tablespoon or two in a large cup and add hot water. It will steep and become thick like pectin. You can add honey or not, and I eat it with a spoon because the thick part tends to sink to the bottom. It has a mild nutty taste and a comforting texture—especially for anyone who is lactose intolerant or allergic to wheat, because we don't get much thick stuff normally.

My experience and I am the canary in the coal mine when it comes to gas and bloating, is that flaxseed has never caused this with me. I may not have eaten enough though—Metamucil destroys me, as does Senna and other vegetable fibers. I have finally abandoned them after many trials. But flaxseed is gentle and comforting.

It can also be cooked, like any other grain or seed. The usual ratio for grains is 1 cup to 1.5 cups of water. With flax, you may want more water.

Come to think of it, the stuff may make great soup base!

From: **Montana**

Nicole Graziano
Prolific Member

Interesting, I made the same discovery this week. I put mine (ground) in yogurt with dried fruit. Tastes good and is helping a ton!

From: **Wharton, NJ USA**

Topic: I need help with Magnesium??

Alexandragirl
Regular Member

I keep hearing about it for IBS-C. Does it help? I need more info please ... thanks.

From: **Texas**

Ghitta
Prolific Member

Magnesium is a natural mineral osmotic: it draws water into the bowels making them loose and runny. There are differences between types of magnesium such as oxide (which I use) and citrate, chelated, magnesium mixed with calcium & zinc, etc., etc. and a good Google search should also help you out. It is necessary to drink a lot of quality water when taking magnesium and also to have kidneys in good shape. G—

From: **Florida**

Laylo
Regular Member

I take magnesium citrate capsules (NOW brand). This type of Mg is easily absorbable, as is oxide. Do not get Mg Malate, which is used for Fibromyalgia.

Magnesium, when used to support IBS, is known for relaxing muscles. It will alleviate constipation, if the dose is sufficient. Try 500 mg caps 2x/day to start. Stay at that for two days. If it doesn't work, go up by one cap per day until you get results. Do not exceed 3000 mg/day.

Be aware that magnesium is antagonistic to calcium in the body. So, taking excess Mg will diminish the Ca that your body is able to intake. This will eventually cause a calcium deficiency. I recommend that you consult with a nutritionist when you start taking high doses of supplements.

Vitamin C also works to loosen stools. It can also cause gas, so be careful if you try it. Do not add this at the same time you add magnesium. It makes sense to only add one supplement at a time, until you know its effects on your body. Start at 1000 mg 3x/day. Stay at that for two days. If it does not loosen your stools, add 1000 mg each day until you get relief. If it makes your stools too loose, cut back by one. Do not exceed 8000 mg per day. (Most people can only tolerate 3000—4000 mg.) Get a buffered Vitamin C with bioflavanoids.

Be aware ... I am not a doctor, I do not claim to diagnose or treat. I am only educating you about the role of these nutritional supplements. The choice is yours what you do with the information.

From: **Santa Cruz, California**

Sharon 24
Regular Member

I have been having a lot of good results with magnesium and Vitamin C. I take 1 gm of magnesium and 4 gm of Vitamin C in the evening. I have results the next morning. This is the best result that I have had in over a year. You will probably need to experiment with the dosage. I read about this combination on the internet and it sure works for me.

From: **Ohio**

LK
Prolific Member

Alexandragirl,

There seems to be a lot of different dosages recommended to you here. So of course, I'll add another ... but hopefully it will clarify things a bit.

The recommended daily allowance is around 500 mg/day. Its best to take about that much, see how it works for you and then ask your doctor if you can up the dosage if you need to. I take 500 - 600 mg every night before bed and that works for me. There are others on the board here that are taking much higher doses, but they should check with their doctors if they are taking this much. While you may be able to safely take up to 3000 mg a day, it is typically not recommended every day, and for most people 3000 mg would give you serious D.

I hope this helps.

From: **Canada**

Laylo
Regular Member

It is prudent to spread out your dosages of either Mg or Vitamin C throughout the day. Take Vitamin C tabs no closer together than every two hours. Taking them all at once will irritate your bowel and you will not possibly be able to absorb them.

Vitamin C is a water-soluble vitamin that is excreted in urine approximately every two hours. Your body uses what it needs.

I highly recommend purchasing a nutritional supplement book for more information about the signs of nutrient deficiency and possible side effects of supplement overdose. A good book is "Encyclopedia of Nutritional Supplements" by Michael Murray, ND.

From: **Santa Cruz, California**

Topic: Question about magnesium supplements

Carla_777
Prolific Member

Hi, I've been taking 100 mg of magnesium for about three months now and I haven't noticed any effect. Should I be taking magnesium oxide or magnesium citrate? I have tried Milk of Magnesia once, but that made me feel really ill. Any ideas anyone?

From: **England**

Megsy33
Prolific Member

Magnesium oxide is a good choice. Try taking more. Go up to 250 mg magnesium oxide (that is only 63% of the daily value). You can safely go up to 400 mg (100% of the daily value). Anything over that, I would check with a doctor first. Make sure you take calcium with it in a 2:1 ratio (calcium:magnesium). So, if you take 250 mg magnesium, take 500 mg calcium citrate or carbonate with it.

From: **MA**

Ty
Very Prolific Member

I agree with Megsy, except about the calcium. When I take calcium, especially in that ratio, the calcium will "override" the magnesium and constipate me even more. With my doc's approval, I take up to 750 mg a day of magnesium oxide. The days I take calcium, it goes to 1000 mg. And I've tried many different kinds of calcium. The carbonate seems to constipate me the worst (would make sense as that's the kind the D-types use to keep their D at bay).

From: **Portland, Oregon USA**

Topic: Magnesium

Ann304138
New Member

I have read about many of you that are taking magnesium. I was wondering about those of you that are taking the liquid form; when do you take it ... morning or bedtime?

This board is really helping me. I have struggled with IBS for many years. Doctors simply told me to take Citrucel; they have been little to no help. It has caused me to not have much respect for doctors at this point. This forum has been more help to me than any doctor.

From: **Waterville, Ohio USA**

Ghitta
Prolific Member

Ann, why not try magnesium supplements in pill form rather than liquid? Please do not confuse Milk of Magnesia with magnesium supplements. I take chelated magnesium in pill form, twice a day with meals, 250 mg per dose, and that seems to be working fine for me, helping me quite a bit. I also take them with other vitamin and mineral supplements. G—

From: **Florida**

Mojosue
Regular Member

Yeah, I'm taking magnesium tablets too—first time round they didn't do much, but I gave them another go. Seems to help—specifically with the monthly constipation. I think its partly because it works as a stool softener, but also because magnesium helps the nervous system, I believe, so I think a tense nerve in the belly is relaxed and the colon works a bit better.

Sue

From: **Ipswich, Suffolk, UK**

Bloated_again
Prolific Member

I take two tablets at night (250 mg each). I have been doing this for so long that I know that this amount works best for me. You will know what is too much by trial and error. The good news is that if you take too much the worse that can happen is you will get D. I would start at the low dose and work your way up if needed. This little pill has changed my life for the better.

From: **Ohio**

Narelle
New Member

Hi

I'm curious about magnesium. My naturopath put me onto the powder form that you mix in water and it helps movement in the bowels within the day. The problems are often back within several days though. I really dislike drinking the stuff; I have almost vomited after drinking. Is it OK in juice?

How does this differ from magnesium supplements? What is Milk of Magnesia?

I'm concerned about taking the above for an extended period of time (have been using for almost three months now, off and on); can the bowel become dependent on it?

Also, off-topic a bit, but people are mentioning flax oil—is that the same as linseed oil? Does it come in tablet form?

And, what does a drinking hot liquid do?

Sorry for so many questions, but I'm SO very glad I found this board.

Thanks,

Narelle

From: **Melbourne, Australia**

Ghitta
Prolific Member

Narelle—in answer to your q's: MOM (Milk of Magnesia) is magnesium hydroxide, whereas my supplements, for example, (in pill form, easy to take and to travel with, as opposed to a powder) is chelated magnesium oxide, more easily assimilated by the body, so they say. Linseed oil (or seeds) is in fact flax, but don't go drinking the mixture one cleans one's paintbrushes with!!!! In French, for example, flax seeds are called "grains de lin" as in linseed. Another thing, that I've already posted on this site, if you are in a crunch and really need to go without using an irritating laxative, you can take a good quality vitamin C supplement in powder form, in juice for example, and keep sipping until you feel the need to go and keep drinking it until your bowels are loose. Excess Vitamin C also provokes diarrhea so … … it may cause slight cramping, depends on the person.

Probably anything, including foodstuffs that we take on a regular basis will cause the body to rely on it—for example, if I stopped using olive oil, magnesium, prunes, etc, I'd probably plug right up. I also use hot liquids (tea, coffee) in the mornings and late afternoon to help me go to the bathroom; the hot (and very cold) liquids help to provoke the bowel to move. Also, caffeine helps a lot of people, but I'd rather be "addicted" to things such a magnesium supplements, olive oil, etc., than stimulant laxatives which can really wreck havoc, as you've read on this site. And yes, flax (or linseed) gelules are available and easier to use as a supplement than the oil itself, which actually tastes pretty lousy to me. However, one should be aware that for females who have experienced breast cancer, (not my case, thank God) there are now new studies that show that flax can contribute to new cancerous growth. However, this only applies to women who have had breast cancer.—Hope I answered your q's, G—

From: **Florida**

Mikeralph
Prolific Member

My preventative medicine doctor only recommends magnesium if is complemented by an equal dose of POTASSIUM, 400 mg magnesium and 400 mg potassium per day.

From: **Cleveland**

Topic: Constipation—How Long To Take Lactulose?

PatriciaUK
New Member

Hello everyone—I would be grateful for any feedback regarding the length of time I should take Lactulose.

It has been prescribed for fairly long-term constipation (which alternates between frequent bowel movements and/or passing only small amounts at a time)

I initially took Lactulose for two weeks, felt okay again, stopped taking the medication, and within six days I am back to being pretty constipated again.

My questions are:

—did I stop taking it too early?
—will longer term use do any harm?

Thank you very much,

Pat

From: **UK**

Kathleen M, Ph.D..
Very Prolific Member

The osmotic laxatives like Lactulose will not cure the constipation—once you stop (unless something else has changed, like you found an amount of fiber that keeps you going), the constipation comes back.

The good news is that as an osmotic laxative it can be taken indefinitely if needed.

K.

From: **Somewhere over the rainbow**

Katiegro
New Member

Took it—gave me a horrid migraine and just more gas and bloating—no movement whatsoever!

From: **Mississippi**

Hyacinth
New Member

I have been using Lactulose for about three years with great success. I take about one and a half tablespoons every evening. It does produce a lot of gas, that is why I take it at bedtime—then only my husband has to listen to the strange sounds!

From: **Minneapolis, MN, USA**

Mushtush
Prolific Member

Pat, took Lactulose for years. It only helped very mildly. I too, had to take it at night since it created intense amounts of smelly gas ... my poor husband. I stopped about a year ago since I couldn't stand the gas anymore. Good luck to you!!!

From: **New York**

Badger1
Regular Member

Hello PatriciaUK,

I have been taking Lactulose for some time, as my other medication tends to cause constipation. It does cause bad wind, but compared to how it produces a decent "poo", I would not be without it.

From: **UK**

Cicelyak
New Member

Does Lactulose cause poor absorption of nutrients, the way mineral oil does?

From: **Long Island, New York**

Kathleen M, Ph.D..
Very Prolific Member

I do not think that it would. It draws water into the stool.

Mineral oil is a problem because fat-soluble vitamins dissolve into the oil and cannot be absorbed.

Two different mechanisms.

K.

From: **Somewhere over the rainbow**

Topic: Need Miralax advice please

2btrue
Prolific Member

I want to try taking Miralax, but am really scared, and wondered if anyone could tell me how long it takes before it starts working.

Also, when is the best time to take it, morning or evening, and does it matter whether it is on an empty stomach or not?

I am extremely bloated and have a lot of trapped gas, and I am scared that the Miralax may make things worse. Hope someone can help.

From: **USA**

Bkitepilot
Prolific Member

I have pretty extreme constipation due to my crazy motility problems. I started on the Miralax not too long ago and it has helped me soooo much. Even has helped pushed gas on through (that's a miracle for me).

I started with a capful in the morning and I guess it wasn't enough, because it took six days to start to work. My GI didn't tell me I could take two capfuls three times a day until my next visit to him. You can't OD on this stuff … you'll just end up with diarrhea (GI said anyway). Once I got cleaned out, I can now manage with 1/2 to 3/4 capful a day. I take it in the morning because my stomach and small bowel are at their best then. (I struggle with vomiting due to a possible bowel obstruction).

Taking the Miralax at bedtime, I feel, makes it easier to get on schedule by training your body to evacuate every morning.

Good luck.

From: **North Georgia**

2btrue
Prolific Member

Does it make you very bloated until it starts working? Do you take it on an empty stomach? How long after, and how long before, a meal?

I can't imagine anything giving me diarrhea, because nothing seems to move in my stomach—even without a colon, it just doesn't make any sense to me.

From: **USA**

Nicole Graziano
Prolific Member

Miralax is a lifesaver for me. I take it at night. I wake up gassy, but it is no big deal. It took about four days to start working. I cannot imagine my life without it. It's really given me my life back.

From: **Wharton, NJ USA**

Bkitepilot
Prolific Member

For me, it makes no difference if I take the Miralax with food, after eating, or on an empty stomach … it still does its bidding. I get a little gassy with it, but the beauty of that is that it passes right on through. How great is that for us who seem to get a cork stuck when gas rears it menacing head?

Miralax is a lifesaver for me too. I don't believe I will give it up ever without a fight.

From: **North Georgia**

Ira
Regular Member

Hi:

My physician prescribed Miralax.

It wasn't clear to me if it's actually a laxative, and if so, what kind?

It was pointed out to me that as long as I have one or more BMs daily I'm not technically constipated. However, I usually feel like I haven't completely evacuated. It's actually this incomplete evacuation which is the most uncomfortable, and often painful, feature of the IBS for me.

I'd like to know a bit more about Miralax before beginning it.

From: **USA**

Bkitepilot
Prolific Member

Yes it is a laxative. My GI told me to increase to two capfuls, three times a day, if I needed to. Good grief, I'd never leave the toilet.

From: **North Georgia**

2btrue
Prolific Member

I'm worried about bloating, because I get really bad pressure/pulling and pain due to the bloating. Has it ever happened that the accumulation of water doesn't come out?

From: **USA**

Bkitepilot
Prolific Member

The accumulation of water with the Miralax has always come out for me. I believe it helped with the bloating by moving things along and helping to pass that nasty trapped gas.

From: **North Georgia**

Topic: A list of things that worked for me …

FinallySolved
New Member

Thanks to people on this board, my perusing of many doctor's opinions about IBS-C, many years of trial and error, time to work on the problem, and a couple of years of "training," I have finally gotten my IBS-C under control. I have had a BM every day, at least a little, for the past several months. Because I know many are suffering with the same problem, I thought I would share my experience with others in hopes that what worked for me will also work for another.

I have read many expert opinions about IBS-C, and throughout my life I have tried to follow their recommendations, to some degree or another. I did not know I was going to have to follow ALL of them and add some more of my own to maintain this syndrome. But, here goes:

History/Background:

I am a 29-year-old male. I have always been within the normal range of weight based on my height. I am not taking any medications. (I never have taken any medications that have—positively or negatively—affected my IBS-C.) I am otherwise healthy. The first time I can remember having problems with IBS-C was when I was 14. I may have had constipation before then, but I remember it becoming a problem at age 14. Basically, the symptoms I experienced were much like what others experience. I would not be able to go for several days. It would not matter if I tried to go most days; I felt like I had to go, but little or nothing would come out. I just had to wait. And, when I finally went, I had to strain. (I never had the combination constipation then diarrhea, only constipation.) Oftentimes there was blood and mucus that came out from straining. The day after, I would have stomach gas and would have to take Alka-Seltzer to help. This pattern went on through high school, college, and my work life. When I became self-employed, and had time to work on the problem, I finally was able to get to the point where I am now.

Here is finally what I found works, starting with the most important:

1) Fiber, and lots of it. For breakfast, I have a bowl of FiberOne cereal. The recommended serving size is 1/2 cup, but I have about 1 cup. I also add Benefiber to my coffee. I use the recommended 1 tbsp. in my coffee. I try to eat something for supper that has at least 15g of fiber in it. I go for whole-wheat breads instead of white. I eat things with raw vegetables in it when I can. I eat half a raw, unpeeled, apple with a slice of fresh, fruity bread from a bakery a day as a snack before bedtime. Totaling it all up, I probably eat at least 50 grams of fiber a day, much higher than the Daily Values recommended by the FDA.

2) Exercise. I wanted to lose weight anyway, so I started a workout routine. I try to do an aerobic exercise at least twice a week and anaerobic twice a week. Sometimes I do a little of both. I use a good elliptical to get my heart rate up to 160 or so for at least 15 minutes, preferably 25 if I have time.

3) Re-training. I guess I never thought about this one until I read about someone recommending it. I have been doing this without thinking about it. And, I guess it makes sense once you think about it. If you have to be toilet trained as a kid, your bowels can unlearn those behaviors and learn not to go every day. And, because your body is slower to change as you get older, it takes longer to retrain your bowels. After my breakfast and coffee, I wait until I feel the

urge to go, which is usually about 30 minutes. Sometimes the urge is strong and sometimes I just need to get my day started, so I go ahead and get on the toilet to get something started. I fluctuate between pushing and waiting. Gas usually comes out and then poop. Push a bit. Wait. Push. Wait. Even with this regimen, I am often in the bathroom for a while, at least 30 minutes.

4) Coffee, regular, not decaf, to make you regular. I think the stimulating effect of the coffee helps. I read some doctors recommending coffee and I think it helps me. I drink several cups in the morning.

5) Water. When I exercise, I drink lots of water. I drink about two liters when I exercise. I don't know if the increase in water helps or the exercise, since they are closely tied together. I do have a harder time going the next day if I have worked out outside and not had the chance to drink lots of water, however.

6) Little cheese. I found out about this one by a misfortune, really. I got a urinary tract infection and had to take some antibiotics. They recommend not eating any dairy products while taking it. So, I cut out all cheese. I noticed a couple of things. One was that I could lose those five extra pounds I was trying to lose, and that I can go every day. Before, when I would eat cheese, I would go most days, but still get constipated every once in a while. Usually I felt full, had to strain, and then I could go. But now, with little to no cheese in my diet, I don't have the initial starting problem.

7) Little fried foods. I don't know if it is related to most of them having no fiber, or if it is the oil and stuff. But, I have cut out almost all fried foods and it has helped.

8) Sleep. I try to get eight hours of uninterrupted sleep a night. It has been a while since I had to stay up all night studying, but I think that if I got only six hours, it would negatively affect my bowel movements.

9) Warm Prune Juice. I have not had to do this one in a while, but it helped me when I needed it. If I did not go completely one day, I would give it until the next day to try again. If I couldn't, then I would drink about 12 oz. of warm prune juice with my breakfast and coffee. I would pour some prune juice into a glass and put it in the microwave until it was warm, but not hot. Usually, I could get in the bathroom and go a little. Then the prune juice would kick in. Prune juice literally runs right through me. It works, but it produces some foul-smelling gas, though.

Those are the things that seem most related. There may be other factors such as standing instead of sitting (my self-employment involves me standing more than sitting), wearing loose clothing, etc., but I can't draw any conclusions based on those factors.

As for what does not help:

I tried magnesium supplements, but could not tell any difference. Chemical laxatives work for a day or two, but unless I follow the regimen above, I am back constipated again in a week or two. I did try only Metamucil, but it was not effective enough to be worthwhile. Going to the doctor did me little good. I know many others here feel the same, but I think this is one of those things that only you can fix. The "friendly bacteria" supplements did no good.

Things I have to watch:

I can have a pizza every once in a while with no problems. Usually, the day after I don't go completely, but if I eat something else the next evening with lots of fiber, I am okay. Alcohol is another one I have to watch. Usually, if I drink a lot one night, the next day is fine. It is the day after that I am a bit slow to go. If I drink a ton of water the night of and the next day, I am okay.

That's about it. Those are my experiences and may differ from yours. I am truly sorry that this syndrome is so unfair. I mean, most people I know can eat an all-fried meat and cheese diet, work 15 hour days and still go whenever they get ready to go. But, as they say, "life isn't fair." I guess it could always be worse. The only thing we can do is try to keep a positive outlook about it and do the best we can. There is hope. It may involve more time and energy than you can put into it, but I believe most people can manage this syndrome.

Again, I thank you for the support and the suggestions. I read your posts and knew I was not the only one. I hope my story helps at least one of you.

Good luck!

From: **USA**

Forum V: Food/Nutrition/Diet/Recipes

"Use this forum to post and talk about food, food triggers, comfort food, nutrition, diet or recipes."

For people with digestive systems that work smoothly, foods are not feared and a person can feel free to eat almost anything they want. Individuals with IBS do not have that luxury. A sensitive GI tract requires that care be taken with the food that is to pass through. The simple act of eating can become quite a challenge. In this forum, Bulletin Board members generously share trials, tribulations and tips regarding food and IBS. As you read through these offerings, you will find many practical ideas to help you to find your way to a more comfortable relationship with food.

Topic: Oh, how I miss COFFEE!!!

Stargirl
Prolific Member

COFFEE AND BEER!!

And wine! I'm so jealous of those who can drink all the coffee they want and not have a D attack … and ooooh martinis and champagne … I miss it all, it helped me relax so much … and be social, and I love the feeling of being tipsy … but the next day or even the same night I get cramps in my stomach … it sucks

I have caffeine withdrawal and alcohol withdrawal … ITS NOT FAIR!!!!!!!!!!!!!!!!!

From: **Montreal, Quebec**

Law
New Member

Yep—I miss milkshakes, pizza, whole glasses of milk, cereals, real coffee, and eating at restaurants.

I also wish I could go for a night out drinking without rushing to the toilet two drinks into it, knowing everyone is laughing at me because I did my usual disappearing act for an hour!!

I'm in the middle of "adjusting" … this includes jealousy at all the people I see eating and not worrying about where the nearest toilet is within two minutes sprinting distance!!

I'm not bitter! LOL!

From: **London, UK**

Mholm999
New Member

I miss it all too. A beer (or three) to unwind after work, a big glass of 2% milk, ice cream or hot chocolate for dessert …

I make chocolate chip cookies but now only my wife and her co-workers can enjoy them. I'm sure that, given a few years, I'll be used to it.

My wife loves all the things I cannot eat, and it is hard for her to see me adjusting to my body's needs. She appreciates, however, that I need to do these things for me and does not mind if, when we do go out for a meal, I just have a glass of water.

From: **Madison, WI**

Heather Eve
Regular Member

Oh—a Corona with a lime—how I miss it!

I think that is one of the hardest for me! That was my favorite summertime beverage.

I have to admit, I am still weaning off the coffee. I used to drink it ALL the time! Now I am down to a smidgen in a warm cup of soy milk in the morning and I seem to tolerate it ok. My b/f makes the BEST coffee! BUT—I have had a very yummy coffee alternative at vegan restaurants and am trying to find someone who knows exactly what it was—I might actually call the restaurant to find out. It tasted just like coffee, without the caffeine or oils that set my IBS into a tantrum!

From: **Kearny, NJ USA**

Calid
Prolific Member

Heather: It could have been "Rocamojo". It's made from soy and is pretty good. I make mochas out of it (Rocamojo is made strong like espresso, using a little carob, ice milk, and honey). It's not like Starbucks mocha, but heck, its close enough.

From: **USA**

Topic: Specific Carbohydrate Diet? Yeast Connection Diet? Low-Fat Diet? Which is right???

California
New Member

I've been perusing the Internet for weeks now and am becoming more confused by the day. I have been using Heather Von Vorous' book "Cooking With IBS", but I am now reading other sites and books about specific carbohydrates and yeast items also causing IBS.

If you combine all of the different diets it seems as though there is nothing left to eat.

Which diets do you all use? Which is more effective or is it a matter of personal trial and error?

From: **California, USA**

Mountaingirl
New Member

What to eat? Now there's a good question!

I don't have "The Answer" but I can offer a strategy. Try to imagine how humans ate for the thousands of years before agriculture took over and changed our eating habits forever, and then eat like that. Number one: eat real foods—green vegetables, potatoes, nice raw nuts like almonds, fruits that work for you (maybe cooked fruits like applesauce would be better than raw?), lean animal proteins, maybe tofu—and eliminate processed, manufactured foods.

Try avoiding your trigger foods (if kiwis hurt your stomach, leave them at the market) and experiment/eliminate the common allergens, especially wheat—baked goods, flour, pasta—which are problem foods for many people, including me, most of the time. (I stay away from most grains, although brown rice feels very good in my tummy, and oatmeal, too.) Steamed vegetables, such as Swiss chard and carrots and beets always feel good for me, as do baked potatoes with flaxseed oil instead of butter, sea salt and a little pepper, or baked sweet potatoes (garnet yams), a very soothing food. (Skip the skin, though.)

Of course, try not to eat too much at a sitting. And allow time between meals, at least three to four hours. Drink plain herbal tea like peppermint or chamomile between meals (since honey can hurt you.)

Sometimes you can put your hand on a food, even when it is in the jar or a bag, and your stomach will tell you if that is okay to eat. You will feel it in your gut, just by touching the food.

You will discover many foods that work for you, and many that don't. Be patient and love yourself through this process. It is not easy to have to say "No" all the time. Sometimes I rebel against my limitations, but who suffers then? Only me and my stomach. This is where I am struggling. I am coming to believe that the lesson in having this IBS problem is to recognize, accept and honor my true feelings, and to give myself permission to love myself. Eating foods that I know can cause distress (pizza, ice cream, even kiwi, strange as it may seem) or eating in a way that I know can cause distress (in the car, on the run, while reading the newspaper) is not loving myself. Finding what works takes time, and what works for one might not work for another. May your healing process be full of hope and discovery.

From: **Montague, MA USA**

Topic: What is the deal with fruit?

MEYoung
New Member

We just bought a bunch of fresh fruit at the store tonight; in addition to some we got the other day (we're trying to eat healthier these days). So we have bananas, strawberries, oranges, apples, grapes, cantaloupe, and watermelon—I think that's all. So is fruit good or bad for IBS-D? Does it make D worse? Are some fruits better than others?

I've been snacking on it all night—especially the strawberries—yum!—and I hate to think I might pay for it tomorrow morning.

Mary

From: **MO**

Karyno
Regular Member

I am a huge banana eater … but I can only handle half earlier in the day and the other half later in the day. I eat mangoes regularly which tend to agree w/me all of the time.

I love strawberries as well, but have to be careful b/c too many mean I'll be stuck in the bathroom for the rest of the night.

All berries have more insoluble fiber (not easy to digest for us IBSers) than soluble fiber … so it's always good to be careful with any kind of berry … try adding them to rice cereal w/soy or skim milk (depending on what you can handle) or eat with rice cakes ... whenever you can, base your snack w/good soluble fiber then add in the fruit ... this helps significantly with digestion.

Just don't over-do it with your fruit intake and you should be okay.

Oranges have never agreed w/me though ... so I definitely stay away from those!

From: **SK Canada**

Kathleen M, Ph.D..
Very Prolific Member

Generally, when people (any people) consume large quantities of fresh produce, especially fruits, it can loosen the stools.

The biggest offenders in that tend to be apples, pears, peaches (and all the peach-like fruits, like nectarines and apricots) cherries and plums (prunes) because they contain goodly amounts of sorbitol (a sugar alcohol used in sugar free gums).

Cooking these fruits reduces the sorbitol.

Your mileage may vary. How much these things affect any given individual can be highly variable. Even among IBS-Ders.

Bananas are on the list of what to eat after an acute bout of diarrhea, so tend to be OK.

K.

From: **Somewhere over the rainbow**

Ems
New Member

Hi,

Bananas give me acid reflux immediately. Acidic fruits also give me problems. Mainly it's the fiber and sugars in fruits that aggravate my IBS-D.

I compensate for my lack of fruit with non-fibrous vegetables and I eat twice as many vitamins as I need to.

Ems

From: **Maidstone**

Topic: What to drink, what to drink?!?

Mikenaber
New Member

I've been diagnosed with IBS C/D for seven years now. As with most of us, I have a list of trigger foods a mile and a half long. But what I'm starting to realize is that some foods that I believed to be "trigger" foods, are only such when accompanied by certain drinks. These can range from water, fruit juices, carbonated beverages and of course, the ever dreaded dairy. So my question is, or idea rather, is let's just throw out some of our favorite things to drink here that seem to not cause many problems. Some speak of Gatorade, but the high fructose syrup gets to me. So, let's start listing and see if we can't balance the drink-speak with the food-speak, because I know I drink something every time I eat, so it should be just as important to look at what I'm drinking as it is to look at what I'm eating!!!

From: **Wooster, OH**

Inafog
Prolific Member

I'm D. Water and decaf tea are the only drinks that don't affect me.

From: **Way to go Ohio**

Sciencegirl
Regular Member

I used to be IBS-D, now am C/D when not feeling good (although I am good most of the time now), but I can drink:

> skim milk
> any tea (herbal, green, black, etc)
> club soda (but no other soda pops, diet or other)
> small amounts of alcohol (about one drink, that's all)

I think beer might be bad, not sure. A friend with IBS said Gatorade helped her but not me.

I thought I could never eat at fast food restaurants again until I realized it was the soda pop that was killing me. Have no idea why diet and regular, caffeinated and non-caffeinated, bother me, but club soda doesn't. (Maybe some evil secret ingredient or else I can't tolerate either aspartame or high fructose corn sugar?)

Good luck and good idea for the BB. I only thought to try the club soda after someone here suggested it. It is nice to have more alternatives, isn't it?

SG

From: **Iowa**

Androsine
Prolific Member

IBS-D: So far I only drink water. But I plan to try a soda in the next couple of days. I get the runs from Gatorade and Propel fitness water. I'm not sure why. I plan to try other things soon. Maybe even coffee (scary!!!). I'll let you know.

From: **Alameda, CA**

Mike NoLomotil
Very Prolific Member

"Have no idea why diet and regular, caffeinated and non-caffeinated bother me but club soda doesn't."

Several possibilities ... corn syrup or extract as sweetener, and/or the artificial colorings used.

Some patients also don't realize until they actually have someone measure it, that the carbonation (which can cause discomfort in the unregulated gut of the IBS victim) is also part of the problem. Ah, "but why does the club soda not bother me", the patient queries.

When behaviors are tracked, it turns out to be dose-related. Club soda does not taste all that good, so they tend to only drink enough to stop the immediate thirst.

Flavored soda tastes a lot better, so they end up drinking much more of it than they realize, compared to how much club soda they drink. When the "gas comes out of solution in the gut" faster than it can be eliminated, it produces pain, bloating sensation, gassiness, and the "volume" can affect the "pressure and stretch receptors" in different parts of the gut (which are unregulated already for other reasons, producing the twitchy bowel character of many IBS patients) and even be responsible for spasm or an all-out episode.

Just some other ideas that patients sometimes don't think of ....

These books can be very helpful:

IBS: A DOCTORS PLAN FOR CHRONIC DIGESTIVE TROUBLES

By Gerard Guillory, M.D.; Vanessa Ameen, M.D.; Paul Donovan, M.D.; Jack Martin, Ph.D.

"FOOD ALLERGIES AND FOOD INTOLERANCE: THE COMPLETE GUIDE TO THEIR IDENTIFICTION AND TREATMENT", Professor Jonathan Brostoff, M.D.. Allergy, Immunology and Environmental Medicine, Kings' College, London

MNL

P.S.

I was a SEVERE diarrheic, with a lot of extra intestinal symptoms as well, for over 30 years, in remission, but have learned the best thing to drink with the least chance of any provocation is lots of plain old bottled water.

I do have an occasional Pepsi or Coke or Sprite or Fruit Punch (actual 100% fruit punch only, not the corn syrup sugar water with coloring that masquerades as punch).

From: **West Palm Beach, Florida USA**

Maloo
Regular Member

Hi, I am new to this, but I have been suffering for three years with IBS/D. I also have chronic migraines to throw in the mix, so my diet has been slashed in half. Caffeine is a no-no, but I can tolerate half-caffeinated coffee in the morning, decaf during the day and decaf soda. However, I think the soda is still bothering me with bloating. Three years into this and things are ever-changing with what I can and cannot have. Frustration doesn't begin to describe how I feel about food and drink. I would rather not eat at all. I hate it!

From: **NY**

Julia37
Very Prolific Member

I used to have pain, cramps, and bloating, and now that I have changed my diet I only drink tea, water, and an occasional Diet Coke.

One of my worst triggers is any form of sugar, so I can only drink diet sodas. Coffee almost always caused pain and spasms. When I was on jury duty they had no tea, so I made do with diluted coffee. I did get a few mild symptoms from it. I think Diet Coke also causes mild symptoms if I drink it too often. I sometimes drink soda water in nightclubs if I want bubbles but no caffeine.

P.S.—That Propel "fitness water" is mostly sugar. The first ingredient is sucrose, which is the chemical name for table sugar. It's a total scam.

If you look at ingredient labels, it's shocking how many foods that don't and shouldn't taste sweet, have sugar added. Crackers, for example, might have three different forms of sugar.

When they were promoting Propel and giving it out free, I tried to talk to one of the marketing yuppies about the way they were misleading their customers, but she said to write to the company and turned her back on me, and I said I already have a job and didn't have time to tell her bosses how to do theirs. Typical corporate attitude.

From: **Chicago, IL USA**

Discussion: What to Eat for Diarrhea?

Topic: I am having a bad attack, what to eat?

J9n
New Member

I was very stupid, ate things I KNOW I can't, but did anyway. Hot dog, French fries, beer. We were celebrating some of my son's accomplishments and of course, teenage boys want hot dogs and French fries. Believe me; I will never do that again. I woke up about 4:00 AM in the most pain I have ever had. I still hurt but D has stopped. I am drinking peppermint tea. I have to go to work tomorrow, just can't miss anymore. I know it is going to take days to get back to normal. Do I even attempt any solids or stick to liquids? I have applesauce, chicken, rice, herbal tea, chicken broth. This is the worse attack I have had.

Thanks so much.

From: **California**

Calid
Prolific Member

Yep, been there, done that. I ate something bad this morning and I'm paying for it now. You are eating the right stuff, just make sure your chicken broth is both non-fat AND no MSG, most of it isn't.

From: **USA**

No. 1 Packer Fan
Prolific Member

I find that plain white rice is okay for me. NO BUTTER!

Saltine crackers are good, too.

Sometimes plain, steamed chicken (white meat) is okay if you are feeling better. I can't even think about this until I am on the mend.

Pedialyte is good if you have had a lot of D. The orange is the only flavor I can stand.

Hope this helps!

From: **Western Wisconsin**

J9n
New Member

Thanks for the advice. Are goldfish crackers okay? I seem to tolerate them. I was really woozy at work today and they helped. I am not getting enough food, but I am trying to avoid the Levsin, it makes me feel funny. I am living on peppermint tea, chicken, rice and goldfish crackers. My stomach still hurts a lot, the pain was brutal.

From: **California**

Michele Brake
Prolific Member

We have all "fallen off the wagon" from time to time! I eat white rice and graham crackers. Hope you feel better soon.

From: **Detroit**

Shira
New Member

Hi everybody,

I too, am in a very bad shape the last couple of weeks. My belly looks like a huge balloon, just waiting to be burst. I'm really suffering. I can't wear anything, and the minute I'm off work, its straight home and stay there.

I've tried everything I can think of. I must say that I was on Atkins for three weeks and the relief was really noticeable, but I couldn't stay on that, it was too difficult, especially because I'm vegetarian. Carbs are no good for us! Is the real solution to just stop eating???

Please help me if you can think of something I can do to relieve my stomach and make the gas go away.

Thanx

From: **Israel**

J9n
New Member

Shira, I know how you feel. Do you know what types of foods are causing your problems? I am not sure myself, but I stay far, far away from high fats, red meats, high fructose, whole wheat, and raw veggies. For me, carbs are good. I usually eat potato (plain, no butter, sour cream, etc), white rice (again plain), sourdough bread, and crackers. I have actually lost 15 pounds, mostly because foods scare me!

From: **California**

KaliP
New Member

I am currently drinking lots of hot peppermint tea. It's helpful to add fresh ginger, too. I make mashed potatoes with chicken broth. I like vegetable broth, too. I get the instant from the health food stores—it has less sodium. I go back to this diet whenever my system is upset. It usually works, but it is hard to keep at it because it's boring.

From: **Minnesota**

Smariecca
New Member

I usually go back to the B-R-A-T (banana, rice, applesauce, toast) diet whenever my stomach is in a rage. I also drink a can of Ensure for the vitamins (it's lactose-free which means I can tolerate it just fine). One of my favorite things to eat though is some rice with vegetable broth (I'm a vegetarian so you could do chicken broth instead). Peppermint tea also works well to calm my stomach down.

From: **Northern California**

Jools
Prolific Member

I find peppermint tea is helpful when I have a tummy ache. Also, Twinings makes a tea which is chamomile, honey and vanilla. I find, and some people may laugh, but bananas are a good food to eat, also pasta, boiled rice, and certain cheeses. I can't enjoy sprouts or cabbage any more, as they make me feel too gassy. Pickles and peppers also aggravate me, so I lay off them now. Citrus fruits, I have found, can be a killer especially oranges. Hope this is some help.

Julie

From: **Scotland**

Schnukie
Regular Member

I am like many others. I have no problems with bread (white) and pasta products. Red meats, veggies (especially raw) and fatty foods are no-no's. I still indulge, but pay later. I try to limit alcohol, but limited beer is okay, LOL. Why all the "healthy foods" are triggers, I wonder. I love a good salad, but it doesn't love me. On really bad times when I bloat and can't eat—my favorite is chocolate Ensure!!! Try it.

From: **Ontario Canada**

Daisysp
Prolific Member

Seems to be a real theme here … … … there is no theme!! Everyone is allergic to different foods and food combinations. You really have to do your own tests on foods, to figure out what upsets your intestines/stomach and what foods will become the calming foods you go back to when you need relief.

If you go off the wagon and feel awful, do only liquids, vegetable juices, and soups for a day or two to relax your intestines.

Get a cleanser that does not bloat you or strip your intestines … like Garden of Life Primal Defense, it's a great one. Also Citrucel works well and does not bloat.

From: **Washington**

Discussion: What to Eat for Constipation?

Topic: How to get rid of constipation

TheEncourager
New Member

How to get rid of constipation.

My gastroenterologist told me to do this to get rid of constipation:

1.   Eat a high-fiber cereal like All-Bran. The goal is to eat at least 20 grams of fiber in the cereal. One cup of All-Bran yields 20 grams of fiber. There are other kinds of high-fiber cereals, but you usually have to eat two cups of cereal just to get the 20 grams of fiber.

2.   Drink 64 ounces (eight cups) of water throughout the day. Try not to let a long time go without drinking water except when you are sleeping.

3.   Sit on the toilet in the morning for at least one hour. Do not strain. If you do not have a bowel movement that day, then wait for the next day.

4.   If you get too many bowel movements or diarrhea, lower the amount of fiber you take, but do not lower how much water you drink. Still drink 64 ounces (eight cups) of water per day.

5.   It should take 90 days (three months) of this diet done consistently everyday to get rid of the constipation. If after 90 days, you are still constipated, this diet may not work for you.

This is not an easy diet to follow. First off, the water causes me to go the bathroom too frequently. So, during the weekdays, when I go to work, I do not drink as much water as I should. Also, water gives me gas (flatulence). The fiber also gives me gas (flatulence) which means I eat less fiber on the days I go to work.

If too much fiber causes problems, you may want to increase the fiber slowly.

From: **Maryland, USA**

Topic: Need diet for IBS-C

Maureen L
New Member

Hi, new to all this diet stuff. But need help working out diet for IBS-C. Any help will always be appreciated.

Maureen from Indiana

From: **Indiana**

Jan LEAP RD
Prolific Member

Just a couple quick things to consider:

1. Eliminate all tea and bananas. Cut caffeine gradually. These all can be very constipating for some people.

2. Be sure your water intake is adequate for your size, exercise and environment.

3. Do yoga daily—can be very helpful.

4. Are you getting adequate essential fatty acids, esp. Omega-3's?

5. Do you get six to nine servings of fruits and veggies and only whole grains in your diet?

6. Do you get enough magnesium from beans/legumes and WHOLE grains (wheat bread is NOT whole grain, unless it's 100% whole wheat.)

7.   Have you tried supplementing with magnesium?

Now, this should all be individualized, but working with a local dietician who specializes in IBS-C should help significantly.

Wishing you well.

Jan

From: **Colorado**

Christie s.
New Member

I've found that Oat Bran is one of the only things that will help me go. Rice and rice cereal make me constipated.

From: **U.S.**

Gonowoften
Prolific Member

Maureen, if you are by any chance allergic to gluten, then oat bran would not be suitable for you. I suggest you try psyllium husks as they come from a non-grain plant called Plantain. They are very cheap and you can scatter a teaspoonful on your toast or cereal in the morning, and not even know you have eaten them. They swell up to eight times that of bran, so they add bulk to your stools by absorbing water from your system, so drink plenty. There are products on the market such as METAMUCIL, & FIBROGEL that contain psyllium, but they also have citrus flavorings and other ingredients to form a fizzy drink and are a lot more expensive.

From: **Melbourne, Australia**

Discussion: What to Eat for Gas and Bloating?

Topic: What to take if veggies and fruit are out

Ganas
Prolific Member

Anyone else out there who can't eat many vegetables or fruit?

Can I take a daily supplement so I am sure to get all the good stuff that veggies have?

What are some choices of vitamins that will give me the essentials without gas?

From: **Michigan**

HipJan
Very Prolific Member

Mannatech (online) has a product that consists of freeze-dried healthy veggies. Probably other "vitamin" companies also have such a thing.

Hopefully, eventually you will also be able to add fresh fruits and veggies back into your diet. Here are non-gassy ones that many people, supposedly, can tolerate: squash, green beans, kale, bok choy, chard, turnips, carrots, peaches, apricots, and pears.

From: **Lone Star State**

Meowsie
New Member

I did not eat any fruits or vegetables for years. I couldn't stand it. I have slowly been eating tiny amounts because I miss them so much. It seems to be okay. I would recommend just eating teeny amounts while you are eating a meal of things that don't bother you. Like four or five raspberries and that is all for the day. Hey, it's better than nothing!

From: **Massachusetts**

Gastron
Regular Member

Hello:

Fruits and vegetables are absolutely essential for a healthy diet. Instead of looking for replacements, you should look for ways that you can eat them that won't trigger an IBS attack.

For people with IBS-D the problem with fruits and veggies usually lies in their high insoluble fiber content. This can be significantly reduced via peeling, chopping, blending, etc. Also, don't try to eat your fruits and vegetables on an empty stomach. Eat them after you have eaten something safe.

Most people can handle small amounts of fruits and vegetables when they're mixed in with other safe things. For instance, I always mix a small amount of broccoli in with white rice and I mix sliced bananas into my hot oat bran cereal.

Gastron

From: **Planet Earth**

Jennifer7
Prolific Member

Juice Plus is the best substitute. There are capsules which contain the nutrients from veggies and capsules which contain the nutrients from fruit. I've tried other brands and didn't get the results as I did with Juice Plus.

Jennifer

From: **Texas**

Mason_M
New Member

Peel the fruits and mash or puree veggies with skins. This really does seem to help.

We need them even if they don't like us very much, LOL.

Taking a fiber supplement a little while before eating seems to be helpful as well.

Mason

From: **Collinsville, VA, USA**

Kathleen M, Ph.D..
Very Prolific Member

There isn't much in most multivitamins that should cause gas, and pretty much all of them have the standard set of vitamins that are in all the fruits and veggies.

The problem is that there are other compounds in fruits and veggies that may be helpful in things like preventing cancer and I do not know if any veggie concentrate would have just those and not whatever is bothering you about fruits and veggies.

With fruits the main culprit seems to be sorbitol and if you cook the fruits that gets rid of the sorbitol. A lot of people with kind of general fruit/veggie problems seem to do better on cooked well rather than raw veggies, so cooking things rather than raw may be helpful. The main culprit in veggies is raffinose in the cruciferous veggies and in beans. Now with beans you can soak the dried ones and replace the water before you cook to limit the amount of raffinose.

Also small amounts, slowly building up what you eat may be helpful.

What seems to be the main problem you have? Because if it is gas, taking a probiotic supplement (if you find the one that works for you) may help reduce volume because these bacteria do not produce gas when they digest carbs. But this is reducing fart frequency. This may not change cramping, bloating, etc that is from something other than gas. Antispasmodics or peppermint tea is one way to limit those sorts if issues for some people.

K.

From: **Somewhere over the rainbow**

Topic: Good carbs vs. Bad carbs

Let
New Member

I recently discovered, quite by accident, that removing virtually all traces of carbs and sugars from my diet gives me relief from gas and bloating. The problem is I did not plan on staying on this restrictive diet for more than two weeks. Right now I eat no breads, rice, pasta, potatoes, fruits, fruit juices or refined sugar. I know they cannot all be bad, but how do I figure out what is safe to reintroduce. Anyone has any ideas of what the typical culprits are? Maybe I can avoid those for a while and start with 'safe' carbs.

Thanks

From: **GA**

Dokii
New Member

Hello there, I have found the same problem with carbs, so I've cut out a bunch myself and found a huge improvement with gas and bloating issues. I think the ones to definitely continue avoiding are breads and pasta. I am totally fine with rice and potatoes, but you could be different. There are some veggies that are worse like corn, peas, broccoli which I avoid, so usually stick with carrots, celery, lettuce, zucchini and I'm fine. Fruits are difficult too. I'm okay with bananas, blueberries and a few others, but many are bad—especially apples—they make me very gaseous. I would slowly introduce one thing at a time back into you diet.

Usually if you try one new thing every two to three days, you will soon find out what doesn't go well for you. It is all individual, so you have to persevere and test each food for you.

Also, there are many alternative products out there so you can avoid bread and pasta. I just have rice bread and pasta instead and find it quite good, even better without all the discomfort.

Cheers.

From: **Toronto**

Kmottus
Very Prolific Member

While diets like Zone Perfect may help with glycemic index issues … that doesn't translate directly to what is good for gas.

Unfortunately some of the carbs that are worst a la glycemic index are the easiest on the gas front because they go straight into your blood raising blood sugar rather than staying in the digestive tract where they get eaten by bacteria (which is where most of the gas comes from in the vast majority of people).

Some of the carbs that are the worst offenders on the gas front are things like starchy grains (other than rice) and potatoes. Some of the starch is not digested by us but is by the bacteria in the gut. Another common offender that can effect everyone is raffinose which is in beans and cabbage family veggies (beans, beans the musical fruit ... after all). Sorbitol and other sugar alcohols are not digested by us and can be an issue for some people.

Lactose and fructose may be issues for certain individuals who do not digest/absorb them well, but may be just fine for others.

The other issue is many of the carbs that may increase gas may also have the fiber you need for your GI tract to work well ... so it can be a balancing act.

My suggestion since this diet relieves your symptoms is to add back the things you would like to add back, one food at a time and see how each effects you. With gas/carb issues, a lot of times volume can be an issue. A small amount may be OK most of the time, but larger amounts are much more problematic (more carbs = more gas that can be made from them). So it may be both: which things and how much of each thing (or how much of a combination of carbs in a day) will work for you, and it is hard to know what that will be before you try it.

For some people, probiotics seem to limit the amount of gas they have because these bacteria do not produce gas from carbs when they digest them. And what they eat, other bacteria cannot use to make gas.

K.

From: **NC USA**

Mcrosby
New Member

I experienced some of the same things when I was on the Atkins Diet. I felt really good, but too much meat was something I didn't like. I am going to try the South Beach Diet and have purchased the book on the internet. This is a diet that discusses the good and bad carbs and it says that white flour is bad and since I have almost eliminated it from my diet I have felt much better. The first two weeks is very limited in the amount of carbs you can eat but after that it introduces good carbs. I learned about this diet by watching one of the news stations that had a special program on it and it investigated the diet to see if it was really safe. They decided that it was pretty good and the people they interviewed said that once they restricted certain items from their diets that they did not crave them anymore. Like some carbs and sugar. It helped them to lose weight, and although the author of the diet developed it to help heart patients, he noticed that people lost weight and were able to keep it off. As with anything, though, do research on it before trying it out and talk with our doctor.

From: **IL**

Mymytummy
New Member

If you go for the lo-carb diet types, it's hard to diet when you have IBS!

Try Healthy Life Lo-Carb wheat bread if you don't have wheat allergies, Boca (veggie) burgers and La Tabla Lo-Carb Tortillas—they're at most major grocery stores, now. That way, you're getting a nice boost of fiber (helps a lot with regularity IF you drink lots of water) without insulin-crazy carbs, and fullness without bloating.

Frozen peas are a favorite, too.

Good luck!

From: **Wisconsin**

M2d&v
New Member

I've been on the South Beach diet for a month and haven't felt this good in a long time. In fact, if I eat something that is a bad carb, I am hurting for two days … Not sure what I will do, but I do know that the diet has helped …

From: **MD**

Discussion: Food Intolerances.

Call them food triggers, food allergies, food sensitivities or food intolerance, they are hotly discussed topics in this forum. Suggestions are offered for identifying and coping with food that might possibly be troublesome. As you will see, some members believe that changing their diet led to a major reduction in their IBS symptoms. Their stories may provide you with some ideas for evaluating specific foods and their effect on your body.

Topic: Type C and D, vegetarian, lactose intolerant: any suggs?

Zoë
New Member

Hi, I very from C to D daily. I am lactose intolerant and choose to live a vegetarian lifestyle (yes fish, no eggs). I am so miserable whenever it comes to mealtimes because of the decisions involved. I was wondering if anyone had some suggestions on what to eat. I eat as little white flour as possible and stick to whole-wheat grains due to my C. I also love vegetables and fruit, although I cannot use dairy products to play them up. Many dairy-less sauces, especially high fat ones with lots of oil, bother my stomach also. I think a lot of it is the spicy stuff which triggers my chronic reflux. Anyway, I would love to hear some recipes to add to my boring diet of cereal and applesauce (plus some nude veggies and some fruit). Thanks for reading.

From: **USA**

Rlipski
New Member

Hi, Zoe!

I am also vegetarian and I have eliminated dairy along with rich and spicy foods due to the IBS. I tend to gravitate towards Asian meals—especially sushi. Sushi never causes problems for me. Also—noodle stir-fries with tofu, tamari and veggies. Being a vegetarian, a lot of the food I eat for protein is gas producing, so it always helps me to take Beano, especially when eating Mexican food.

Good luck!

From: **USA**

NDT27
New Member

I am also a lactose intolerant vegetarian but I eat eggs and don't eat fish. I have been experimenting with my diet lately and have found that homemade veggie soup doesn't bother me and is delicious, with a baked potato or whole-wheat bread. I just use water, tomato juice, vegetable stock and salt/pepper as the base and throw in whatever veggies I have on hand including carrots, cabbage, peas, green beans, celery, onions, and potatoes. After you throw them in the base they just need to cook for about an hour. The soup keeps well for a couple of days (and is even better on the second day). I have also had success eating lentils and corn tortillas. Have you tried soy milk and similar products?? I haven't, but know that many other lactose intolerant people that enjoy these often. I hope this helps.

From: **USA**

Uva
New Member

I have lactose intolerance as well. You can get a lactose tablet at the drug store or use the lactose-free milk, which I get in the supermarket.

From: **USA**

Nytebugg
Very Prolific Member

Well, I sure know how it is. I am a vegan (no meat of any kind, no eggs, and no dairy). I have a ton of low-fat vegetarian and vegan cookbooks. Most vegetarian cookbooks have recipes that are high in fat, but the ones that are more geared to a vegan lifestyle are usually much healthier.

Also, if you don't already use soy milk or rice milk, try it, it isn't all that bad. The hard part is finding a brand that you like. It took me about three different brands. You might also ask at your local health food store which brands of dairy-free things they like.

Joanna

From: **Washington State**

Tummyrumbler
New Member

I too am a vegetarian, lactose intolerant, yes fish, but I also eat eggs.

The web is a wonderful resource for recipes (search for vegan) Also, I'd subscribe to Vegetarian Times or a similar magazine, they are very useful.

My favorite foods include lots of the Morningstar farms products (burgers, chicken patties, hot dogs …). I also do a lot of soy cheese, but don't care for the soy milk. Tofu is great in recipes calling for ricotta or cottage cheese—I make stuffed shells with silken tofu, and even meat-heads can't tell the difference!!

I also really enjoy firm tofu in stir-fry dishes, especially when it is sautéed in oil until lightly browned and crunchy. If you have never had bean curd General Tso style, ask your local Chinese restaurant to make you some—sweet, spicy, crunchy, and soft, all at the same time. If you can't take spicy food though, it's not for you.

I also have found that the Moosewood collective cookbooks are great. My all-time favorite recipe book is a big orange bound one—I can't recall the title, but it has recipes for every vegetable you can find, and tells what herbs and other dishes complement each veggie. Very useful, especially for spur-of-the-moment cooking, which I tend to do a lot of.

From: **USA**

Topic: Going gluten free for gas problem

StressedOut
Regular Member

Hi all,

I've been suffering with IBS for nearly a year now and I've tried doing lots of things with my diet (cutting out dairy, caffeine, etc.) but as yet I have had no relief from daily bouts of intestinal gas (no odor though, unless there's gonna be a D attack), belching, stomach ache and stabbing pain in my guts when I have a D attack.

My last three D attacks have been after eating pasta and bread, but even when I cut these out my symptoms don't ease. Although maybe this is because wheat products are in most of the food I eat and I don't know about them?

I've been through lots of prescriptions from my GP with no relief and I've recently been seeing a homeopath. Her prescriptions have (as yet) made no improvement, but she recommended me going gluten-free, not just cutting out bread and pasta.

I've been doing this for five days now and I've spent three days with a headache! I'm finding this diet very restrictive and I'm wondering how long before I should start to feel the benefits? Two weeks, a month ...?

Anyone been there and done that or am I wasting my time!?!

From: **UK**

Mrysgrl
Prolific Member

Hi,

I hope you can find a way to get tested. Know what you mean about that doozy of a headache. Barley, wheat, and oat were on my list, so I eliminated gluten. I thought of the headache as a good sign. After about a week, it stops. I hope you can hang in there.

From: **USA**

StressedOut
Regular Member

Just an update for ya …

I am still on the whole no-dairy, no-sugar, no-wheat thing, but have had no change in symptoms. Is there a light at the end of the tunnel!?! Can't believe such a major change in what I'm eating hasn't made a difference.

Am I not being patient enough?

From: **UK**

Echris
Prolific Member

Stressed out:

I was on my gluten-free/lactose-free diet for about two months before the D stopped. I haven't had the big D in about seven or eight months. After 25+ years w/D, the wait was worth it for me. I don't know that I noticed ANY improvement in the first two weeks, so I don't know how realistic it is, if you really are gluten intolerant or gluten sensitive, to expect a big improvement after just two weeks.

Sorry if this isn't what you wanted to hear. After trying all different kinds of medications and diets over the years, I had almost given up on seeing any improvement.

Now I can go to the theater, plays, travel, fly, etc. It's kind of nice to be getting my life back.

From: **USA**

Kathleen M, Ph.D..
Very Prolific Member

Food is NOT in any way the SOLE AND ONLY trigger for IBS symptoms.

SOME people may be able to eliminate most symptoms with diet, but NOT EVERY person with IBS.

Now some "diet cures every ill known to man" types will tell you that if diet isn't fixing you then you are either: a) cheating or b) have to be on it for months/years/decades but it WILL eventually cure you.

I don't believe this.

If dietary changes aren't making any difference at all in one to two weeks (now for true celiac it may be somewhat longer, depending on how long it takes the small intestine to heal/how damaged you were ... but there should be some change in the first little while, it may take longer to have full effect). My opinion is either:

a) you are making the wrong dietary changes and these foods are NOT the ones responsible for YOUR symptoms (no matter HOW many other people on the planet get relief from eliminating A, B or C).

b) You probably ALSO have NON-DIETARY triggers, and for those, for the most part, no matter how much you jiggle your diet, you aren't going to fix them with food changes alone.

How is the overall fat content of your diet? Some people when they eliminate the low-fat, high-carb foods, they end up eating an overall fattier diet and HIGH FAT not JUST various carbs can trigger IBS symptoms in some people.

K.

From: **Somewhere over the rainbow**

Topic: Vegetarian with gluten intolerance

Sarah29
New Member

Hello, hope somebody can offer some words of wisdom.

I have IBS which is usually not too bad but much worse when I eat foods containing gluten. Any kind of bread, pasta and even potatoes can affect me.

My problem is that as a no-meat, no-fish vegetarian, if I cut out wheat, rye, pasta, pizza, etc, then I'm basically left with fruit, vegetables and cheese, which doesn't make for a very interesting diet!

Mealtimes are not too bad although they can get a bit boring, but I'm at a loss to find things that replace snacks such as toast or muesli. I'm bored with raisins and bananas

Any ideas would be much appreciated. I really don't want to start eating meat/fish again as I've been vegetarian for 20 years and don't like the taste/texture of meat.

Does anyone know if you can get gluten-free pasta?

Thank you.

From: **UK**

California
New Member

Sarah: Yes, they make numerous pastas made with rice that are gluten-free. Check online and you can find many choices of not only pasta, but many mixes and other good foods.

From: **California, USA**

Vicky19
Prolific Member

I've been vegetarian since I was four and don't eat meat or fish. I have cut out a lot from my diet because of IBS, including wheat, gluten, and starchy foods such as potatoes and rice, and try not to have anything with dairy products in it.

Have you tried goats cheese and goats milk? They are really nice. I eat a lot of salad and am trying a low-starch diet at the moment, but for the past week since starting it I've had pretty bad diarrhea, so I'm at a dead end at the moment too. I love sweets and crisps but they are a no-no for me.

Corn contains starch and so do a lot of veggie alternatives as that's what binds the ingredients together. I've been told to try tofu though, so I might give that a go. Also, bananas are pretty starchy and I've just stopped eating them as they can cause stomach problems. I've had constant tummy pain for five months since the IBS symptoms started up, so I'm trying to reduce the pain. I'll try anything!

From: **Birmingham, England**

ExIBS
New Member

Hmm.

I'm lactose intolerant, gluten intolerant, suffer from hypoglycemia, and have been vegan for eight or so years ...

And I smoke.

I guess that's worse.

Rice, water, and cigarettes?

From: **USA**

Topic: Fructose Intolerance Food Advice

Caitijean
New Member

Does anyone know of a recent list of foods that do not have sugar? Splenda has caused big problems for those of us suffering from fructose intolerance. It has replaced the other sugar substitutes & I do not know where to turn. Splenda is "sucralose"—too close in makeup to fructose and so it causes a severe reaction.

I was diagnosed when I was 15 with IBS. Just this year it was determined that I had fructose intolerance & not IBS. I had gone to tons of doctors. My life got to the point where I did not know if I would make it to the bathroom in a public place. I am convinced that fructose was the problem. My life has improved—I no longer have to run to the bathroom UNLESS I have fructose.

As I've removed fructose from my diet, my life has improved tremendously. The setback is that now that I have removed fructose, when I do have a little bit my reaction is more immediate.

From: **Iowa**

Julia37
Very Prolific Member

Hi everyone! It's been a while.

I have fructose sensitivity and I've found the only sweetener that agrees with me is aspartame (also called Nutrasweet). I had a similar bad experience with Splenda.

I have to be careful not to eat Equal too often because the maltodextrin in it can disagree with me also.

The only thing to do is check all ingredient labels and shop at health food stores for truly sugar-free foods like crackers. The trend right now is to put corn syrup in everything; hopefully they'll stop before the whole country becomes diabetic.

From: **Chicago, IL, USA**

Topic: My diet—which has really helped!!!

Ems
New Member

Hi all,

I have been following my diet for six months and I feel alive! OK … I get pain now and then, but no bloating and very few bouts of diarrhea (only when I've been out drinking!).

I have cut out wheat/gluten. Most food companies show allergy advice on the back of foods, so it's easy to cut out. Most supermarkets in the UK stock a good selection of wheat-free alternatives, i.e. wheat-free pasta, and you cannot taste the difference! Wheat is in nearly everything, so a lot of us have become "intolerant". There are many books available explaining this issue.

I also avoid spicy foods, beans, and lentils, (typical windy foods!) High-fiber vegetables and foods, rye bread, etc, cause my symptoms to worsen.

I also have soy milk in my rice pops for breakfast but eat low-fat real cheese. Therefore, I haven't cut out all dairy. Dairy can often cause sensitivities in people. Fat also, apparently makes your intestine spasm, so lean meats and low-fat foods help.

I personally can't eat fruit. The fiber and acid leave me in a lot of pain. I eat extra vegetables to compensate for the lack of vitamins. I have also found that high iron hurts my tummy. I have sought a lot of nutritional advice and my diet contains twice as many vitamins as needed (except iron), so I do not take multivitamin tablets.

I also find probiotics and bio-yoghurts give me chronic pain and diarrhea. Coffee and strong tea also have this effect. Caffeine is a diuretic, i.e. makes you go to the loo. I drink peppermint tea; peppermint has been proven to help IBS.

I drink about three liters of water a day and take regular low-impact exercise. Classes like yoga and tai chi help to relax and as we all know the more stressed we feel, the worse our symptoms are!

You may find by cutting out stuff for a while you may be able to re-introduce it back slowly. I am not a doctor, so you must seek professional advice or really research this topic before you dramatically change your life or eating patterns!

I hope this helps!!

Ems xx

From: **Maidstone**

Dlt647
Prolific Member

Hi EMS. I, too, have stopped eating all wheat/gluten products as well as all dairy. The dairy showed up positive in my allergy testing last year so I haven't had that in a while. I recently stopped eating wheat/gluten products and have noticed a huge difference. I buy gluten-free products from my local health food store. Occasionally it bothers me that I can't just eat what I want, but most times I'm okay with it. I bought some gluten-free cookies this week and didn't notice there were some dairy products in it.

I also started taking calcium at the recommendation of my OB/GYN and had some significant gas and bloating. Once I stopped, though, I'm back to normal. I have to stay away from anything this causes gas. I have the inability to pass gas very easily so it sits there causing discomfort. I have had many abdominal surgeries over the years and think adhesions may be a part of this (from what I read adhesions can cause the inability to pass gas). Other than that, my constipation has pretty much gone away and the pain/bloating has subsided with this diet.

I know you are supposed to be checked for celiac before starting a gluten-free diet, but I didn't want to go through that. I just thought it was worth a try to go on this diet and, amazingly, it worked. That is all I care about. Good luck and glad to hear you are feeling so much better.

From: **Pennsylvania**

Discussion: LEAP

Many Bulletin Board members use this forum to discuss their experiences with a program called LEAP (www.nowleap.com). LEAP involves blood testing and food trials as a systematic approach toward identifying food intolerances.

Topic: What's up with LEAP?

Alongtin
Prolific Member

Hi, I'm pretty new to the board, and I just heard about LEAP for the first time. I went to the LEAP site, but I would very much appreciate the expertise of someone who has done it.

I suppose that my biggest question is cost. Will it break the bank? There's a chance it could help me, but I need to be able to afford it!

Also, is it like the diet I've heard of where you only eat, say, chicken, rice and pears, then add a new food every week?

Sorry for the ignorance, I hadn't heard about this until this morning!

Thank you!

Amy

From: **Inverness, FL**

Bobby5832708
Prolific Member

Amy,

I started the LEAP program about three months ago. I've had IBS-D for over 30 years and have had many tests, all finding nothing wrong. The LEAP tests found which foods I can and cannot eat, and this has led to a dramatic reduction in my IBS symptoms. I am not sitting on the toilet most of the time anymore and I have reduced my consumption of medicines (Bentyl and Imodium) to about a pill or two a week. The results, for me, are truly amazing.

The cost is, I believe, about $700. It is a very small price to pay to feel better.

Very basically, this is what happens: They take some blood from you and test it in the lab. They then tell you what food ingredients you shouldn't even look at, what food ingredients you probably shouldn't consume, and which food ingredients are safe to eat. Based on that information they put together a diet plan where you start with a select few foods and gradually add the other safe ingredients over time. This way you can easily tell which foods cause a reaction and you always know a 'safe' diet to go back to if an added food causes problems. This is just a very basic description as I see it. All I care is that it really works!

The program has been easy for me because I want to feel better and I'll do whatever it takes. I had to completely change my diet. Some people might not have to go that far. We are all different and what is good for me may be really bad for you. That's what this test does—it finds out exactly what YOU can and cannot eat and does it very accurately.

Gofer it!!

Bob

From: **Winter Springs, FL USA**

WashoeLisa
Prolific Member

Hi!

Just to add to what Bob said (Hi Bob!), the diet is very minimal at first, but you don't eat the chicken, rice, etc. You eat the least reactive foods to YOUR body and that is different for everyone. For me, the beginning diet was cod, lentils, onions and celery. The reason for adding foods slowly is to test them. Every test has a failure rate and this is a way to find the things that may have been missed OR to find the foods that trigger a different immune system component that LEAP isn't designed to test for. The great thing though is that you still find out ALL of what you can't eat.

I am at two years on LEAP now and it has been more than worth its cost.

Let us know what you decide!

Lisa

From: **Carson City, NV, USA**

Alongtin
Prolific Member

I have severe C/D, and I'm really scared that I've been getting diet info that doesn't work for me personally. I've been following the Heather Van Vorous "Eating For IBS", so on really bad days, it is pure soluble fiber no matter what, like white bread and rice, but what if wheat is my problem? There never seems to be any way to tell! So LEAP sounds like the thing for me.

Could some of you (thank you already WashoeLisa!) share the foods you had to start out LEAP eating? I, of course, realize that mine will be completely different, but I sort of want to know what I'm getting into before I spend the money. I want to know that I could do it, whatever foods come up on my list!!

Thank you all for your help!!!

Amy

From: **Inverness, FL**

AnnieL
Regular Member

AMY,

I've been on the LEAP program since two months and it has worked very well for me.

My insurance paid about $368.00 because I had my blood drawn at my doctor's office. I opted to work with the LEAP dietician because I had 35 reactive foods. However, I would have paid it all myself because of the difference it has made in my life as I was always looking for bathrooms.

I started off eating chicken, pork, crab, cauliflower, onion, asparagus, barley, amaranth, cow's milk, butter, sesame, peanut, watermelon and honeydew. These were my safest foods. After one week I could add one new food each day.

After two months I am eating a fairly normal diet and try to rotate my foods so that I don't eat the same things day after day. I have also lost 12 pounds and am now at my ideal weight

I think that you should try LEAP. Good luck

Annie

From: **Seven Lakes, NC**

WD40
Very Prolific Member

My first phase foods were garbanzo beans, salmon, sole, turkey, codfish, red snapper, buckwheat, rice, wheat, quinoa, cucumbers, celery, broccoli, carrots, apples, honey melon, pineapple, papaya, Swiss cheese, cottage cheese, sunflower seeds, ginger, leek, garlic, cane sugar, and cayenne pepper. Each phase lasts about a week and with each phase you add new foods everyday. The first phase is only hard because you have to get really creative with the allowed foods with the allowed spices. As the phases progress the daily menus get easier and easier. During the phases it is very important to stick to your lists. Also during Phase One some people feel a little funky as the body tries to readjust itself. Days Four and Five hit me pretty good, and it was all uphill from there, minus the days where I cheated and regretted doing so. Good luck to you, and I highly recommend the program.

From: **California**

Ohnometo
Very Prolific Member

I think the others said it very well. It works but you have to work at it. I haven't been in the hospital since last November with IBS—that is a miracle because I was going to the ER and doctors many times last year. First you need to go to the web site and fill out some information to see if this is something that might benefit you. I was told many years ago to stay away from all of the food they say to stay away from when you have IBS and didn't get any better. This is why it is so nice to work with LEAP because they will tell you the exact things to take out of your diet. It could be a food or it could be a chemical …

Good luck.

From: **Wild Wonderful West Virginia**

Discussion: What to Eat to Gain Weight?

Although weight loss is not a typical symptom, some people with IBS do experience a dramatic loss of weight because of food avoidance. Overcoming that avoidance and finding foods that are comfortably digested can be difficult. The following posts offer some answers:

Topic: Need a High-Calorie Recipe

AD
Very Prolific Member

I desperately need to gain weight. I am an 18-year-old male with chronic excessive bloating, nausea, and IBS-C. At 5'3", I weigh only 68 lbs. and am looking for a recipe that is high in calories. I cannot stand drinks or shakes that taste like milk. I would like to find something high in calories that won't make me too nauseated, bloated or stopped up.

From: **North Texas**

HipJan
Very Prolific Member

Hi and welcome!

I've also had a terrible time with my weight (dropped really low, probably due to mal-absorption). But sounds like you have it worse than me. Unfortunately, what food works for one may not always work for another. But I'll try to summarize how/what I eat. Sorry, I don't use recipes, per se ...

1) I have to avoid gluten (wheat, barley, rye), so I eat a lot of rice products. I have a sizeable bowl of hot cream of brown rice cereal (w/soymilk) for breakfast; it's good with ground almonds and/or ground flaxseed sprinkled on it.

For snacks, I have rice cakes (no, not so many calories by themselves) and/or rice bread (lots of calories) spread with almond butter (easy to digest, healthy, and lots of calories). I also might have brown rice as a side dish with my dinner or lunch. Sometimes I might have rice pasta.

2) One easy-to-digest dish you might try is brown rice mixed with split peas ... again, more calories! Also, split pea soup. If you're interested, let me know, and I'll type in my versions of those.

3) I have four servings of fresh veggies each day, one, maybe two of them being root veggies (more calories). Sweet potatoes/yams are very good for us—and high in the calories; try them baked or roasted (cut up in little pieces, drizzle a bit of olive oil and seasoning over them, and stick them in the oven at 375 degrees for 35–40 min.).

4) Sorry, you don't like milk-like products, but I do have a glass of rice milk (or sometimes soy) for a snack; to it can be added ½ piece of fruit (then beat up) and/or 1 tsp. Ultra Clear Sustain (nutritionist-recommended protein powder; wouldn't try just any).

5) I'll sometimes drizzle olive or flax oil (maybe w/lemon or lime juice and basil or something) over my veggies. Those two oils are good for us—and they add a few more calories.

6) Fruit—unfortunately, I can't have too much of that, but I do at least have an apple, peach, plum, or pear each morning before breakfast—sometimes other times as well.

7) Protein—Salmon's great for us and has quite a few calories! I also have lean chicken (gotta avoid animal fat, despite the loss in calories!)—you could sometimes sprinkle ground almonds on it for extra calories.

8) Oil supplements—Many of us don't get the proper oils in our diets, esp. omega-3 and possibly also omega-6 and that can really have a negative impact upon our health. Those of us who are really low in weight may have a particular (critical) need for such essential fatty acids. You might check out fatty acid supplements such as flax oil capsules and also ground flaxseed.

KEY: Eat little meals approximately every two to two-and-a-half hours throughout the day. Unfortunately, our IBS diets don't usually help us add the calories.

But, I will say that I've been very patient and diligent and, finally, over the past four months I have gained 13 much-needed pounds. Good luck!

From: **Lone Star State**

Topic: An IBS diet for gaining the weight back

Ronr
Prolific Member

Just wondering, I hear lots of people trying to lose weight with their IBS, but is there a good IBS diet to help people who have lost weight from this IBS to gain it back? Any foods that will pack on the pounds but not the IBS? Thanks.

From: **USA**

MariaM
Prolific Member

I'm dealing with the same problem. I'm really thin—5'7" and only 103 lbs! (I lost 12 lbs from a bad IBS attack). I almost had to go in the hospital for tube feeding (yuck!). I have read Heather Van Vorous' "Eating for IBS" book and I try to follow some of her guidelines. The doctors and nurses keep telling me to drink Ensure drinks between meals or else add them to a milkshake. Of course, this goes against what a lot of books advise about eating for IBS. Most books advocate eliminating most or all dairy. I've been able to tolerate the Ensure pudding better than the Ensure drinks. So far I've managed to gain a few pounds, but it has been a slow process—about a pound per month.

From: **Tabb, VA**

Christiana
Prolific Member

To gain weight, try IBS "junk food". Here's a recipe that's totally IBS safe:

Chocolate-pudding Cake Recipe

1 cup flour
2/3 cup sugar
2 Tbsp. cocoa
2 tsp. baking powder
1/8 tsp. salt
1/2 cup water
2 Tbsp. applesauce
1 tsp. vanilla
2/3 cup brown sugar
1/4 cup cocoa
1 3/4 cup hot water

Mix first EIGHT ingredients together, pour in sprayed baking pan.
Mix brown sugar and 1/4 cup cocoa and sprinkle on top of batter.
Pour hot water last on top of the mix.

Bake at 350 degrees for 45 minutes.

The hot water sinks to the bottom to make a pudding at the bottom. Do not freeze. Its kind of like a fudge brownie

---

Ronr
Prolific Member

I thought cocoa causes D?

From: **USA**

Christiana
Prolific Member

No, no, no. Cocoa is perfectly FINE for IBS. I mean just plain cocoa ... nothing added, not processed, not alkalized, etc. Cocoa also has soluble fiber. I have had bad IBS-D and cocoa stabilizes me just fine.

From: **USA**

Cindy from Texas
Prolific Member

Been there, done that. With all my food aggravations, I lost a cumulative 22 pounds over a six-year period. I started at 112, lost 10 pounds in some 12 weeks when I first got IBS, and each year for every two or three pounds I'd gain, I'd lose four or five. By last April, I was down to 89 pounds!!! I'm 5.4 so that's pretty thin. I started doing a controversial form of acupuncture called NAET last Mayish. The first four to six weeks I went once a week. My husband and I first noticed I started filling in around my collar bone/breast bone. I had started gaining weight!! We were so excited. Buoyed by the results I started going twice a week. By late August, I found I'd gained 10 whole pounds. By Christmas, I was up to 108. Wow. After Christmas, I have been having a flare-up, and am now down to 103, but that's a lot better than where I was. I now only go every two weeks, but it has really helped me a lot. I wish I could go once a week, but that's all I can afford right now. The range of food I can eat has really improved. I have also heard probiotics has worked wonders with IBSers having weight loss issues. I hope to look into that at some point, but for now NAET has worked so well that's where my money's going for the moment. It's about $65 a session here in Austin. Best of luck.

—Cindy

From: **Austin**

Topic: Ensure Plus for gaining weight with IBS-D?

Mbz
New Member

I have trouble gaining weight with my IBS-D and was wondering what things others have tried that worked?

I am also curious about taking Ensure Plus as a supplement to my meals in order to gain weight.

Does anyone know if this is "IBS safe"?

Thanks! Mike

From: **AZ**

Lexi_Con
Very Prolific Member

Hi Mike.

I am IBS-D with GERD, and the D hits with extreme urgency.

I also am very sensitive to MSG, which seems to be prevalent in many foods and food products. Often it is not even clearly identified, so it becomes even more difficult to avoid. I tolerate dairy fairly well.

As to your question about Ensure:

I have resorted to a similar product called Boost at times when I cannot digest anything, and fatigue and exhaustion mean that I have to get something to stay in my guts.

I have never had a problem with the Boost.

I don't know if Ensure has MSG, or not, but I would check the label carefully.

Hope this is of some help.

Take care … from Lexi

From: **Winnipeg, Manitoba**

MariaM
Prolific Member

Ensure pudding has helped me to gain back ten pounds. I personally find the pudding more tolerable than the drink. You have to special order the pudding by the case through a pharmacy.

From: **Tabb, VA**

Julia37
Very Prolific Member

I wouldn't touch that stuff—dairy and sugar, two of the more common food sensitivities. I think you should only try it if you're certain you don't have sensitivities to the "foods" in it.

I've looked at a few of those diet/weight gain/nutritional drinks and my impression was they're made mainly of sugar, soy, milk, and chemicals. Better to eat real food—bread, potatoes, nut butters, olive oil, and pasta—find some French fries you can tolerate and eat them every day, weight gain will not be a problem! Wish I had that problem. Try gourmet potato chips. Have to go, I'm getting hungry!

From: **Chicago, IL USA**

Sillyface
Prolific Member

I wouldn't go near Ensure, but I can't tolerate fat, and it has something like 9.6 grams per serving. This is the "fatty food" they gave me when I went for my HIDA scan so that my gallbladder would empty.

However, before I had IBS I had an eating disorder. Back then, when I was learning how to eat again, I started with Slim Fast and moved up to Ensure. At least I could be sure I was getting some good nutrients that way.

From: **Saskatoon, SK**

Linda C
Regular Member

Ensure has gotten me through many a rough day …

There actually is no dairy in it. I checked that very carefully before I had it since I am lactose intolerant. I believe it says "dairy free" on the label, but I could be wrong. Anyway, I've never had any problem with it and find that it is often the only thing my system can handle and it takes away that empty feeling.

From: **Toronto, Ontario, Canada**

DrDahlman
Prolific Member

Ensure certainly does have dairy in it. It contains whey protein concentrate. If you are having IBS, it's worth it to find an alternative source for calories. Anyone who has a dairy sensitivity or fructose sensitivity needs to be careful. Additionally, the soy in it can increase gas and bloating. I usually participate in a different thread, but saw this and wanted to say that I take this product away from all my patients.

I am a chiropractor with a degree in nutrition.

From: **Cincinnati, Ohio**

Ibsed
Prolific Member

My husband has very low weight after a colon operation to remove a tumor and is in chemo (which can cause diarrhea, of course). His intestines are extremely sensitive but he is taking two Prosure drinks every day on the recommendation of his dietician—and having no extra problems of D.

The possible reactions to dairy, soy, etc. surely will depend on whether the person has a sensitivity to those things in the first place? If you don't, then I would have thought it would not be such a problem.

Sorry, just realized I have confused Prosure with Ensure—the dietician actually favored the former as it also contains Omega-3 fatty acids. She prescribes it for many of her underweight patients who have difficulty gaining weight through normal eating.

From: **Switzerland**

Julia37
Very Prolific Member

I'm biased because I'm sensitive to soy, lactose, and other sugars, but I don't think it's healthy to eat over-processed "meal replacements" for anyone. Too much sugar especially isn't good for anyone. Soy has hormones in it, "phytoestrogens", but it's added to many foods. There are lots of things not known about foods, like undiscovered vitamins and minerals, and people who eat over-processed and fast foods aren't getting the balance and nutrition they need. When I was growing up I was raised on the traditional Midwest diet, the unhealthiest in the world. Too much meat, white bread, cheese, milk, pastries, sweets, no vegetables, a few fruits. People eat like this and then wonder why they're heavy and don't feel well. Whenever I leave Chicago and go to smaller Midwest towns, it seems like every adult I see is obese. There are news articles about how unhealthy our nation is and how obesity and diabetes are epidemics. Gee, I wonder why.

From: **Chicago, IL USA**

Daisysp
Prolific Member

Try Goatein, which is a goat's milk protein drink that seems to be easy to digest with few, if any, of the side effects we are all suffering from. There is no sugar in it, no flavor at all actually. If you make it into a smoothie, try this recipe, it's nutritious and tastes great!

30 grams powdered Goatein (can get this online or from a health food store, brand is Garden of Life)
1 zucchini
2 carrots
1/2 banana (if you can eat those)
1 tsp almond butter (better than peanut butter)
1/2—1 cup rice milk
water and ice to blend

I add 1 to 2 tsp granulated fructose to mine.

Eliminate sugars, artificial products and dairy from your diet to feel better!

IBS-D (used to be C) for 8 yrs.
No Grain, No Pain!!

From: **Washington**

Topic: Need to Gain Weight!!

GodHasNotForgot
New Member

Does anyone have any suggestions for gaining weight w/IBS-C? I have suffered from excessive gas, and as a result have cut back on numerous foods: dairy, wheat, starch, red meat and sugars such as fructose. As a result, I have lost 25 lbs ... would have been great if I was overweight ... however I'm 5'8 and now 125 lbs.

What stops me from eating is not so much the constipation but the gas (which I imagine is caused by the constipation).

Example diet: cornflakes w/rice milk and almonds; rice noodles with grilled chicken; salmon w/brown rice; kiwi/papayas & water; wheat-free/milk-free/gluten-free cookies. (also take daily multi-vitamin and calcium supplements)

Please advise.

From: **USA**

Birdingal
New Member

Try the rice dream ice creams—they are delicious and full of nice fat to plump you up. You can also try tofuti which is obviously made from tofu, and also has loads of calories. What you need are calories.

Good luck!

From: **Berkeley, California**

GodHasNotForgot
New Member

I tried this ice cream recently ... yes it was delicious ... however it contains carob bean ... which does not help me because of intolerance to beans (they even mentioned this on their web site) … I was truly disappointed since being an avid ice cream lover in the past … same with the tofu ….

I have added more wheat-free products and more 'mini' meals … I've gained 5 lbs … Just seem to be having a little trouble from here …

I do thank you for your advice … perhaps I'll try it again w/Beano.

From: **USA**

Julia37
Very Prolific Member

Calcium supplements cause gas, as I was reminded when I accidentally bought "enriched" oat milk. Stop them, I bet it will make a huge difference. And no enriched products either.

Instead of that, I eat spinach and broccoli and make oatmeal bread with whole rolled oats, all of these have calcium.

If you still have trouble you could try cutting out all forms of sugar. I have fructose sensitivity and I've noticed sugar can sometimes cause gas.

For weight gain all you need are French fries and potato chips. Find some you can tolerate and eat them every day. Weight gain will sooooo not be a problem! I only have to indulge a few times before the weight starts coming on. I love potatoes, they're tasty, nutritious, and the starch soothes my tummy.

From: **Chicago, IL USA**

Polly6034
Regular Member

An easy way to increase the calories in your diet is to add fats and oils (if these don't upset your IBS) … e.g. fry your chicken instead of grilling, olive oil dressings, etc. Also, increasing the serve size of high calorie foods—almonds, rice, etc. Drink fresh fruit juice instead of water.

Has cutting out all those nutrients actually helped your IBS? If not, perhaps it's time to start adding them back into your diet?

Polly

IBS-D with nausea, and occasional gas and cramping

From: **Brisbane, Australia**

Discussion: What to Eat to Lose Weight?

The opposite issue, working toward the goal of weight loss, is difficult for most people. Adding IBS to the mix can be daunting. Here are some ideas from people who struggle with the need to lose weight and still eat foods that are soothing for their IBS:

Topic: Serious Weight Loss Needed3

Cofaym
Prolific Member

I need to lose at least 100 lbs, although I lost 80 when I first changed my diet to an IBS-safe one. I haven't lost weight in months and have in fact gained 30 lbs back. I am trying a 1200-calorie diet with yoga in the evenings. It consists primarily of sourdough bread, soy cheese, and applesauce. Has anyone else found a way to safely lose weight in more than minute amounts? Don't want to throw my stomach out of whack!!!

From: **San Diego, CA/USA**

Bad girl
Regular Member

I enjoy yoga, but I also like to ride the stationary bike. It's easy on your joints and it burns lots of calories. Exercise is the best form of weight loss I've found. And it boosts the endorphins too!

From: **Rolla, MO**

WD40
Very Prolific Member

I'm on a weight upswing as well. I did the Atkins for a couple of months and lost about 12 lbs., but I've gained it all back. I got a really bad attack of IBS and just never went back on the diet. Now I'm eating carbs like crazy, because it makes my stomach feel better, but I'm now 40 lbs overweight. Ack! My aunt did Weight Watchers and lost 90 lbs in about a year. I'm thinking of doing that but I don't have a lot of extra money right now. I'm on Elavil and that does NOT help.

I've never had such a hard time with my weight as I have since I've been on this doggone drug, but if I don't take it I'll be nauseous 24/7 with D every other day. I feel like I'm stuck. I know which foods to eat and which foods to avoid and I don't tend to overeat because it triggers an IBS attack, and exercise causes GERD attacks as well as headaches and nausea, so I don't know what to do anymore (and to think I used to be an athlete!!!)

From: **California**

Kdathrt1
New Member

I am right there with you guys. I need to lose about 60 lbs. I've done Weight Watchers in the past and it does work, but not really in the budget at this time. I have no problem with exercising, but I get frustrated when it isn't coming off. It's hard trying to find what to eat and what not to eat with IBS. Atkins is impossible when we need fiber. I'm at a loss. If you guys find anything let me know.

From: **Newnan, GA**

Julia37
Very Prolific Member

I think maybe if you try different forms of exercise until you find one you're comfy with that would help. I eat a lot of carbs also, but I walk a lot living in the city. My commute is 11 blocks of walking each way, and in addition I walk to run errands. I also ride my bike and dance as often as possible. Maybe something low-impact and not so strenuous would help you exercise.

After I took the sugar and fruit out of my diet I lost 40 pounds, everyone says I look so good. I eat a lot, but I suppose it's mainly the commute that's keeping me (relatively) thin. I hope you find an exercise you're comfy with and feel better.

From: **Chicago, IL USA**

Topic: IBS food and dieting: Possible?

Peanuttface
New Member

I have recently been diagnosed (well, after many tests and drugs, that's what they THINK it is!) with IBS. Since I've been having all these problems, I've gained about 7 or 8 pounds. Mostly water gain and inability to exercise due to pain or discomfort. But my question is to you all that are familiar with the SCD (Specific Carbohydrate) diet. I have been on it for about a month now and it helps. But how do you lose any weight with such high-fat flour (almond flour) that is in almost everything? Lunch and dinner I can usually stick to lean protein and a veggie or salad. But breakfast gets boring with eggs EVERY SINGLE DAY! I like the bread and muffins and such but they seem so incredibly high in calories and (good) fats. Anybody have a suggestion? I want to eat (now that I can!) But I have got to start losing some weight so that I can fit back in my clothes again. What do ya'll think?

Oh, I'm IBS C and D, alternating between stressful situations and diet.

Thanks!

From: **Germany**

Smurf1
Regular Member

First: start thinking outside the box. Eat lunch or dinner type foods for breakfast instead of eggs every day. Just eat smaller amounts. A food that is safe to eat in the afternoon and evening is safe to eat in the morning as well.

Second: starches are always at risk of causing one to gain weight because if they are not burned off quickly, they are converted into fat. High-fat starches are even worse. They are both high-carbohydrate AND high-fat.

The SCD diet is more about keeping your body/digestive system happy than it is about losing weight.

Maybe eating more meals that are primarily lean meats and vegetables, without the starches, could help you lose weight. It did for me.

From: **Phoenix, AZ, USA**

Isobel707
New Member

Hi Peanuttface,

I didn't do SCD or whatever, but I did start a similar, low-carb regimen almost two years ago to lose weight, and the pounds just fell right off. A few months into the diet, I was probably eating at least 100 g. of fat per day (mostly good fats, from olive oil, soy, flax seed, and nuts). I completely avoided garbage like donuts, muffins, etc. Anyways I lost something like 10 lbs in the first six weeks I was on the diet, which was really good for me (I wasn't that overly fat to begin with, so I didn't have much to lose). Note that on a low-fat diet, I didn't lose a single pound, and constantly felt hungry and deprived.

So yeah, I know you are really skeptical about eating things that are high in fat. I was too, which is why I did low-fat diets for a number of years before finally giving up. I finally convinced myself that fat was not the "enemy," but those non-nutritious refined carbohydrates that not only screw w/your blood sugar but (at least for me) aggravate IBS symptoms.

So go ahead and use the almond flour—I love that stuff. I use it along w/flax seed meal and soy flour to make waffles in the morning … yummy! Yes, it does have a lot of fat, but (1) it is unsaturated ("good" fat), (2) it tastes better, in my opinion, and (3) it is MUCH more nutritious that that Bisquick instant-mix crap (sugar, preservatives, hydrogenated oils, other bad stuff) that would wreak havoc on my digestive system.

Anyways, I initially did the low-carb thing to lose 10 lbs, but I lost 20 and now I am actually struggling not to any lose any more (see my other posts). Ironically, however I still follow low-carb eating because it drastically reduces my IBS symptom and is a lot healthier. If I eat one of those big store-bought muffins or eat a bowl of pasta, I am bloated like a balloon for *days*, and have more gas that one can imagine.

P.S. For me, exercise (jogging, doing Stairmaster, doing aerobics, etc.) really helped the gas pains and discomfort. Others on this BB have said the same. Yes, I know IBS can feel like you're getting stabbed in the stomach sometimes, but for me it always got WORSE when I would stay at home and just sit there in pain. 100% of the time that I exercise, I get relief in some form of another.

—Izzy

From: **Cambridge, MA**

Smurf1
Regular Member

I 100% agree with Izzy. Fat is not the enemy.

For years I ate low-fat, high-carbohydrate. I ate meals with no taste in the hopes of losing weight. In addition to ruining my stomach, I wasn't losing weight the way I wanted.

Since making the switch away from the refined carbohydrates, I am eating a lot more fat then I used to. Guess what? I am not gaining weight. I am losing weight. The funny part is I am not trying to lose weight. I am only trying to keep my stomach happy.

I also feel extremely bloated when I eat pasta, breads, and sugars. I do not feel this way when I eat meats and vegetables only.

From: **Phoenix, AZ, USA**

Peanuttface
New Member

Thanks Izzy and Smurf for the encouragement. This "IBS-thing" is the strangest thing! I had raw cauliflower today and it was delicious. But I almost had to go home due to the PAIN and bloating at work. I absolutely wanted to die. Also, I wondered about the honey on the SCD diet plan. If I eat too much of it (or too many nuts), I can be really sick with bloating and gas. Is that because of the carbs in both or what?

I agree with you Smurf. When I have had the dynamite willpower to stick to protein and veggies (a little cheese and occasional fruit) all day, by Day 2, I feel pretty darn good. I am the happiest person.

One more thing I was wondering … does HOW MUCH you eat bother you as much as WHAT you eat?? I eat the smallest meals in the whole world! Like 100 to 150 calories and my stomach is almost distended. And then it takes FOREVER to digest. Just wondering … I thought I had read somewhere that this may be a possible side effect.

Also, I was wondering Izzy, with your weight loss due to the low carb regiment, how low did you go? Was it like the Atkins? Would you mind posting a normal day's menu for me for reference? I'd love to try it. I have found that it also curbs my sweet tooth after several days. The first days are hell though!

Thanks again for all y'all's help.

Peanutt

From: **Germany**

Isobel707
New Member

Well I didn't go as low as the Atkins diet (in induction period, it calls for no more than 20 g. carbs per day). I actually did the opposite, I gradually decreased my carbs as I went along (when I started, I had to use up all the juice, bread, and pasta left in my kitchen). I got a lot of recipes/ideas from that Protein Power book written by the Eades. Their plan calls for 30 g carbs/per day in phase I, and then 55 in phase II or something like that.

Anyways, since I only had wanted to lose a few lbs, I think the lowest I would go is 30–40 g per day. But after a few months or so I had to increase it since I had already lost enough weight. (Plus, I would get terrible leg cramps due to low potassium levels, which can be a side-effect of low-carb diets.) Nowadays I probably do around 70–100 g. carbs per day or something like that.

And as for a typical day's menu, I eat three square meals a day, about 500—600 calories each. For breakfast, I might have some cottage cheese w/berries, and some Fiber-One cereal and a protein shake … or sometimes I make almond-flour waffles or three-egg omelets w/cheese. Lunch is something like a salad and some almond butter on a Wasa cracker or a veggie burger w/cheese and unsweetened ketchup. Dinner I might have stir-fry tofu & bell peppers w/chicken apple sausage. Or I might just grill some chicken and eat it w/peanut sauce. For desserts I usually have fruit or sugar-free Jello or pudding. Drinks are usually water or club soda and I drink soy milk (I don't like regular milk).

P.S. and yeah, the first few days of low-carbing *are* hell, at least for me anyways. I think I had a headache for like two days (due to sugar withdrawal). But don't get discouraged, you'll feel tons better in time!

From: **Cambridge, MA**

Forum VI: <u>Medications</u>

1. Diarrhea specific

Lotronex (*alosetron*), Zofran (*ondansetron*), and Kytril (*granisetron*);
Remeron (mirtazapine)

A relatively new class of medication has been developed for the treatment of the symptoms of Irritable Bowel Syndrome, medications that work by targeting the receptor sites of certain neurotransmitters found in the gut. Neurotransmitters are chemicals within our bodies that allow impulses to pass from nerve to nerve. In the intestine, these neurotransmitters are responsible for the process of digestion and affect the working of muscle contractions, secretion of mucus, and absorption of fluids. Acting on specific neurotransmitter sites, medications in this class work to improve IBS symptoms.

The 5-HT3 medicines are used to treat diarrhea-predominant IBS. These medications prevent serotonin (a neurotransmitter) from attaching to 5-HT3 receptors, resulting in a slowing of colon contractions and therefore reducing diarrhea, urgency and lower abdominal pain. The following discussions cover members' experiences with Lotronex, Zofran and Kytril.

<u>Discussion</u>: Lotronex

When Lotronex, a 5-HT3 blocker first came on the market, it was hailed as a godsend by some IBS sufferers. Unfortunately, for others, particularly individuals with a history of constipation, the medication proved to have serious (and in some cases, fatal) side effects. The medication was then pulled from the market, to the great distress of those individuals who felt that the medication had given them their life back. Lotronex has since become available again, but with many restrictions on its prescription, most notably that it is *only* approved for use by women, to treat diarrhea-predominant IBS.

Topic: Lotronex started Saturday ... when should I be going to the bathroom?

Kaylis9d9
Regular Member

I took my first pill Saturday night and have only taken one pill each day, at night. I really haven't gone much at all since then. I am not in pain, which is great. However, I am worried because I am not used to not going to the bathroom. Note that I am IBS-D only and that I had a fairly bad episode before I started taking Lotronex ... did anyone experience something similar after first taking Lotronex? I have never in my life been constipated. What symptoms would I display?

From: **New Jersey**

Nath
Prolific Member

Lotoronex makes me C also. I would suggest not letting it go for too long. If I hadn't gone for three days, I'd stop taking it for a day or two, just till you have gone again. I think it's about working out your own balance, changing your dose and increasing fiber until you get the right combination.

From: **Australia**

Kaylis9d9
Regular Member

SO, I went from Saturday night until Thursday without going too much. So I stopped taking it Thursday night ... been two nights now. Haven't gone much still. I am just shocked one pill a day did so much for me. My working theory was that since food is staying in my body longer than five seconds now, my body needs to get used to it.

From: **New Jersey**

Nath
Prolific Member

I think that is the major problem, we are so used to D that we have no idea what normal really is. It just takes some time and practice.

From: **Australia**

Luna
Very Prolific Member

If you started the Lotronex after a bad D episode, you wouldn't have a lot of junk built up inside yet, so it could be a few days and that would not be abnormal. Way back when, before I had IBS-D, I used to poop every two to three days.

With the Lotronex, if you go three days without so much as a teeny little poop, I'd skip a pill or take half pills until you go. It really is strange going "normally" when you are new to Lotronex—solid stools, regular BMs ...

From: **Ohio, USA**

LUCIA
Prolific Member

I personally think it is really bad to take a pill every day. You should wait until you have a BM before taking the next one. Also, try just taking half if possible. You could get a serious constipation problem. Plus, make sure to get all of your refills, even if you don't need them, as you go along with taking them. I get the feeling that one day it may be taken off the market again. I plan to stock up because it really works for me. Try to be conservative in using Lotronex.

From: **GLENDALE, CA. L.A.COUNTY**

Verna Eileen
Prolific Member

Lotronex is not a "take as needed" prescription but, you DO need to find your own dosage. We're each different.

I started out immediately on two a day when it first came out and did beautifully. Yes, I was constipated from time to time, but dealt with that by eating fruit, spinach, anything else I couldn't eat before, because it was like instant Drano. Like prune juice. Call me crazy, go ahead, but I like it. Watermelon was real effective, too.

Now I take half a pill in the AM and a whole one at night. Occasionally I skip one or the other for a day or two just to get a good clean out. You'll have to keep toilet locations in the back of your mind until you find the correct dosage for your body, but smaller amounts and much less frequent BM's are to be expected. That's kinda what 'normal' is all about, or as close as we can get to it. Good luck and just listen to your body; it'll tell you if you're on the right track.

From: **St. Joseph, MI, USA**

Luna
Very Prolific Member

I agree, if you get too stopped up all it takes is a little bit of forbidden food and you'll be cleaned out again. I can eat a lot more things when I'm on Lotronex, but there are still some things I can't eat much of and some others I can't eat at all.

Everyone is different and responds to Lotronex differently. When it was first out, I took two a day and needed that. I would often skip one on a weekend or otherwise be careless and forget, so that might have helped me be a little more regular. My stools were really hard with that dosage. Now I'm on the one a day dose and take one and a half in times of extreme stress or other times when I need more. My stools are formed but not as hard as they were before, and if I eat something that disagrees with me, I get soft stools or even D. With two a day I got D only ONCE in the five months I was on it. I think one and a half might be a better dose for me overall, but my doc is more comfortable with me being on one and is hesitant to prescribe for two a day. My IBS isn't as severe as it was when I first was on Lotronex, too.

I really notice if I miss my Lotronex, so it is definitely not a take-as-needed drug for me. Often the effects are delayed a little ... This week I was taking my pills at odd hours thanks to weird sleeping habits, and I think I missed my Lotronex completely one day. My stomach wasn't as good and then I got D today. I really need to keep a constant minimum level of Lotronex in my system in order to get the best results.

From: **Ohio, USA**

LUCIA
Prolific Member

We all need to find our own dosage level but I find that taking it as needed works for me. Drugs work on me right away. I don't like getting constipated, so I try to keep the dosage at a normal level for me.

I got constipated when I first took it, so I decided to take it every other day and I also cut it into a half when I feel I didn't need to take a whole one. I have told my doctor how I take it and he agrees with me and approves my method of taking it. We are all different in our levels of IBS-D.

From: **GLENDALE, CA. L.A.COUNTY**

Topic: Lotronex and GAS … Help!!

Pisces65
Regular Member

Anyone experiencing bad gas from Lotronex? I am a long-time user and just now being affected so bad that I had to stop taking it. I've been off five days now and still no sign of relief. I'm assuming Lotronex stays in the system quite some time. Just curious if anyone else has experienced this. I have been on Lotronex for the second time around, with no problems the first time, back on since the reintroduction and now this is happening—very upsetting since it's always worked so well and still is except for the gas. I just can't go on like this. Anyone???

From: **NY USA**

Kathleen M, Ph.D..
Very Prolific Member

I'm not sure the gas is directly from the Lotronex.

More likely you have had a shift in the colonic flora to species that produce more gas (not known if drugs will do this or not, it can shift on its own) or what you are feeding the bacteria you have.

I would try adding probiotics even IF the bacteria shifted from the Lotronex (BIG IF). These shifts wouldn't just go back to what it was overnight anyway. Like I said, they can shift on their own for any number of reasons and may not shift on its own back (I assume you mean you are farting a lot, not just you suddenly have more pain??)

Probiotic bacteria (Acidophilus and others) produce no gas from the digestion of the carbs that we cannot digest (starchy foods, sorbitol, and for some, fructose and lactose).

K.

From: **Somewhere over the rainbow**

JuliaNYC
Prolific Member

I second Kath's recommendation. I solved the gas problem by taking a probiotic with my morning Lotronex. The one I use is called Culturelle. I have also used Schiff's milk-free acidophilus when I couldn't get Culturelle. The Schiff's works too, so probably any probiotic would. Curiously, I don't need to take one with my evening Lotronex. It may take a day or two for the effect to take hold, but it's worth a try.

From: **New York, NY, USA**

Pisces65
Regular Member

Thank you both so much for your replies. I am running right out to get the probiotics. How long do you think I should take them?

Is it possible that I will always have to take it? I will definitely start the Lotronex back up. My life is just not the same without it.

Thank you again. I will let you know how things are going in a few days.

From: **NY, USA**

Kathleen M, Ph.D..
Very Prolific Member

When I found a brand that worked for me, I had to take it regularly for a few months to keep the benefit. Now I take some a few times a month, sometimes missing a month altogether.

The bacteria do grow in there and if you can get a good amount going they can keep going for awhile, but you are always being re-seeded with something, so you may need them periodically for awhile.

Some people find that ones that have "prebiotics" like FOS can increase gas for awhile, and some even have that issue with plain ones. I've not had that problem … usually with me either they work well or nothing. DA-IBS seems to be one that works well for a lot of people (Digestive Advantage-IBS).

In any case, if you aren't getting relief with a brand after two to three weeks, you may want to try a different one.

K.

From: **Somewhere over the rainbow**

Pisces65
Regular Member

JuliaNYC and KathM … you two are the best!!

I'm so much better. If you hadn't answered my post, I'd be off Lotronex and suffering terribly from gas and diarrhea. I can't thank you enough! I am taking Nature's Bounty Probiotic Acidophilus, 10 mg, which is 100 million active, just in the AM.

I can't believe my Gastro didn't mention anything about bad bacteria in my system, or how to remedy it, and just told me to go off Lotronex to see if it made a difference. It really makes you wonder about these doctors sometimes.

Again, thank you both from the bottom of my heart!!!!

From: **NY, USA**

Discussion: Zofran and Kytril

Zofran and Kytril are 5-HT3 inhibitors that have predominately been prescribed for the treatment of severe nausea and vomiting in cases of chemotherapy or surgery. When Lotronex was taken off the market, many physicians recommended Zofran or Kytril to their patients as an alternative.

Topic: Lotronex vs. Zofran

PAWS79
New Member

Hi All,

I have been taking Zofran since July, and I have been, for the most part, better than I was in the past, but by no means normal. I still get a lot of gas, cramps and D. My doctor suggests I switch to Lotronex because Zofran is not meant to be taken for long periods of time and he is concerned about long-term health damage. He has sent all the info to GSK for approval, but hasn't received the stickers in the mail yet or any other information. I have Celiac disease and am only 23. I was wondering if anyone could tell me the difference between Zofran and Lotronex and how they affect different parts of the body. I would really appreciate any help that can be afforded. Thank you and good luck to everyone

PAWS79

From: **USA**

Gasgirl
Very Prolific Member

Hi, Paws, I had been using Zofran in place of Lotronex until recently. I found the Zofran was very binding, but this effect didn't last as long as the Lotronex does, so it was hard to get consistent results with it. It also got rid of my queasiness. It had little or no effect on gas, pain, or bloating. In fact, it was often painful to have a bowel movement.

Lotronex is longer lasting, not quite as binding (I get closer to normal consistency BM's rather than hard rocks followed by too soft BM's) and it definitely helps the pain and hypersensitivity. It also helps gas and bloating for me, if I can get the dosage right. These two symptoms remain the most vexing for me, but I am making progress.

Hope this helps.

From: **Cambridge, Massachusetts**

Debbie Benning
Very Prolific Member

All Zofran did for me was constipate me and then I would have explosive D after a couple of days. Very ugly cycle. I had very bad gas and pain throughout.

From: **USA**

Jennifer7
Prolific Member

Actually, the Zofran works better for me than Lotronex. It hasn't been working quite as well in the last month, however. What is the dosage of Zofran you have been on? I've been taking 2 mg/day. I forgot to say that I've read that the difference in Zofran & Lotronex is that the Zofran works in the brain & Lotronex works in the gut. Both inhibit serotonin from reaching the brain in the gut. I really don't see why Zofran would be bad long-term, but Lotronex wouldn't.

Jennifer

From: **Texas**

Gasgirl
Very Prolific Member

In line with what Jennifer said, my doctor didn't see anything wrong with taking Zofran long-term; it is in the same class of drugs as Lotronex—that is, a 5-HT3 inhibitor.

My health insurer, on the other hand, explicitly discourages long-term use because of the exorbitant cost. They still covered it, though.

From: **Cambridge, Massachusetts**

Kodiakgirl
New Member

Let me ask, are any of you on Lotronex and Zofran together? I have been on Lotronex 1 mg/day and Zofran as needed, which has been up to as much as 8/mg 3x's/day. My nausea is pretty bad and Zofran doesn't even touch it some days. My doctor swears by Lotronex and I am in my second week of taking it. Seems to be helping—D has stopped and only going once per day. But what to do about the nausea? I am having a hard time eating and desperately need to gain weight. From what I am reading—being on the two together doesn't seem like a good idea.

From: **Home**

Marilyn Naylor
Prolific Member

Kodiakgirl—I was on Zofran before Lotronex—I wouldn't take both of them together. 8 mg/3x's a day is a lot of Zofran. I used to take 8 mg/day and thought that was a lot. Are you sure the Zofran isn't causing the nausea? It did for me in the beginning. I haven't heard where Lotro causes nausea. I've been back on Lotro for about two months. In the beginning I took Imodium with it if necessary. The longer I'm on Lotro, the better it seems to be working—haven't gotten my full confidence back yet though. I'm taking .5 mg a day.

Good luck!

From: **Baton Rouge, LA, USA**

Mtk
Prolific Member

I have been taking Zofran for 15 months now and it has been working quite well. I cut the 8 mg pills in fourths and take a fourth every day. It works as well as Lotronex, if not better. I do have some bad days every now and then, but even normal people who do not have IBS have bad days. I just switched insurances, so I'm hoping my new insurance will cover the Zofran. If they don't, I will just have to pay the price. The thought of going back to the way I was before Zofran is unbearable.

From: **Hoffman Estates, IL, USA**

JMC
Regular Member

Kodiakgirl

I take Lotronex, Remeron, and Zofran (4 mg), but the Zofran is only to be taken when I'm having severe bouts of nausea, not as a preventative. I have some other meds I also use for nausea; more for preventative measures (nausea and D are my two biggest IBS problems). I rarely use the Zofran, only when the nausea is debilitating.

JMC

From: **ILLINOIS, USA**

Topic: Zofran vs. Kytril?

Verna Eileen
Prolific Member

Hello All,

My insurance is making a fuss over filling my Mail Order prescription for Zofran, which is now finally a successful drug for me. They OK'd the first 15 tabs at the pharmacy but are now balking at additional through the mail. They have suggested Kytril as an alternative. I found some info online which has me puzzled. Another 5-HT3 receptor antagonist? I need some other opinions to present the most info to my doctor who tries very hard to work with me on this.

From: **St. Joseph, MI, USA**

JuliaNYC
Prolific Member

Verna,

I am by no means an expert in the intricacies of Kytril (granisetron) and Zofran (ondansetron). All I can tell you is that both are 5-HT3 receptor antagonists, like Lotronex (alosetron) and Anzemet (dolasetron). However, I was working in a cancer hospital during the Phase 2 and Phase 3 trials of Kytril and Zofran, and what I noticed then is that Kytril was tested in much younger children than was Zofran. I looked them both up tonight and saw that Kytril is considered safe for use in children as young as 2, but Zofran is not recommended for children under 4.

The list of possible adverse effects is similar. The usual dosage of Kytril is lower (2 mg daily as opposed to 8 mg daily for Zofran; these are the dosages for chemotherapy and radiation therapy related nausea). If insurance is recommending Kytril, it may be because 2 mg of Kytril is cheaper than 8 mg Zofran (that's definitely true), and we all know that insurers like nothing better than saving money.

Julia

From: **New York, NY, USA**

Jeffrey Roberts
Member # 1
Founder

Kytril has shown slightly better efficacy than Zofran for sufferers of IBS, but the cost is outrageous.

Jeff

From: **Toronto, Ontario, Canada**

Verna Eileen
Prolific Member

Thank you all so very much for your rapid response.

The slogan here "You are not alone" is right on the money. That's why I came here and that's why I stay here.

Thank you again.

From: **St. Joseph, MI, USA**

Discussion: Remeron

Another 5HT-3 medication is Remeron, an antidepressant that works by targeting neurotransmitter receptors in the brain. Due to its positive effect on intestinal symptoms, it might be prescribed to an IBS patient who also suffers from depression.

Topic: Remeron users

Humanistguy
New Member

Anyone out there who is currently using or has used Remeron successfully to treat IBS discomfort, I would be interested to know what dosages you found maximum relief at. Also, if you've found Remeron to be an unpleasant experience and had to move on to other medications, please feel free to speak out! I'm looking at this drug as a possible treatment option for IBS-D. Thanks kindly.

From: **Seattle, Washington**

Crampyjo
New Member

Hi Humanist:

I started on Remeron three months ago, so it's still pretty early in the game. However, I can tell you that the resultant changes in my sleep quality (on 15mg dose) have dramatically eased my GI pain (as I told my doctor … pain's gone from a scream to a whisper). I could feel a difference within just a few days.

I also have fibromyalgia and got relief from muscle pains for the first two weeks, but that has recently changed (muscle pain is back with a vengeance, so perhaps I need my dosage adjusted).

As to side effects, be prepared to sleep A LOT especially for the first few days (I slept 13 hours the first night). Also, my appetite really soared (wanted to eat anything that wasn't nailed down for first two weeks) but that seems to have normalized now as well.

In general, I'm VERY pleased. Haven't had this level of relief from any other meds I've tried over the past year.

Good luck with whatever you try!

Crampyjo

From: **Ottawa, Ontario Canada**

LotronexLover
Very Prolific Member

Remeron worked GREAT. No side effects. It was one of the best drugs I have ever taken! I highly recommend it. Just be sure to give it a few weeks. The effectiveness on the intestine is a few days. However, it will make you REALLY sleepy for the first few weeks. So sleepy that you may not want to keep taking it. I promise you this does go away … just wait a few weeks. Good luck!

From: **Cherry Hill, NJ USA**

Digest Dan
Prolific Member

For Your Info. I had a bad reaction to Remeron. I became lethargic and depressed for two weeks when it was tried. When I stopped it, I felt immediately better the next day. Just so you know. My doctor explains that everyone has different reactions to antidepressants and you never know. I am going well now on Elavil and Lotronex … You never know how an individual will react unless you try … Dan

From: **New York**

StayStrong
Prolific Member

I've been on Remeron for about three years at 15 mg. I tried 30 mg, but didn't notice any difference and went back down. It's not going to be a miracle drug, but it does help to firm stools without severe constipation.

I was also on Lotronex when it first came out and it didn't work for me. I guess I should mention that I'm male and 6'1, 200 pounds, so just because you are big doesn't mean you need a higher dose. You need to try and get eight hours of sleep a night or you'll really feel tired all day.

Good luck.

From: **Las Vegas, NV**

2. Constipation specific

Zelnorm/Zelmac (*tegaserod*);
Amitiza (lubiprostone)

Discussion: Zelnorm/Zelmac

In contrast to the 5-HT3 drugs, which work to block serotonin from being absorbed at the receptor sites in order to slow down the colon, Zelnorm is a medication that was developed to act like serotonin in *stimulating* the 5-HT4 receptor sites to speed up colon contractions. Although not a cure, clinical studies have demonstrated that it is effective in relieving the symptoms of chronic functional constipation and the bloating, abdominal pain and discomfort that go along with it. Zelnorm is *not* to be taken by individuals who suffer from diarrhea-predominant IBS.

Topic: Normal for Zelnorm to stop working so soon?

2btrue
Prolific Member

My doctor suggested I try Zelnorm because I have been very constipated since having my colon removed. It seemed to work for two days and now it does nothing.

Has anyone had the same problem?? I find it real hard to believe that it can only work for two days. My doctor thought this would be the cure-all for my problem, but he obviously doesn't know too much about Zelnorm, or is it just me?

From: **USA**

Bada Shanren
Very Prolific Member

That's actually very odd. If you read other posts here, the problem seems to be that it takes a week to six weeks to start working. What do you mean it stopped working?

Bada

From: **Murfreesboro, TN 37130**

ITeachKids
New Member

Apparently, Zelnorm isn't the answer for everyone. I took it for a week, one tablet twice a day. Nothing. My doctor told me to take TWO twice a day. Still nothing. I was soooo hopeful. I guess it's not the miracle drug I was hoping for.

Cynthia

From: **Georgia**

Ganas
Prolific Member

Just constipated me, except for the first time I took it.

From: **Michigan**

Bada Shanren
Very Prolific Member

Ganas.

That might be because you are a male? The first two times I tried it that happened, but this third time around it has been all diarrhea. Melissa said that hypnosis does the same type of restructuring that Zelnorm does, so this time I'm going to try them together.

Bada

From: **Murfreesboro, TN 37130**

2btrue
Prolific Member

I'm not male and I have heard that it stops working after about six weeks, so one would think that it should work at the beginning. I think I have actually become more constipated and the pain is real bad. Surely it would be risky to continue taking it?

I guess this medication has been such a disappointment for so many of us, I do wish they would come out with other options and that there would be more competition amongst the drug companies, that way we could get help and they'd make money which would be a win, win situation. Oh well, we'll have to wait and see I guess!

From: **USA**

SharonJoann
New Member

I have been taking Zelnorm since January. It is a miracle drug.

Initially my doctor put me on 6 mg twice a day. After about six weeks, it seemed to "stop" working. In other words, my BM's were about two to three days apart again, although the bloating was GONE!

I cut the dosage in half … after reading a lot of success stories on this site. I started taking 3 mg twice a day … once when I get up and then at bedtime.

This works well for me. The consistency is still a little like D. When I have to go, there is NO time to think about it and it is very liquid and loose, some of the time. Most others, it's just VERY soft and somewhat explosive.

I don't care.

I go every day … usually two to three times a day. I am not bloated. I am losing weight again (I had stalled out when I couldn't poop!). I feel better. I don't feel like I am going to have a "blow out" when I am shopping thus necessitating that I stay close to a toilet (although, as I said, when I have to go, it's not a drill).

Over the past month I started to take the 6 mg again—once a day, and skipped the weekends. Over the course of the month I got bloated, VERY constipated, and miserable. I am back to my 3 mg twice a day and I am regular.

This drug is NOT a laxative. It's meant to make your gut and colon more like normal. To take it and expect "laxative" results is inappropriate. Take it the way it is prescribed and if you feel your dosage is not correct, remember with Zelnorm, at least in MY experience, less is more.

My doctor is thrilled with the results and plans to keep me on Zelnorm indefinitely. He is aware of my dosage change and fully concurs.

Sharon

From: **Jeannette, PA**

Cheryl HH
New Member

I was so happy when my doctor gave me samples of Zelnorm … thought my life might actually return to normal!!!

It worked great for about three weeks, and then became less and less effective. The doctor only allowed me to take it for 12 weeks due to uncertain side effects. After a month I was totally miserable, had missed five days work at a new job. He told me to start it again, that it should work like the first time. No such luck. It's not helping at all. Guess I'll try lowering the dosage and see if that might help.

So much for hoping for a miracle.

Cheryl HH

From: **Work**

Babydoc_au
Prolific Member

If you are constipated, you could try taking regular magnesium (Epsom salts will do, as it is cheap)—I found this made a huge difference for me. I guess you should check with your Dr if this is OK first. I felt worse before I felt better with Zelnorm, but I persisted and after about four to five weeks I improved. I also take fiber with it, and now take only 3 mg twice a day.

From: **Australia**

H8_IBS
Prolific Member

Interesting that cutting it in half actually helped more. I never would have guessed that. Thanks! I am going to give it a shot. It helped me incredibly with bloating and pain, but made C worse.

I do have to add that it did absolutely nothing for me when I had foods I couldn't eat before I went on it. I was enjoying having a flatter stomach and no pain until I had something with milk in it. I have always had to avoid milk, but I felt so good I thought I could cheat. Nope. I paid for that for three days!!!!

If Zelnorm hasn't made any difference in any of your symptoms, perhaps try modifying your diet a bit.

Kari

From: **NJ**

Topic: HAS ANYONE TAKEN ZELNORM MORE THAN SIX WEEKS?

Golden67
Regular Member

HI I HAVE BEEN ON ZELNORM FOR SIX WEEKS. AT THE BEGINNING, IT MADE ME VERY SICK. AS WEEKS WENT BY, I FELT A BIG IMPROVEMENT. THEN AFTER SIX WEEKS, I WENT OFF IT BECAUSE THE PAMPHLET SAID IT WAS RECOMMENDED FOR SHORT-TERM USE. A WEEK AFTER I STOPPED, MY OLD SYMPTOMS CAME BACK, CONSTANT CRAMPING AND BLOATING, 24 HOURS A DAY. I WENT BACK TO MY DOCTOR AND HE SAID TO GO BACK ON THE ZELNORM. SO I DID AND I AM SICK THE FIRST WEEK, WITH THE D AND CRAMPS. HAS ANYONE BEEN TAKING IT ON A REGULAR BASIS? I TAKE 6 MG A DAY. WHEN I HAVE BAD CRAMPS, IS THERE ANY SPECIAL DIET THAT HELPS? THANK YOU.

From: **New York**

Haglips
New Member

My main complaint was bloating and constipation, not too much cramping, just hard, lumpy stools. I just started taking Zelnorm and the results are unbeliev-able. It worked for me within 24 hours. My doctor said a lot of people stay on it long-term.

From: **Illinois**

Jeffrey Roberts
Member #1
Founder

You might be interested in a successful study conducted by Dr. Gervais Tougas at McMaster University in Hamilton, Ontario that followed patients on Zelnorm for one year. He concluded that Zelnorm was safe to take longer than what the indication suggests.

Jeff

From: **Toronto, Ontario, Canada**

Jules1199
Regular Member

I am a 23-year-old Female; IBS-C diagnosed two years. I have been on Z for a year and half. It gives me D only if I don't eat enough with it or drink alcohol or too much caffeine. I was VERY sick for the first 10 days I was on Z. I was weak and had constant D. Food was moving right through me in a matter of a couple hours. I couldn't keep anything in. However, with any medication, it takes time for your body to adjust. Personally, two weeks of hell was worth a year and a half of relief.

From: **Rochester Hills, MI, USA**

Tiss
Very Prolific Member

I'm on my third day and have not experienced the terrible diarrhea like I did on the first day. Not normal BMs, but it seems to be working anyway. My question is this: what in the heck is the point to get on something that works, only to be taken off of it after a few months or a year? I have had problems with C my whole life and I'm 47, so I hate to take something that eventually I'll have to go off of! Also, how does this work differently than a laxative? Sure feels like a laxative at work to me. Does your body get dependent on it?

Tiss

From: **Mid USA**

GailSusan
Very Prolific Member

Tiss, I started Z six years ago in a Phase III clinical drug trial. I was off it for a while after the study ended until I was able to get the FDA to make an exception and put me back on the drug. I've now taken it every day for almost three years. I've had no adverse side effects, other than the D (which being C, I don't even THINK of complaining about). I can build up a resistance to the drug very easily (in less than a week), so I only take a small dose in the AM so I can have a BM (D mostly, but what the heck, it beats the alternative). I lived in pain 24/7 and had two operations due to impacted feces, so to me the Z is a miracle drug. It doesn't work for every form of constipation. Constipation has many causes. For certain kinds of constipation, Z works better than anything out there, but you have to play with the dosages over a period of time to find out what works best for you—once a day, twice a day, 3 mg or 6 mg, etc. (I take 3 mg once a day in the AM when I first get up.)

From: **USA**

Sally-p
Regular Member

Hi All:

I have been taking Zelnorm for two and a half years. I first got it from Switzerland before it was approved in the US. I have always taken one dose in the AM, about 4 mg, little more than half a pill. I started not getting good results in Dec 2003, and today is the first day I have gone without it. I am not sure where this is going, whether it is a break hoping I can take it again, or a permanent stop. I started getting more abdominal pain and my gut felt like it was frozen stiff. Nothing would "soften" it up. After reading the latest information about the possibility of decreased blood flow, I became concerned enough to stop for a while. So, I am taking a wait and see attitude.

From: **Virginia**

Cinna
Regular Member

I've been taking Zelnorm for about five to six months now. Not once have I had diarrhea with it. I take 6 mg twice a day with a stool softener. And I go at least once every two days, I try and eat lots of fiber and drink lots of water, but I'm still so very constipated. Also, whenever I have a BM, I have intense pain in my lower abdomen and I seriously scream because it hurts so much, I guess because it's so hard. I take two capsules of my stool softener; it's the most I can take.

The side effects I seem to get from Zelnorm are dizziness, being light-headed, and headaches.

I was on a bland diet before, but I kept losing too much weight, so now, I'm on a different diet. Problem is, the foods I can eat make me sick, but if I don't eat, then I'll just lose more weight and that sure isn't healthy.

From: **Canada**

JennyBean
Regular Member

I went on Zelnorm last November (I think) and I took it for a couple of months ... 6 mg twice a day, and it worked wonders. Then I decided to stop taking it because I get sick of popping pills, and my IBS was still very controlled. Every now and then I get pains after eating something that doesn't agree with me, and I'll get bloated and constipated, but nothing like it used to be. I went completely off of the Zelnorm after those initial months for a few months and was doing fine, and then when my IBS-C symptoms started to be bothersome, I started taking the Zelnorm again, and then I felt better again. So since November, I just take it for a little while until I start feeling better and then stop it and continue to feel fine for awhile.

Maybe it's my mindset and I've gotten over a lot of the anxiety that came with the stomach pains, the bloating, and not being able to go to the bathroom, so the IBS is a lot easier to deal with now that the Zelnorm helped so much with my symptoms.

I don't think "short-term" means that you can take it for six months and then go off of it forever. And doctors seem to have a different idea about how long you can stay on the pill. My doctor gave me a prescription good for a year the last time I was in there, and he did tell me to initially take 6 mg twice a day, but then I could take a lower dose, even once a day, if I felt a lot better.

From: **Southern California**

ITeachKids
New Member

I've been taking Zelnorm for almost two months now, and it's just begun to make a difference. I'm so surprised to hear that people get immediate results, side effects, and/or laxative-like effects! Is it normal for it to take a while to work in some people? I guess everyone's different. Sometimes even WITH the Zelnorm, I have a BM once or twice a week some weeks, and one every day other weeks. This is kind of the story in all areas of my life ... consistent inconsistency.

Thanks,
Cynthia

From: **Georgia**

Cjsm
New Member

Does Zelnorm make anyone else hungry? I was starving the whole time I took it. Also, I was only taking 1/4 of a pill and I still felt bloated after having a BM. Any suggestions?

From: **Brevard, NC, USA**

KitKat
New Member

I've been on Zelnorm since Oct 2002. It worked for me right away. I only take 6 mg in the morning every other day. If I take it more than that, it doesn't work. It makes me very hungry, but I can live with that. Zelnorm has changed my life. I can't imagine not having it. This is something I plan on taking for the rest of my life, provided it's not taken away from us.

From: **Vancouver, BC, Canada**

Zanne
New Member

I'm a 41F, I've had IBS-C for over 20 years. Primarily severe pain, distention, bloating. Through diet I've been able to control it to some extent. Bad episode recently, no matter what I put in my mouth, my gut would go into severe spasm. Dr put me on Zelnorm 6 mg twice a day. I've been on it four weeks, helped with distention, did nothing for pain. Two weeks ago went on Levbid .375 mg twice a day. Wow! The combination of these two drugs has been amazing! Of course I still have to stick to my strict diet. But this is the first Thanksgiving that I did not have a belly full of pain after dinner. Very pleased with the combo!

From: **Upstate New York**

Topic: Zelnorm side effects

NancyG
Regular Member

Has anyone taking Zelnorm had weakness and fatigue?

From: **Oak Park, Calif. USA**

Tiss
Very Prolific Member

Yep, I feel pretty tired too, but I've felt tired for years, so I don't think it's the Zelnorm (for me anyway). I have noticed that I have more racing, sort of obsessive thoughts, trying to go to sleep. My doc says it's not the Z, and I tend to be pretty obsessive about everything, so maybe it's not. If it's helping with C, I guess you have to make a decision on whether the good outweighs the bad. I'm sticking with Z at this point as it has worked well for the C (knock on wood) so far.

Tiss

From: **Mid USA**

Princesshannah
New Member

To anyone who has taken Zelnorm for the recommended time: Do you feel better now? Or does the medication just work until you stop taking it?

From: **Australia**

Sweetypie1216
New Member

Hi Princessshannah,

I've been on Zelnorm for over a month now and have noticed a change in my bowel movements—but I'm still finding that I have quite a bit of gas and bloating, along with abdominal pain. I'm going to give it another month or so to see if that goes away.

I really like that I'm going to the bathroom more—I just wish the pain would go away. Mind you, I really should be watching what I'm eating—that probably doesn't help!

From: **Ontario, Canada**

Guts for Garters
Regular Member

I find I go through different stages with this drug:

Start off on half a tablet twice a day and it works really well for a week or two. Then, the effect tails off. So, I go up to one tablet twice a day, go to toilet every day, but not like at the very beginning—stools are long and thin, and I go a few times during the day. Still bloated, despite this! Also, I start to get very tired (I'm in this phase now) as if my body is being overworked inside or somehow depleted of nutrients—like stuff is being processed too quickly. I have no energy and any stress leaves me feeling wiped out. It is unpleasant and depressing.

The trouble is if I stop the drug, or reduce the dosage, I just go back to having C, which is also depressing!

Anybody else experience a similar cycle of reaction?

From: **Switzerland**

PoohNP
New Member

I have been on Zelnorm for two and a half years, and although it involved a lot of trial and error with dosing and meals, my IBS is definitely better. I can tell a difference when I do not take it. The fatigue and headaches I initially felt when beginning it, have become a distant memory.

From: **Syracuse, NY**

Texasgirl
Regular Member

I have been taking Z for 11 months. One tablet twice a day. I have regular BMs and no pain. The bloating is still there for me, but not as bad. I have experienced the same cycle as Guts for Garters. However, the fatigue is gone.

To: Princesshannah & Sweetypie1216 …. Don't give up yet. The pain will go away. Give your body time to adjust to the medication. Give yourself a couple of more months, not just one month. Z is the best thing that ever happened to me. Hang in there, it will be worth it.

From: **Texas, USA**

Discussion: Amitiza

Amitiza was recently approved for treatment of chronic idiopathic constipation in adult men and women. This medication works by activating specific chloride channels (proteins that transport chloride) in cells lining the small intestine, with the result of an increase in fluid secretion and intestinal motility, thereby easing the passage of stools and alleviating symptoms associated with chronic constipation.

Topic: Lubiprostone Approved by the FDA

Tiss
Very Prolific Member

How does this drug differ from Zelnorm?

Tiss

From: **MidUSA**

Flux
Very Prolific Member

Zelnorm is a partial 5HT-4 agonist that works at a higher level to induce secretion of water into the intestinal lumen than this new drug, which acts directly on chloride channels to open them. Putting chloride into the lumen brings water into the gut lumen via osmosis.

Zelnorm also has direct effects on motility through its 5HT-4 agonist effect. Specifically, increases in peristalsis (frequency) in the small bowel as well as changes to motility, both increasing phasic contractions in the colon to facilitate transit.

From: **NY**

Atrain
Prolific Member

If Zelnorm also attempts to promote motility, will this new drug be less effective than Zelnorm for the people with severe chronic C?

From: **USA**

Kathleen M, Ph.D.
Very Prolific Member

There are other parts to the equation than just what it does.

What your body actually needs, how you as an individual process the drug, etc.

It is really hard to guess if drug X doesn't work as well as drug Y will.

The clinical trial data I saw summarized looked like this new drug works for a fair number of people. But I've seen no comparison studies (which normally are not done prior to approval) or information about who it worked for with which drug histories they have.

K.

From: **Somewhere over the rainbow**

3. Antidepressants, Antispasmodics, Antidiarrheals

Elavil (*amitriptyline*), Prozac (*fluoxetine*), Paxil (*paroxetine*), Lexapro (Escitalopram Oxalate), Effexor (*venlafaxine*); Bentyl/bentylol (*dicyclomine*), Levbid/Levsin (*hyoscyamine*); Imodium (*loperamide*), Lomotil (*diphenoxylate*)

Not all medications have the same effect on everyone. Side effects which are non-existent for some may be unbearable for others. Many individuals with IBS are forced to try a variety of medications to find a regimen that works best. Here is a sampling of Bulletin Board discussions regarding a variety of medications routinely prescribed for the treatment of IBS symptoms.

Discussion: Antidepressants

As the name suggests, medications of this class are generally prescribed for the treatment of depression, but may be prescribed to IBS patients due to their beneficial effect on IBS symptoms. This positive effect is thought to be due to the fact that antidepressants reduce activation of certain brain pathways during times of stress or pain. By acting on the central nervous system in this way, the sensation of pain is blunted, and other physical symptoms of IBS which are exacerbated by stress are reduced.

Topic: AMITRIPTYLINE ANYONE?

Sparkle*
Prolific Member

Hey, I've been on a baby dose of amitriptyline for nearly 18 months, 20 mg every night.

I was prescribed it after years of quite debilitating IBS, and it is the only thing (alongside diet change) that has helped ease my symptoms.

I'm 22, and have had IBS since my early teens, and imagine I will be plagued by it for the rest of my days, but I'm concerned that I'm not going to cope if/when I have to come off this medication.

Is anyone else taking amitriptyline or similar tricyclic tablets, who can offer me any advice/share their experiences? By the way, when my doctor prescribed this (as a large effort) he failed to mention it was an antidepressant ...

From: **London/Kent**

NancyCat
Very Prolific Member

I take it and it has worked well for me. The dose I take, 30 mg/day, is really small and would never help someone who needed it for depression as the dose is too low. I didn't want to even try it at first since I knew it was an antidepressant and thought that said something bad about me. I have gotten past that. In addition, I also take a low dose 20 mg of Paxil that my gastro feels will help with the anxiety and allow the Elavil to work better, as I reported that it wasn't working as well. So far I'm pleased with the results.

I can't think of a reason why you would need to stop taking it, unless you are trying to get pregnant. Whatever you decide, don't stop taking it cold turkey—you need to taper it a bit before you stop or you can get rebound pain. Hope this helps.

Nancy

From: **Massachusetts**

Susaloh
Prolific Member

Hi,

I agree with everything Nancy says. I've been taking a 25 mg slow release capsule of amitryptyline every night now for more than a year and it has made me regain some weight, fitness and a normal lifestyle. I feel brilliant now even though I still have some symptoms, I still can't eat many things and I still have to lead a very disciplined life. But I've gone back to work, and I'm so fit that I haven't had as much as a cold this winter yet.

I asked my doctors about how long I will be able to take this medication and they said basically there's no time limit. People have been known to take amitryptiline for 11 and even 30 years. Apparently it doesn't even damage your liver in such low doses.

I think I will enjoy life as it is for now, but if I feel very fit and safe, I may eventually try to wean myself off it, but I won't hesitate to take it for a long time if I have to. I understand when you're only 22 you don't particularly like the idea of taking a medication for the rest of your life, but the rest of your life is a very long time and things may change in between, or you might find out more about the reasons for your IBS—like I when I found out that I have a very strong dairy intolerance, even stronger than I thought at first, and this has been responsible for part of the problem. Good luck anyway!

From: **Kiel, Germany**

Magnolia
New Member

I've been taking Elavil for years ... probably five or more. I started at 10 mg per night and have worked up to 30 mg ... 40 mg if I'm having a bad flare-up. According to my doctor, you can take this medication for years. I did a lot of research and am not worried. The drug doesn't appear to have any long-term negative effects.

It has helped me SO much; I can't imagine NOT taking it. And, don't stop taking it to see what will happen. I've done that and the symptoms come back and sometimes are worse. Just keep taking the dosage to control it and you should be fine.

Good luck!

From: **NYC**

Topic: Does anyone take Prozac/Fluoxetine???

OldWifeyNo2
Prolific Member

Hi all,

I have been taking Fluoxetine for two weeks now. The first week was terrible, felt sick, couldn't stay out of the toilet, and kept having panic attacks!! This all seems to have calmed down now, but I still don't feel any happier. How long do these things take to kick in?? I'm only taking 20 mg per day and I am thinking of asking the doctor to up the dose! Would be great to hear stories from anyone else taking this drug. Thanks.

From: **UK**

RT
Regular Member

I have been taking Fluoxetine/Prozac for three weeks now. The jitteriness and shakes sometimes associated to it could be causing your panic attacks. It has given me almost an out-of-body or euphoric-type sensation at times, which makes me panic a little, but I was told that the side effects usually mellow out around the four-to six-week mark. I am also on the 20 mg dose. I would think if you were to ask your doctor to increase the dose for you that your symptoms might worsen. I did have a four-day period where I was practically pissing water out of my rear end. I know this sounds gross, but I can relate to your frustration of having to run to the bathroom. Your symptoms could also be related as much to the trauma

IBS attacks do to the body. I have felt run down, weak, shaky, and stressed for the last six weeks since the onset of my latest flare-up. Between the diet changes and the Prozac in for the last three weeks, I have just barely noticed an improvement over the last two days. Give it some time and keep in touch with your doctor or pharmacist. Good luck. Keep your chin up.

R.T.

From: **Portland, Oregon**

OldWifeyNo2
Prolific Member

FINALLY! I am in my third week on Prozac and everything seems to be settling down. I feel a lot better myself and my bowel is more or less behaving!! The only things I am slightly concerned about now are that my temperature is a little high and my urine is quite dark in color. I have read that a side effect of taking Prozac is flu-like symptoms which could explain the high temp, but I'm baffled with the dark urine, could this possibly be an infection of some sort? I have no pain though, other than the usual IBS pain which is settling down anyway. Any ideas?

From: **UK**

Jessica28
New Member

I have been on Prozac now for about three months and I WISH it would make me sit on the toilet, since I'm IBS-constipated!! I have had no problems at all with it. I finally have found something to ease my anxiety and allow me to sleep through the night.

From: **Phoenix**

Paul762
Regular Member

I wouldn't take this drug for anything. I am still having side effects from this drug one year after stopping it. I was given it for depression but I think it is what has caused my IBS-D, as I had no health problems before starting this drug, now I am housebound. A coincidence? I think not. The reason I don't think it is a coincidence is because I'm still having the same side effects now as I had when I started the Fluoxetine, and like I said I stopped taking them over a year ago.

From: **North West**

Gottogo
Prolific Member

I have been on this drug for about five years now. It really helps with depression.

My doctor told me that it's not a magic pill that will give instant relief.

I really have not had a lot of side effects, which surprises me since I am one who suffers from taking some meds. It comes in a patch form, too. I tried that and I started to gain weight. So I went back to taking it in pill form.

It takes about six weeks for it to really start working. Talk to your doctor about it. Hope this helps.

From: **Ohio**

Topic: Paxil

Bluesclues
New Member

Anyone had any negative side effects from taking Paxil?

From: **Nova Scotia, Canada**

Irritable_IBSqueen
Prolific Member

Yes, I had no sex drive for almost a year, so I stopped taking it. Also my IBS-D acted up again and it wasn't worth increasing the dose of that med.

Cindy

From: **MA**

Zayaka
Very Prolific Member

I had low sex drive during the first weeks and then it changed. The only long-term effect that I complain about is the weight gain. Other than that this med has given me my life back.

From: **Puerto Rico**

Jetfan20
New Member

Paxil has given me my life back. I swear by it. It worked immediately from day one on IBS-D. It has been six months since I started using Paxil, and the only problem that I have is that I put on 20 pounds because I am eating everything in sight.

David

From: **Los Angeles, CA**

MDN
Prolific Member

Is the weight gain in EVERYONE? My brother has been on it for seven years and has not gained a pound. He is in terrific shape, however, he does not take it for IBS, does that matter? I am thinking of switching to it for IBS-D, because Lexapro isn't cutting it.

Is there any way to avoid it? My diet is great, but what causes the weight gain?

THANKS!

Mike

From: **New York**

Jetfan20
New Member

I personally feel that the Paxil is not causing me to gain weight, but not having to worry about what type of food I'm eating and/or at what time of day I'm eating is the culprit. After 21 years of having IBS-D, I have been given a "Get Out of Jail Free" card. I went from a too-thin 185 pounds to 219 pounds (about 12–14 pounds heavier then my target). But I would gladly make the weight for IBS-D trade any day of my life.

David

From: **Los Angeles, CA**

MDN
Prolific Member

Jetfan—Did you try any other antidepressants for IBS-D besides Paxil? I am on Lexapro and it isn't strong enough, so we are either going with an older tricyclic antidepressant (TCA) like Elavil or Pamelar, and if not, another SSRI, which will be the Paxil.

After reading these posts, it almost makes me want to skip the TCA trial and jump onto Paxil!

From: **New York**

Jetfan20
New Member

I did try Elavil, it did nothing for my IBS-D, but it made me exhausted and zombie-like. Paxil worked on my IBS-D right away, but I did have to deal with some side effects, like sweating and waking up in the middle of the night, but the side effects went away within a month. I would definitely try Paxil, it has been a miracle for me.

From: **Los Angeles, CA**

Snickers32471
New Member

As soon as I started taking Paxil, my IBS-D when away. Before Lotronex came along, I didn't have a life. It was filled with constant bathroom anxiety to the point where I couldn't even go food shopping. When Lotronex was taken off the market, my world was shattered. I had to find something else that would help me! Finally, someone else that I worked with who had severe IBS-D suggested I try Paxil. What a miracle I thought it was!

Since trying Paxil, I have some side effects like night sweats (I'm drenched when I get up in the morning) and weight gain (25 pounds). But you know what; I'll take the weight gain and the sweating over the horrible IBS-D any day!!!!

Good Luck!!!

From: **Philadelphia**

Topic: Doc wants me to try Lexapro …

Tamgirl21
Prolific Member

… I told him no way! I went to the GI asking for something to help my IBS-D. Thank goodness I kinda know my stuff b/c I have read numerous times that a side effect of Lexapro is D, am I right? Why is it that you go to the doctor for stomach meds, they try to put you on antidepressants? Whether I am calm at home or out, I have D almost all the time! Can't they just prescribe something for that?!

From: **New York**

Kathleen M, Ph.D..
Very Prolific Member

Most of the antidepressants have BOTH constipation and diarrhea as side effects and can act very differently in different people. Any of them may work for any given person with IBS regardless of which symptoms they have (it is very idiosyncratic, and it can take working through several antidepressants to find the one that works)

Usually in IBS, what is causing the diarrhea or constipation and pain is the nerves in the gut acting up. The antidepressants balance out the nerves in the gut. Tricyclics are usually a bit more prone to constipation than diarrhea, but it is not 100% with them either.

Prescription antidiarrheals are not necessarily any more effective than Imodium. Lotronex is for IBS-D, but not all doctors did the paperwork to prescribe it.

From: **Somewhere over the rainbow**

Tiss
Very Prolific Member

I have IBS-C and I take a small amount of Lexapro (5 mg). It has not affected my IBS at all. The only thing I don't like is that I have no appetite and I've lost some weight, something that I cannot afford to do. It is the only SSRI that I've been able to tolerate. I am sleeping better and overall have less anxiety. Maybe you could try it. You could always go off of it if it makes your IBS worse.

Good luck,

Tiss

From: **Mid USA**

Chixpix
New Member

I also have only IBS-D (never constipation), and my doctor put me on Lexapro. It has worked GREAT! It helps with the pain, bloating, cramping, diarrhea, etc. The only problem is that it might be giving me INCREASED anxiety, so I am going to talk to my doc about that. Very weird! They can do different things to different people so there's no way telling how you will react until you try it out. I will tell you from my experience though, that it helped tremendously with the diarrhea. I also tried Paxil before which was also great for the IBS, but it affected my libido too much.

From: **Peoria, IL**

Karen3480
Regular Member

I was on Celexa first, which is Lexapro's cousin … the first one to two days I did have D but as your body adjusts to the medicine, things will get better. I'm on Lexapro right now, it's awesome. I no longer have cramping, and I've only had D one time in three months, I think it was because I ate something bad. My doctor is talking about stopping the medicine in December because she feels I'm fine now, I never want to go off this stuff, I've gained 15 lbs and I do believe it's from the Lexapro, but I rather be fatter than sick every day.

Karen

From: **NJ**

Zanne
New Member

I have IBS-C. This is what I am currently taking.

I take 6 mg of Zelnorm, .375 mg of Levbid, 150 mg of Wellbutrin XL and 10 mg of Lexapro in the morning before breakfast. I take 6 mg of Zelnorm and .375 mg of Levbid before dinner. I then take 20 mg of Lexapro before bed.

I don't like to take all these meds, but at the moment it appears I don't have much of a choice. And it is helping. And not being in severe pain is worth it.

From: **Upstate New York**

Topic: Effexor

Rach
New Member

My doctor prescribed Effexor for my IBS-D. I haven't taken it yet because the potential side effects and withdrawal symptoms scared me. Has anyone taken this, and if so, did it help?

From: **Ohio**

Vamplady
Regular Member

I have been on Effexor XR for a year. I was up to 75 mg.

Well, I decided to try life without meds. So I did the wean-down. If you do it SLOWLY you will have low withdrawal side effects.

However, I found that with my persistent anxiety, I needed something to keep me calm. So I went back on my Effexor at 37.5 mg and I have been here for three months now.

It to me is a good antidepressant/anti-anxiety medication. I suffer from GAD (Generalized Anxiety Disorder) and this one has had the least effects on my brain, as far as feeling tired and stupid. It also has a constipating effect and with my post-gallbladder D this helps.

Good luck!

From: **Illinois**

LyndaG
Prolific Member

I've also been on Effexor XR for about a year or so.

For me, it's been the best antidepressant I've been on. (I'd taken Luvox quite a few years ago, but there are much better ones now … then I tried Remeron … horrid experience for me.)

I say 'for me', because everyone is different, so meds don't all work the same for each person.

My doctor has told me though, that Effexor is one of, if not the most, frequently prescribed of the antidepressants.

When you first go on any antidepressant there are side effects which gradually go away after about two to three weeks … this is due to your body becoming adjusted to the drug. Then once those wane … things become pretty much normal, at least it was for me.

I'm on 75 mg, started out at 37.5 mg and worked up.

And Vamplady is right about the gradual withdrawal if you stop the meds (with your doctor's advice).

Good luck … hope you feel better soon.

Take care,

Lynda

From: **Toronto, Ontario, Canada**

Dlt647
Prolific Member

I've been taking Effexor since October 2004 and have found it quite effective. When I first started, I had horrible side effects such as panic attacks. My doctor prescribed Klonopin for several days until I got through the initial period and I have had no problems since. I am currently taking 75 mg. I suffered from anxiety and some depression and the Effexor has really helped. I no longer experience the anxiety feelings and the depression has gotten a lot better also. The only problem I have noted is some weight gain. I have started a regular exercise program which I hope will help with this. I had unfortunately gotten pretty lazy before from the anxiety/depression.

From: **Pennsylvania**

Rowe2
Very Prolific Member

I am also on Effexor, but I take the extended release form. I take 75 mg before bedtime. It has reduced my spasm pain 90%. I'm much calmer, too. I don't have to take anything else with Effexor. Good stuff. I'm very seldom constipated anymore. I still have some loose stools, but not runny D.

From: **Georgia, north of Atlanta**

Sage1979
Prolific Member

Hey, I'm a 25-year-old male and I've been taking Buspar with Ativan as needed. I don't think Buspar is as effective as I initially thought. What would Effexor do for me and my problems with D and anxiety? Would it help with those things? I have to go back to the doctors soon and am interested in this drug, thanks.

From: **East coast**

Vamplady
Regular Member

Sage1979,

One of the side effects of Effexor is constipation. Everyone is different though. It is a good medication for anxiety, post traumatic stress, general anxiety, obsessive compulsive, etc., as well as depression. The list goes on.

I found it helped a lot.

From: **Illinois**

Discussion: Antispasmodics

Topic: calling all Bentyl users ...

Diamondgirl
Prolific Member

Hello all ... long time since I've posted here. I've been having some flare-ups of my IBS-D, and rather than take Imodium on a daily basis, I went to my doc and he prescribed 10 mg of Bentyl, to be used as needed. Anyone recently used this that can give me some heads-up? I appreciate it!

From: **PA**

Christiana
Prolific Member

I take Bentyl three times a day, and I'm sorry to say that it does ZIPPO for me. I hope you have better luck with it.

From: **USA**

DirtBikJ
New Member

I used Bentyl for a short period of time. I still keep some on hand. Dosage was one every six hours, as needed. It worked great for me for about six months, but now seems like it lost its effect of controlling the spasms. Not sure, maybe my body is used to it.

From: **Utah**

Mom2One
New Member

Bentyl made me feel really loopy. I switched to Levsin and that works much better for me, plus it doesn't give me any side effects.

From: **Arizona**

Godj88
New Member

I take it! I love my "blue pills"! They make IBS more tolerable. I also take Imodium. They do make me very tired, but besides that, I love 'em!

From: **Tampa**

Diamondgirl
Prolific Member

Reporting back. Bentyl is just not cutting it for me. It seems to make me dry-mouthed and loopy in the head. Plus, it doesn't seem reliable. It seemed to work okay yesterday, no major D issues, but today, when I took it before dinner, I still had D afterwards. I think I'm giving up on this and just taking Imodium Advanced until I get to my GI doc.

From: **PA**

Kyymee
New Member

I took Bentyl for two years … at first it worked but I think I started to become "immune" to it. I was taking it every six hours. I was extremely dry mouthed … I would wake up in the morning feeling like I had swallowed a desert. After awhile … it really didn't work for me. I am now taking Lotronex one each day … it works great. Hope this helps … Kim

From: **New Hampshire**

Topic: Levsin
Missytoe18

New Member

Well, I was just diagnosed with IBS two months ago and my doctor put me on Levsin (the kind that dissolves under your tongue) It started out working fine, but things have recently went downhill with it. It doesn't help the cramping as much as it used to ... and I'm experiencing some crazy, not-so-fun side effects. After I take it, I get really dizzy and my heart rate gets faster. I feel like I'm having a panic attack or something. Is this normal? I'm wondering if I should go to the doctor again and see what he thinks because I really don't like these effects.

From: **NC, US**

Sage1979
Prolific Member

Levsin, Bentyl, basically they are useless and don't do anything to help you. I've been on both and I must say they're of no help.

From: **East coast**

Rowe2
Very Prolific Member

Couldn't do without my Levsin. I use the same kind. What mg are you taking? You might need to decrease, but it sounds like you are having a reaction to it. The only side effect it gives me is a bit of drowsiness, but it sure calms the gut.

From: **Georgia, north of Atlanta**

Missytoe18
New Member

I am taking .125 mg of it. I usually end up taking two of them ... because my cramps are horrible (one to two tablets every four hours are my dosage instructions).

I did go to my family doctor. He too, was afraid I was having a reaction to the medicine. He told me to stop taking it and visit a gastro doctor this week. So we will see soon.

From: **NC, US**

Kathleen M, Ph.D..
Very Prolific Member

Anticholinergic drugs can affect heart-rate and stuff. Taking double doses will increase the chances of these sorts of side effect. I tend to get increased blood pressure and heart rate from these types of medications.

You might try peppermint (I use Altoids) to see if it helps while waiting to see the doctor.

K.

From: **Somewhere over the rainbow**

Waldo
New Member

I began taking Levsin .125 mg, four times per day, but it made me too constipated. I've reduced to taking it twice a day, every day, and it really helps prevent diarrhea. If I eat something that disagrees with me now and have that "urgent" feeling, it comes out as a regular BM, rather than the explosive diarrhea that I had in the past (thank God!). I haven't had any other side effects, but everyone reacts differently.

From: **USA**

Discussion: Antidiarrheals

Topic: The Dichotomy of Imodium!

Cricket
New Member

Hi.

Does anyone else have a fundamental problem with the way Imodium helps IBS-D? I have!

I should say that I am IBS-D, with the major problem being urgency brought on by anxiety at (specifically) not being able to find a loo in time.

When I take Imodium, I want it to act quickly: say in two minutes! Now, I know this isn't possible, but I would have thought perhaps 30 minutes would be reasonable?

For me, Imodium takes around 24 hours before it starts doing anything. Fine, you say, then take it 24 hours before a journey or other tricky event. Well, on rare occasions I do. The reason I don't take them every day is that I don't want to be bunged up all the time. When I know that I haven't gone at all for three days, my anxiety is worse when I have to go out, since I know there is so much waiting there to come out!

Also, say I take a pill (or two) 24 hours in advance ... When I get up the next day I really want to evacuate as much turd as possible. It makes me feel better. However, I often can't, as my Imodium has started kicking in! Then, three days later, suppose I have some other stressful event—I can still barely go to the loo but I'm majorly anxious because I know I have a lot inside me that would really like to get out some point ...

I suppose I am trying to say that the point at which I am coming down off the Imodium induces more anxiety than it helped in the first place.

What I really want is a tablet I can take which acts like Imodium, but taking about five to ten minutes to start and lasting for about two hours.

My main point after all that blathering is that if your IBS is based largely on anxiety, Imodium is a double-edged sword, and one that I, for one, can't really use.

I'd be interested to hear of other peoples' thoughts on this ... Perhaps everyone who swears by Imodium would like to put the boot in!? But I'm interested how people deal with that Imodium comedown and the inevitable need to poo sooner or later!

From: **Lichfield, UK**

Shorty
Regular Member

I have been on three calcium a day for about four months, and I also take one Imodium every morning. The calcium has helped my diarrhea quite a bit, because mine is caused by anxiety mainly. I still have a BM at least every other day, even with taking one Imodium, and with the calcium my BMs are very firm. I haven't had diarrhea for a long time. I still get anxious & have anxiety at times, but the calcium is slowly getting rid of that. I think my brain is starting to have more confidence in going out and doing more things. Have you tried the calcium?

From: **Orem, UT**

Peony
Regular Member

I have the same issues with Imodium. It blocks you up for days, which is nice in a way, but bad because you don't know when it's coming or how much is coming. However, you know its coming and the anxiety that brings is terrible. I know exactly where you're coming from.

From: **Boston**

Cricket
New Member

Thanks Peony. I'm glad that someone can identify with what I'm saying. You said it so much more succinctly than me!

I find that I very rarely use Imodium because I don't want to deal with the after-effects in a few days time and because I usually need relief NOW, and Imodium just can't do that (for me).

From: **Lichfield, UK**

Jackie-G
Very Prolific Member

Wow, I can't believe this thread popped up now. My son just had a bout of diarrhea, which has never happened. He took Imodium, and now, three days later, he's having a problem with feeling like he has to go and can't, and more pain than usual. How long does it take for the effects to wear off? And what do you take for quick relief? Thanks.

From: **NJ**

Cricket
New Member

Hi. Yeah, that sounds similar to what I get after taking Imodium. I don't get that much pain, but a definite feeling of fullness.

In answer to your questions though, JackieG, I can only comment on my reactions to Imodium. I never take more than one, and then it starts working about 16—24 hours later and lasts for around 48 hours. I'm not sure what would happen if I took two or more, but I'm reluctant to give it a go.

As for quick relief, I haven't found any medication that helps for that. The only thing I can do is get to that toilet and purge!

Having said that, I find that I can accept Codeine Phosphate tablets (15 mg, my doctor said they MIGHT help with urgency/diarrhea) more easily. I can take one of these in an evening and it helps me for most of the next day and not much beyond that. Not ideal, but I prefer it to Imodium.

Hope that might be of some help.

From: **Lichfield, UK**

LotronexLover
Very Prolific Member

Try taking the Imodium in capsule form instead of tablet. I think it dissolves into your system much faster. I get mine through my doctor—$15 a bottle. It is under the name Loperamide, not Imodium, when done under the counter.

From: **Cherry Hill, NJ USA**

Topic: Lomotil?

Irritable_IBSqueen
Prolific Member

Has anyone had any luck taking Lomotil or is it just like Bentyl? The reason I ask is that my doc wrote me a script and I picked it up in case I need it. He said, it's good to take it before the onset of D, but D happens so fast. Does it do any good for the spasms and pain afterwards?

I see my GI doc on Wednesday. My Psych doc has done just about all he can do for my IBS at this point. Psych doc increased my Valium to three pills per day, so 30 mgs per day, to be spaced out, but at least the pain won't be there. Then I take a lovely 1000 mgs of Depakote ER for what my bad mood swings do to my IBS, so you can see what a mess I am.

I called the nurse at my GI doctor's office today, crying, begging to get into the office before I have to return to work, and I am fortunate to get in on Wednesday.

The nurse did advise me to take the Lomotil like my Psych doc suggested. What are you all doing, going crazy?

I'm so depressed; I'm tired of fighting this IBS.

From: **MA**

Leroy
New Member

I take Lomotil. I take it only when Loperamide (Imodium) is not doing the job. I take it to shut down "D", not before. It seems to work well.

From: **California**

3fans8
Regular Member

I take Lomotil in the morning; one is all I need for all day. Been on them for 20 years. Then I got worse, felt I had to use the restroom all the time, was only okay if I was at home. Suffered like that for over a year. Had a colonoscopy done, it was fine, then went back to the doc, was tired of living that way. Well, it was depression. Was put on Paxil, best thing that could ever happen. Except I've gained weight. (Going to try Wellbutrin to see if it will work and I can lose weight). My doc says IBS and depression go hand in hand. I thought he was nuts, But I feel better.

Good Luck!

From: **IN**

4. SIBO (small intestine bacterial overgrowth) specific

Xifaxin (rifaximin), Neomycin

New research has focused on an overgrowth of bacteria in the small intestine to be a cause of IBS symptoms. This research opens the possibility of new treatments for IBS, namely using specific antibiotics to reduce the overgrowth and thereby provide symptom relief.

Topic: A New IBS Solution by Dr. Mark Pimentel

Jeffrey Roberts
Member #1
Founder

A New IBS Solution, Mark Pimentel, M.D. Health Point Press, January 2006.

Rating: Five Stars—This book merits your attention. It could likely explain the cause for your symptoms.

Dr. Mark Pimentel is the Director of the Gastrointestinal Motility Program at Cedars-Sinai Medical Center in Los Angeles, California. The purpose for writing this book was to declare a unifying hypothesis for the cause of IBS. Numerous research studies performed by Dr. Pimentel, and duplicated by many centers world-wide, point to an overgrowth of bacteria as being the missing link which explains the symptoms felt by 10–20% of the population. He does an admirable job at explaining the background for this new theory, along with treatment options. After reading this book you are more than likely going to want to discuss its findings with your own physician.

From: **Toronto, Ontario, Canada**

Topic: About to Start Rifaximin ... ... should I???

Daisysweetpea
New Member

I was about to start the protocol, but haven't read the book. Been following some of the discussion online here and have been talking to my doc about it. I have IBS-D, but that's been self-created because I hated being IBS-C ... now I don't know if I should take Neomycin or Rifaximin or both????? Please someone give me some informed opinions about this? I certainly do feel better being on antibiotics, but yes, in the past the symptoms have returned once I am off them. I do take probiotics, but they seem to bloat me. Fiber causes too much bloat and gas. What feels best? Not eating????!!!!

Daisysp

From: **USA**

SpAsMaN*
Very Prolific Member

You should get a breath test for lactulose. If you are methane producer, I would go with Neomycin, especially if you feel constipated.

From: **Quebec, Canada**

Daisysweetpea
New Member

I have my doc prescribing me both Neomycin and Rifaximin ... not sure which one to take though. Wasn't able to get a breath test done; we don't have one locally and it's not covered on my insurance.

I know the protocol for the Rifaximin, but what is the protocol (i.e. mg and dosage) for the Neomycin?

Also, wasn't there a part of the original protocol that maybe considered using one or both of these for a year to kill all possible? Done of course, with a regimen of probiotics also? Ugghh, any help would be great, I want to start, but don't want to waste time or money. I have insurance for a very limited amount of time right now, and these are very expensive items!

Daisysp

From: **USA**

Fberry1916
New Member

How did you find the protocol for Rifaxamin?

I would get a great smokies test (comprehensive stool analysis) to see if you have an infection that could be causing your symptoms & let that guide your antibiotic choice. It has been well worth the money for me. I spent tons of money fighting my yeast infection with Nystatin, when my yeast was resistant to Nystatin & sensitive to Diflucan.

My real problem (& possibly yours) is lack of normal flora, & taking the wrong antibiotic can make you worse off than you are now.

My current problem is Citrobacter freundii, which is why I'm asking about the Rifaximin.

Thanks!

From: **USA**

Daisysweetpea
New Member

Thanks for your feedback. I am in an odd situation, working with my primary care doc instead of the gastro doc as he was such a horse's private part! My regular doc said he'd go ahead and prescribe me what I wanted to try; I am doing as much asking as I can. I am also on a very limited time line with how long I will have insurance to cover all this ... ... to tell the truth, I feel better on any and all antibiotics! I have had four bladder infections in the last four years and two incidences of having teeth worked on that required antibiotics ... not all were the same (mostly sulfa for my bladder though) ... feel good while on them, then I back it up with acidophilus.

Anyhoo, checked today about getting Neomycin added to the Riflaximin protocol and can't get it approved till the 20th (doc is on vacation!). So, either I go ahead and try the Riflaximin or wait ... dang it!! It's been nine years, maybe I ought to be patient, but I don't think any one of us is with finding the crux of our issue.

Daisysp

From: **USA**

JenEbean
Prolific Member

Daisy,

I have been on the Rifaximin for about two months now. It has cut down on the frequency of the diarrhea, but not cut it out completely. I had the breath test which was positive. Next month I start on Cipro the first week of the month, nothing the second week, Rifaximin the third week, and nothing the fourth. My

GI said I am pretty resistant to getting rid of the overgrowth, so I will alternate the two antibiotics until I see the new GI in April. My GI is moving ... waaaaa I loved her. My advice is to go ahead and try the Rifaximin, I have had absolutely no side effects from it at all.

From: **USA**

Topic: Why I Am Going Through Antibiotic Treatment

Surfboar
Prolific Member

About four years ago, I was in a bad stretch and had dropped about 20% of my body weight. I looked like a skeleton. I hurt 24/7 and even had exploratory laparoscopic surgery (which found nothing of course). I didn't want to do anything except curl up in a ball. My doctor was beside himself trying to help but was not really up to speed on IBS.

He suggested a psychologist (waste of time) and seeing a urologist. The urologist found a prostate infection and while he said that wouldn't be causing all of my symptoms, I should treat it. So he put me on a three month course of antibiotics ... ... Doxycycline in my case. Anyways, I started feeling better all over and regained all of my weight and the IBS symptoms stopped completely after eight years of this terror. It was almost a year of bliss before the IBS came back.

The point is that after meeting Dr. Pimentel in Los Angeles and participating in one of his breath analysis studies for diagnosed IBS patients, I began to see the connection between bacteria and IBS. I actually chatted with him for about 15 minutes and related my experience with the treatment for the prostate infection. He told me that he hears that constantly from his patients that their IBS symptoms improved during periods of taking antibiotics for other ailments.

I know that there are people here that attribute their problems to antibiotics, and I can see the connection between a previous episode of antibiotics causing the initial problem. In my case, I think I picked up food poisoning somewhere and that was my initial trigger.

This past summer, I showed my doctor the breath test results from my participation in the clinical trial and he decided to try me on Flagyl. I did three 10 day courses of Flagyl and each time, the IBS went away completely, but would come back a few days later. What I think was lacking was the follow up treatment with Zelnorm or some other pro-motility agent that would restore the wave functions of the small intestine. Without that, the normal bacteria in the colon was somehow backing up or refluxing into the small intestine and recolonizing it.

I have since moved from SoCal to Florida and am now taking Neomycin as suggested by Dr. Pimentel in his book. I am on day 5 and I already feel so much better. This time though, I will start on Zelnorm after I finish the Neomycin. It will be a low dosage, 2—3 mg at night before going to bed to restore the small intestine cleansing wave function and to avoid the contents of the colon from backing up and messing up the small intestine again.

I honestly believe that IBS will go the way of ulcers after the medical community finally accepted that H-Pylori was the cause and not stress. IBS will be routinely diagnosed from a small intestinal bacterial overgrowth and treated successfully with gastro-specific antibiotics such as Rifaximin and Neomycin. There is, of course, the underlying condition that allows SIBO to happen and that may be the role of Zelnorm or other drugs that promote the wave function of the small intestine. Perhaps there is an underlying anatomical reason that some people are prone to SIBO while others don't have the problem. Or perhaps the SIBO was caused by exposure to a nasty bug that took up residence in the small intestine.

You don't have to agree with my theory, but I think everyone would agree that lactulose breath testing should be part of the battery of tests that doctors should be using when dealing with IBS patients. It is a hell of a lot easier and less expensive than colonoscopies.

Good luck to everyone, I have faith that we will all beat this and it will be sooner rather than later!!!!!!!

From: **Tampa**

5. Probiotics

Align (Bifidobacterium infantis 35624), Digestive Advantage
IBS, VSL#3

Probiotics are dietary supplements that contain helpful bacteria. These "friendly" bacteria appear to aid the intestinal tract in maintaining a healthier bacterial balance and thereby reduce IBS symptoms.

Topic: Probiotics

Terrig
Regular Member

I know that there have been many discussions on this, but I don't have the energy to go searching for them, sorry!

I am being treated with Paxil & Metamucil now, would like to get off the Paxil due to side effects, but am not willing to go back to the daily IBS problems.

Has anyone had success with probiotics? I am IBS C/D and very annoyed because I am going through a bad IBS spell right now!

Thanks.

Terri

From: **Pennysylvania**

Kathleen M, Ph.D..
Very Prolific Member

Success varies, but some people get good results.

A fairly new brand, Digestive Advantage IBS, seems to work for a good percentage of people and may be worth checking out.

Other brands people seem to like:

Culturelle, VSL#3, Jarrodophilus, and PB8 are what come off the top of my head.

The quality of the supplements varies across the spectrum of them, and some people need to try a couple of brands to find one that works well for them.

K.

From: **Somewhere over the rainbow**

Lagomorph
Regular Member

I have read the many posts on probiotics and I have decided to try them out, along with the continual use of calcium carbonate for my IBS-D. I'm on day two—we'll see what happens. I am on a lactose-free version, but I'm not feeling too confident about the product. I may try another brand or I've also read that some people have tried yoghurt (with the proper bacteria) with much success.

From: **Canada**

Talissa
Very Prolific Member

Like Kath said, DA IBS has helped some people, including myself. I am taking much more expensive ones now as well, with no noticeable difference like I had w/the much less expensive DA IBS. (Am probably wasting my $$$ on the others). DA IBS enabled me to eat fructose again … w/the exception of anything with high fructose corn syrup. But that's OK, who needs the processed junk anyways?? Hope you find what works for you.

Talissa

From: **Nevis, Eastern Caribbean**

Topic: Bifantis—Proctor and Gamble Align

Funny Gutz
New Member

I have been seeing some changes during the last few days, but I won't jump to the conclusion that they are solely the result of my probiotic concoction. I want to see the changes persist and hopefully improve how I feel. In the spirit of that I've decided to continue my probiotic supplementation for a minimum of three months, and even try some VSL#3 in the mix.

There is one difference I think is due to the probiotics. Things are a bit smellier than usual, if you get my meaning.

Specific observations follow for those that are interested.

My cramps are still around and as urgent and painful as ever, but my residual pain level is a bit better. I'm going to the bathroom almost as much, but I was doing well on that front since I just got over an IBD flare from October. I may have less urgency first thing in the morning, but I'm not entirely sure if this is a fluke. Movements seem to be more productive, less liquid. And I'm passing more gas; I almost want to say a lot more.

The changes so far aren't all that helpful (if they are even attributable to the probiotics) but they could be a stepping stone to better health overall, so I have no problem sticking with it.

From: **USA**

TriciaB
New Member

I have been taking Align for three weeks now. I have IBS with constipation switching to loose stools. I can let you know this has been a wonderful three weeks. I feel like a normal person, it's something I will not go without.

Tricia

From: **Wisconsin**

DireWeeYah
Prolific Member

It has been two weeks since the first dose. I don't want to give unwarranted hope with such a short time-period but this is working for me. Your mileage may differ.

After five days, stools were still loose, but urgency that day and since then have been WAY decreased. For the past few days, stools have alternated from "somewhat loose" to "Lincoln-log beautiful." In fact, for the holiday, I went to visit my folks by car 330 miles away. THIS IS A FIRST: I didn't even stop once for any kind of break on the way there! That was awesome.

After over-indulging on turkey and the fixings, I didn't have to go that whole night—that was a bit surprising to me. The next day, after eating way too much delicious Greek fast-food, I did have a semi-urgent need to use the potty. It wasn't one of those "uh oh, I better drive 100MPH to the nearest market restroom" but I will still classify it as urgent nonetheless. However, no D. That has been the only urgent episode so far.

I drove back on Saturday and only stopped one time and that was to pee. What a reversal!

So far the most significant positives are way less urgency (my biggest symptom) and less frequency. I have not experienced any negative effect from the product.

Again, this is just one man's account. Until I have had at least two months experience on this product with consistent decrease in my IBS symptoms, I am not going to give the blanket thumbs-up yet. Unless something extra good or bad happens before then, expect another report from me in about two weeks or so.

—John

From: **Las Vegas, NV**

Stomachio
New Member

I started taking Align about a week ago and can report some good news. For the first four days I was sticking with Imodium, but when the weekend came I stopped the Imodium and didn't have any problems. In fact, my stomach felt so normal that I didn't even notice it at all—which is only weird because its been a long time that I've had that feeling (or lack thereof).

Went to work on Monday, ate at some restaurants that usually upset the stomach, and had no problems. So thus far I am cautiously optimistic. It has only been six or seven days.

I think I may be noticing that I am more thirsty than normal. Also, though D is apparently gone, now I am closer to C. No pain or anything like that, but I'm only going to the bathroom in the morning and it a bit of struggle to get everything out. Well, I'd rather that than urgency … but we'll see if things adjust as my system gets used to the stuff.

In general I feel much better, and so much so that I am already walking out of the house without taking the stuff, and only when I'm halfway to the car remember and have to run back.

Also curious about the interaction of Align and alcohol. Will have to test this in the future.

S.

From: **USA**

Wornout
Regular Member

Today is my tenth day on Align. I had three or four good days starting on about the fourth day, the improvement being a diminished amount of gas and bloating. But yesterday, I had gut pain all day which culminated in D in the evening. So, it's a wash, so far.

From: **Oakland**

SteveE
Very Prolific Member

I'm now on my 15th day of Align. I've had two days that I'd rate myself as feeling pretty bad (today happens to be one) and the other was the day after Thanksgiving. I haven't noticed any days where I feel substantially improved yet. However, there are three important things to remember at this stage:

1. The package says it can take six weeks to really see improvement and some of their alleged testimonials indicate this as well.

2. My eating habits have been a bit abnormal recently with the holidays happening.

3. My wife seems to think that the two days out of the 15 that I complained about feeling pretty bad didn't *seem* bad from her perspective. In other words, she's seen me look a great deal worse and wonders if the Align may be minimizing symptoms that would be quite a bit worse had I not been taking it.

She may have a point. Today, for example, I did have some gas, felt bloated, had two urgent trips to the bathroom, but the cramping was not as bad as I'd expect given these other symptoms and I didn't feel chills or light-headed or any of the other stuff that sometimes goes along with a major attack. The trouble is, there's really no way to know what those days would've been like without Align.

What I do know is that it's clearly not harming me in any way, so I guess I'll continue to take it for at least eight weeks and see what happens.

Best wishes,
Steve

From: **Illinois**

Topic: Digestive Advantage

Feisty
Very Prolific Member

Has anyone tried Digestive Advantage? Did it work for your constipation, gas, and bloating?

From: **USA**

RailFan
Regular Member

I just started on it this week. For me, it's worked WONDERS ... so far. I've got IBS-C, and I'm still taking Levbid/Hyoscyamine once daily. (The pharmacist said it was OK to take DA and Hyoscyamine together.) I still take psyllium fiber every few days, too. DA has greatly reduced my C, as well as gas buildup and bloating. I'm feeling better than I've felt in the last several months!

What I am still unsure about is whether or not DA is safe long-term.

From: **Kansas**

Tiss
Very Prolific Member

How many do you take and do you take it AM or PM? Also, are you strictly C?

From: **Mid USA**

RailFan
Regular Member

Hey, Tiss!

Yeah, I'm pretty much strictly C. I'm following the dosages recommended on the package. They tell you to take two chewable tablets the first and second days, then one tablet daily after that. I take the DA in the mid- to late afternoon. I'm blown away by how fast it kicked in! I felt a difference the very first day, and I don't feel like I've lost any ground having gone down to the single tablet dose.

From: **Kansas**

Tiss
Very Prolific Member

I took my first two tablets last night and I had LESS gas today. I started Lexapro last week (5 mg) and it was upsetting my stomach and causing horrible gas, but today I was better and I think it was because of the Digestive Advantage.

From: **Mid USA**

TypeO
Regular Member

Hi guys, can you explain exactly what this does? I've looked it up on the internet and it said it's for lactose intolerance, is that right? So if a person doesn't eat much dairy is it worth their while to try this? I'm at a loss here with deciding to try it or not. I am strictly C and don't eat much dairy at all. The results you are telling about are great, I hope it keeps working for you all.

From: **USA**

RailFan
Regular Member

I am feeling like I've had a setback of some sort. The tabs worked great all this past week, but today (the fifth), I'm back to feeling the way I was. Then again, my stress level is increasing, too. I may try increasing to two tablets to see what happens.

I'm still worried about whether or not this product causes dependency, and the web site doesn't address that. Does anyone know?

From: **Kansas**

Kathleen M, Ph.D.
Very Prolific Member

I think there are two products: the Lactase enzyme one and the DA-IBS which has probiotic bacteria.

Um ... there is nothing about either probiotic bacteria or lactase enzyme that would cause dependency. Neither is a stimulatory laxative or drug with addiction potential. Now if it helps you and you stop it, things may go back to how they were.

Probiotic bacteria often do not colonize people that permanently, so if the bacteria help you, it may require taking them fairly regularly to maintain the effect.

K.

From: **Somewhere over the rainbow**

Tiss
Very Prolific Member

I wonder if good yogurt does the same thing as a probiotic since it is bacteria. Or is yogurt considered a probiotic?? I am confused!

From: **Mid USA**

Kathleen M, Ph.D.
Very Prolific Member

The bacteria in yogurt are often the same kind you get in probiotics. The best way with yogurt to make sure you have live bacteria is to make your own.

Basically you take some plain yogurt with live cultures in it, add it to warm milk (most people heat the milk to near boiling to kill off any bacteria that are in it—let it cool to lukewarm after heating it, so you don't kill the bacteria in the yogurt) keep it in a warm area for a while (usually in the oven with a pilot light on or turn the oven to warm, then turn it off and put the yogurt in there)

After a few hours it thickens up and you can save some of it for the next batch (you may need to restart every so often if it get contaminated or loses potency).

Basically if you make it yourself and eat it fresh you know the bacteria are alive and well.

K.

From: **Somewhere over the rainbow**

6. Over the Counter (OTC): Fiber Supplements, Alternative Medicine

Benefiber (partially hydrolyzed guar gum), Citrucel (methylcellulose), Equalactin (*calcium polycarbophil*) Metamucil/ Perdiem/Prodiem (psyllium);
Calcium;
Peppermint Oil

Discussion: Fiber Supplements

Topic: Fiber Supplement—Psyllium!!

Hdog
Prolific Member

I have had Gastro problems for many years. It has been my experience that with the current modern diet we eat, we just don't get enough fiber in our diets, and I think that has been well documented. I have found that supplementing your diet with a psyllium product is just a good healthy thing to do. It is a water-soluble fiber—a bulk stool-forming agent and it's safe to take daily. I have found it works as well for diarrhea as it does for constipation!!! Psyllium does break down intestinal bacteria, and generally does produce some gas when you first start using it, but the gas will go away as your system gets use to it.

Your GI tract has to have some form of FIBER for it to properly function. If you don't get it in your diet then you have to get it somewhere else.

Any better ideas???

Hdog

From: **Charleston, SC**

JenS
New Member

I like FiberCon tablets. Two each morning when I wake up, with a full glass of water.

From: **Florida**

Vikee
Very Prolific Member

I have found that Metamucil works well too, but produces too much daily stool volume, which needs to be eliminated daily or it gets too wide. It must have to do with my intestines and age. I'm 59. This didn't happen years ago with Metamucil.

I have found that two caplets of Citrucel, two times a day, with lots of water works much better. The Citrucel powder produced sticky-ish stools. Probably was caused by the other ingredients or something else. It (Citrucel Powder) may work now, but I'm not ready to experiment because the caplets and water work! Not perfectly and not all the time, then again, nothing does!

From: **PA, USA**

Jeanine
New Member

Hi All,

I'm new to this forum but had to mention what I use for fiber—Perdium. This stuff is great. It's weird to take, but you get used to the little pellets that you swallow with a full glass of water. Once or twice a day and I stay regular—somewhat. It's not as gassy as Citrucel or Metamucil.

From: **Maryland**

Topic: Benefiber

Dc2002
Regular Member

I am a male suffering from IBS-C for more than two years. I have been taking the generic brand of Metamucil for the last one and a half years and it has worked great. However, in the past four months, it really is starting to slack off. I'm frequently becoming constipated while taking 3 tsp/day each day at same time. I often feel the urge to go around the time I take it, often wondering to myself if I'm really gonna go or not.

I'm considering changing over to another fiber supplement. My question is which one works the best for IBS-C? I've read good things about Benefiber and Citrucel both. I need a powder fiber that will allow me to 'go' closer to the time I take it, and more comfortably, too. Also, to go daily instead of one or two times per week when I've got C. One last thing. Looking for the fiber which keeps urgency to a minimum during the course of the day. (I currently take it at 3:00 PM. because that's when I get home from school). Anyone want to share their comments on the best fiber?

From: **Steelers Country/USA**

Tiss
Very Prolific Member

I like Benefiber the best and I've tried them all I think.

I am IBS-C only, and it helps with the constipation. Also, it does not give me any gas like Metamucil did.

Have not tried the tablets but I use 1 tablespoon in the a.m. and 1 tablespoon in the eve. I use the powder. You can use more if needed.

From: **Mid USA**

Teach
Prolific Member

Will that dose give you the runs? I usually get so gassy from the others. Does Benefiber do this?

From: **PA**

Popp
Prolific Member

Fiber works both ways. If you're loose, it will help firm it up. And if you're constipated, it will soften stool to pass it.

From: **USA**

Topic: Citrucel or Metamucil? Which one?

Kimmie
Prolific Member

I was wondering if there is a difference. I know Citrucel has methylcellulose and Metamucil has psyllium husk. Do they work the same or is one better than the other? Thanks for your input!

From: **Ohio**

Kac123
Prolific Member

Hi Kimmie,

Citrucel was much, much better for me than Metamucil. Metamucil, being psyllium, is a fermentable fiber and causes bloating and gas—and for me lots of discomfort. Citrucel is made from a non-fermentable fiber, so there is no bloating and I've never been uncomfortable from it (in fact, taking it when my stomach did hurt a little usually helps things).

Everyone is different though and finding the right fiber for your body takes a little trial and error. Just remember no matter what type you use that you drink lots of water—fiber without water does nothing.

Hope you are feeling well today!

Kac

From: **Philadelphia**

Maxson
Regular Member

I've just started taking fiber for the past five days or so and I can't believe what a difference it has made for me. I haven't had to take any meds at all since I've started using it. I am using Benefiber from the makers of Ex-lax. It is all natural and the pharmacist recommended it. It has no taste whatsoever, which is amazing. You can sprinkle it on any food or beverage you want. It is sugar-free, grit-free, and non-thickening. I highly recommend it. Now, my problem has been IBS-D and it has totally controlled my problem. I assume it would also help if you have IBS-C. Give it a try! Thanks for the tip on drinking extra water, I haven't been doing that, I will start!

From: **Illinois**

Kimmie
Prolific Member

I'm IBS-D also and my doctor put me on a new medicine for my PCOS and it has made my D even worse! It is supposed to get better, but anyway she told me to start taking fiber and I want the best one that won't make my problem even worse. Thanks for any advice.

From: **Ohio**

LaurieAnn
Prolific Member

If it is any consolation I take Citrucel and have had no problems with it yet. I also have PCOS. One of the ways I know it's flaring up is when my hands look dirty. (PCOS causes skin pigmentation changes for those of you not familiar with the wonderful syndrome.) My hands started getting dirty yesterday and today they look splotchy like I have been rubbing them with newspaper. Oh, but that's not what this is about. The End. With the Citrucel I have found that it's not gassy, doesn't send me to the toilet all the time (I had never taken a fiber supplement before so this is a first for me and I was s-c-a-r-e-d!) and I have actually felt a little better each day. So I'm rooting for Citrucel and wishing you the best of luck.

From: **Illinois**

Robbin
Regular Member

I have been taking Citrucel for two weeks and it has been helping with BM's and not gassy like with Metamucil. My question is this: I started taking a minimal dose. About 1/4 scoop of the clear mix powder in 8 oz of juice, and I was having a BM every day. I did this for a few days and then went to the full dose, one scoop in the same 8 oz of liquid, and then I didn't go every day anymore, I almost felt constipated again. Label says to take one level scoop in at least 8 oz of liquid. Is it possible that 8 oz of liquid is not enough with the full dose? Maybe I need to adjust the powder/water ratio. How much water or other liquid is actually necessary. Is it possible to cause constipation if not drinking enough liquid with it? Wouldn't a full dose work better then 1/4 of the dose? Thanks!

From: **New Jersey**

Kac123
Prolific Member

Robbin,

From my experience, the more water you can drink the better off you are. My doctor told me that I should have two liters of water as my MINIMUM intake and do what I could to go over it—and I try to do that … I feel like I'm floating around most of the time, but its better than the pain!

Also, the amount of fiber you body needs from supplements may vary—I've been taking Citrucel for two years now and very rarely to I take more than 2 or 3 capsules of it, which is nowhere near the normal dose. If I go over that, my body doesn't respond as well to it.

So, the short version—keep experimenting with the fiber/water—you'll find out what works for you.

From: **Philadelphia**

Topic: Equalactin question?

LucieS
New Member

My doctor told me to take Equalactin to help with my IBS-D, but when I got it home and read the package, it says it is a laxative. That is the last thing I need right now. Does anyone know if this works and if I should try it?

Help!!!

From: **California**

Kathleen M, Ph.D..
Very Prolific Member

Fiber generally gets labeled a laxative, but soluble fiber is not a stimulatory laxative.

It regulates the amount of water in the stool.

Thus it can be used for either IBS. In IBS-C it holds water in the stool; in IBS-D it absorbs the excess water.

They call it Equalactin because is should equalize the water in the stool. For those that it works for, of course.

K.

From: **Somewhere over the rainbow**

Spasmodic and proud
New Member

I like Equalactin. I'm an IBS-A and it works a little for everything.

For me, it takes a couple doses to start working (over the course of 24 hours or so), but when it does, it is a relief. I've been taking it in conjunction with my anti-spasm drugs, which tend to make me a little constipated.

Good luck!

From: **Wisconsin**

Topic: Metamucil

Kjzg
New Member

I've been using Metamucil two times per day for almost one year. I started after a terrible attack of spasm/bloating/constipation/diarrhea. It took me a few weeks to get used to the Metamucil, and since then I have not had any problems! (Thank God!)

My question is this ....

I've contemplated trying to switch to Fibercon Caps. They just seem a bit more convenient. Does anybody have an opinion on this?

Has anybody ever "switched"?

What kind of results did you get?

Looking forward to your answers!

Thanks!

From: **USA**

Frostbite
Prolific Member

I've never tried the Fibercon Caps. In fact I just started back using Metamucil last week. I wished I'd stuck to the Metamucil when I was first diagnosed. I always remember the old saying 'If it ain't broke, why fix it?' In other words, if Metamucil is working so well for you, why change?

Did you know that Metamucil is available in wafers? They are a lot more convenient, but I wasn't very impressed. They stuck to my teeth and you still need to consume a glass or more of liquid. If you do try the Fibercon, please post what you think of it.

From: **Canada**

Islandsue2002
New Member

Years ago I learned that Metamucil and Fibercon are almost the same thing, but Fibercon is so much more convenient to take, so I don't take Metamucil anymore. Just this month my gastroenterologist put me on Citrucel, which although a synthetic fiber, is supposed to be better than Fibercon for constipation. He also has me on Lactulose. I am getting some relief, but not from the bloating or gas pains. Not yet, but hopeful.

From: **Chicago**

Marym
New Member

I switched from Metamucil to Fiberchoice. I like Fiberchoice better because of the convenience. Those chewy tablets stick to the teeth though. And the gas is about the same. I never could take Citrucel; it didn't do a thing for my problems of C and D.

From: **Kansas**

Sue Baker
New Member

Seems to me that taking a fiber supplement alone is not where we all need to look for our answers.

Fiber supplements are designed to assist with regularity and firming up stools (for D sufferers) and softening them (for C sufferers). In themselves, they will not eliminate what triggers your IBS. Other associated problems need to be investigated, e.g. intolerances to food chemicals, imbalances (acidic foods). Look beyond your fiber supplements for the answers to gas, pain, bloating, etc.

I have found a returning normalcy, by using Metamucil and discovering my food chemical triggers. I no longer eat tomatoes, citrus, or other acidic foods. It's just not worth it! Of course, I take vitamin supplements to counter their loss. And I eat plenty of other "safe" veggies. Keep working hard to discover your triggers—don't rely on quick fixes. Living with IBS is hard-work!

From: **Australia**

Cloverleaf
Prolific Member

Just a note to remember: Fibercon and other calcium polycarbophil fibers have less fiber per dosage. So you may in fact have to take six Fibercon to get the same dosage of one tablespoon of Metamucil. I find it's not really effective for my constipation.

Docs should not be telling anyone that any fiber is better than others. You should try to find what works for you. Everyone reacts differently to fiber, although it seems that most people find that they get the most bloating and gas from Metamucil.

Perdiem is a good alternative to Metamucil, because it is psyllium fiber but you don't dissolve it in water. It makes me feel much less bloated and gassy and seems more effective. Another added benefit is that one tablespoon has four grams of fiber.

Citrucel is methylcellulose, and it makes many feel less gassy. On the other hand, one tablespoon is only two grams of fiber, compared to three with Metamucil, so that may be one reason why people feel better on it. I find it's not particularly effective, but I use it every couple of days to mix up my fiber supplements.

The key is to find what works for you, and to understand how much fiber you get with each dose. Lots of tablet-type fibers have only .5 to 1 gram of fiber. You'll have to take more of them.

From: **Wisconsin**

Discussion: Calcium

Topic: My Calcium Success!!

Mdbiggs
New Member

Just had to share with you all that Caltrate has helped me in ways that I could not have imagined! I feel like a NORMAL person again. I have been taking half a pill 3X a day and after the first dose I have only had one D attack (due to my own overindulgence) and I feel great. No longer scared to go places and I even went to a concert and enjoyed myself. Just had to share and hope that many more people in the future find relief from this simple remedy.

Melissa~ who is for now D free!!!!

From: **USA**

Shawn Herron
New Member

Yep, that's been my experience as well. Calcium has, quite simply, worked wonders! I have an occasional "spell," but absolutely nothing like what I used to have, and even then, I can usually attribute it to something in particular.

My doctor is fascinated by it, and has recommended it to several other people to try.

I don't take Caltrate; I take a Walgreen's equivalent, by the way, without magnesium.

From: **Louisville, KY**

MarkinCA
Regular Member

If you have D, it's important to avoid magnesium at all costs.

Last year I tried one form of Caltrate for weeks without any effect. A few days ago I tried the most basic Caltrate 600, without ANY extra ingredients, not even Vitamin D (which by aiding the absorption of calcium may be leaving less to do its job in the gut). The benefit was almost immediate.

If you have severe D, you may not have to worry about getting C, and the things that might cause C in normal people, may not cause it in someone with IBS-D. I WANT something to be a little C as a way of counteracting the D. Therefore I'm taking the calcium without the added magnesium, and I think that's what's making the difference.

So far I'm taking six a day—two tablets, three times a day—which is a lot. But if it continues to help, I'll try taking less to see if the benefit holds.

Mark

From: **USA**

LNAPE
Very Prolific Member

Thank you all for posting your successes. We are all a bit different and what form helps one may not be the best for another. At least you took the time to try it and not give up so quickly if it did not help right away and tried a different form until you came up with the right dose.

There are a lot of variables to taking the calcium. If you take other meds, even OTC stuff, they can affect the way it works.

Taking a regular dose every day is a must. Taking it with food also is necessary. I had diarrhea almost every day for 23 years and I still need the calcium with the small amount of magnesium to keep me on track. Now if I take my dose too close together, the magnesium will have an effect so I watch for that.

Other brands work also, not just the Caltrate, but I always mention that one because it can be found most places. You can compare labels and get the store version of Caltrate Brand.

Continued success, and maybe someday a study, will conclude that calcium does help and it will be made known to the many suffers who now do not know.

Linda

From: **Hamilton, OH, USA**

MarkinCA
Regular Member

I regret to report that the burst of enthusiasm I had recently has evaporated. After a few days of apparent success, the benefit I thought I was getting from the calcium just stopped, and things went back to how they were before. Oh, well ….

Mark

From: **USA**

LNAPE
Very Prolific Member

Mark,

Do not give up, even normal people have times when they get diarrhea from a bug or bad food.

When you had an attack this time, was it as bad and as long as it used to be? Try to stay with it and hopefully you will feel better again. This does happen from time to time.

Linda

From: **Hamilton, OH, USA**

Twocups424
Prolific Member

I also tried the calcium to no avail. Hey everybody, try it though. Everyone is different and it may just work for you. I think that calcium soaks up excess stomach acid but not bile; at least that is what my Doctor told me. He said that aluminum works better to soak up bile (which is a major cause of irritation to the bowel if you have too much) without magnesium, of course. I use AlternaGel. It helps to a degree.

From: **PA**

Marianne
Very Prolific Member

When Linda posted her success story on this board I tried the Caltrate Plus. It takes six tablets a day to control my diarrhea. But the WONDERFUL thing is that the Caltrate Plus does control it. I have one bowel movement a day, right after I eat breakfast. If I forget the Caltrate Plus, I am in trouble again. I have been taking C+ successfully for almost three years now. I use the CVS or Walgreen generic. Walgreen gets very high ratings for the integrity of their generic products.

I also eat three slices of Branola Bread "The Original" every day. This bread has a lot of soluble fiber, and I believe it soaks up the extra fluid in my gut and bulks up the stool.

Linda, I've told you before how grateful I am to you, but I don't think I can ever say it enough. What a difference you made in my life.

From: **New York, New York**

Kristian
Very Prolific Member

Hello to Linda and all:

I've also been having great success with Caltrate. Taking half with lunch and half with dinner. I haven't had one episode of D since I started.

I'm home sick from work today with a cold. How wonderful to be home from work and have it not be because of IBS! Crazy, huh? To those who are still suffering, have you tried upping the dose? Linda has been really great at sorting this stuff out with people who need help.

I'm going to see my boyfriend's parents for the first time next month and I think I may be able to eat like a normal person for once ...

From: **New York City**

Discussion: Peppermint Oil

Topic: Try Peppermint Oil!

Ltlt
New Member

About a year ago, after being sick non-stop for months and losing a lot of weight, I was finally diagnosed with IBS-D. The doctor gave me Bentyl, which helped if I took it BEFORE I ate, and then didn't mind missing the rest of the day sleeping. Not a good alternative! I started researching and kept seeing the recommendation to take Peppermint Oil. IT WORKED FOR ME!! I took the capsules religiously three times a day, and carried the pure oil in case of emergencies (a drop on my tongue gave instant relief). One word of caution—while I was sick, I completely gave up alcohol. After a while on Peppermint Oil, I felt much better and resumed things like coffee and a drink now and then. Turned out that, at least for me, Peppermint Oil and alcohol don't mix—I got hives (luckily painless) all over my face and neck. The really happy ending is that, after some lifestyle changes (job stuff), I've been one of the lucky ones where the symptoms have subsided for the most part. I still get flare-ups, but the peppermint oil still works. I hope this helps somebody, I'll never forget what it was like ….

From: TX

Rick UK
New Member

It works for me too. It also stops butt-burn, as it cools everything down.

WELL WORTH trying.

RICK

From: **Merseyside UK**

Spoon
New Member

I tried peppermint oil, turned me out completely, and I was sicker for a couple of days.

They do say that some people's bowels can't take peppermint oil.

From: **New Zealand**

Coping the best I can
New Member

Where do you the peppermint oil that everyone is talking about? And does it come in capsule also?

From: **Virden IL**

Gasgirl
Very Prolific Member

Coping,

You can get peppermint oil capsules at health food stores, just be sure you get the enteric coated ones or else they will give you heartburn. If you have GERD, peppermint oil might not be a good idea.

I tried them, but they didn't help me, and burned coming out the other end.

From: **Cambridge, Massachusetts**

PeacefulHart
Prolific Member

I opt for organic peppermint tea because I can control the strength of the peppermint, which for me is very important. Too much causes me problems. I've obtained some very good relief by using peppermint tea occasionally.

From: **USA**

Forum VII: <u>Cognitive Behavioral Therapy and Hypnotherapy</u>

"Use this forum to discuss Cognitive Behavioral Therapy (CBT) as a coping treatment for IBS, and/or associated Anxiety or Depression, and Hypnotherapy as a coping treatment for IBS."

Numerous research studies have found two forms of psychotherapy to be effective in treating IBS symptoms—Cognitive Behavioral Therapy (CBT) and Hypnotherapy (HT). These treatments provide a reduction in IBS symptoms without the side effects that can result from taking medication. This forum offers a place for members to learn about the benefits of these therapies and to share their experiences, questions and concerns.

<u>Discussion</u>: Cognitive Behavioral Therapy (CBT)

Cognitive Behavioral Therapy (CBT) is a form of talk therapy that helps people to change unhealthy ways of thinking and unhealthy ways of behaving so that they feel better. Cognitive strategies include calming self-talk, identifying and modifying irrational beliefs, and the use of distraction. Behavioral strategies include assertiveness, progressive muscle relaxation, and biofeedback. CBT has been shown to be an effective treatment for a variety of disorders, including IBS, depression, and anxiety.

For the IBS patient, CBT focuses on teaching techniques to reduce overall and anticipatory anxiety, strategies for reducing excessive attention and vigilance for symptoms, and ways of challenging irrational thoughts that contribute to excessive emotionality and exacerbate physical symptoms.

The following series of posts offers a selection of discussions regarding irrational thoughts that are commonly experienced by IBS patients. For each thought, members responded with suggestions for healthier, more helpful ways of thinking. You can incorporate their responses into your own ways of thinking about yourself and the disorder. This will help you to keep your body calmer and reduce the stress on your digestive system.

Topic: Irrational Thought of the Week

BBolen Ph.D
Prolific Member

One of the main tenets of Cognitive Behavioral Therapy is that how a person feels is directly related to what a person is thinking. As we all know, we don't always think reasonably and rationally. Our thoughts can be distorted by our emotions, our past experiences, lack of information, etc. When we think in a distorted manner, we are likely to experience emotions that are overblown or unnecessary. CBT helps people to identify, challenge and replace thinking errors, thus reducing excessive, unhealthy emotionality. This helps a person to handle situations more calmly and effectively.

Dealing with a disruptive physical disorder such as IBS can be stressful (how's that for an understatement?). As emotions are stirred up by the disorder, thinking errors are common. As a new feature to this forum, Eric and I thought that it might be helpful to post a common irrational thought each week, and ask board members to challenge the validity of the thought and replace it with a healthier, more rational thought. This replacement thought can then be used as what we CB therapists call "calming self-talk".

If anyone wants to add an irrational thought to the list, just let us know.

So, here is the first irrational thought:

"I am only assured of feeling well if I stay close to home."

From: **Farmingdale, NY USA**

Br-549
Very Prolific Member

Dr. Bolen, I agree with your statements completely and would be glad to participate in this program.

My instant thought on your suggested irrational thought is an old saying that goes "Home is where the heart is". To me that means peace and happiness comes from internal and not external. We can be happy and secure anywhere we go if we believe so. We can also be insecure and miserable in our own home if that's the decision we make.

From: **The Hills**

AZmom1
Very Prolific Member

"I am only assured of feeling well if I stay close to home."

NEW:

"I may not be 'assured' of feeling well as I go farther from home, but I know it is healthy for me to practice doing it." Each time I go out of my area of comfort, I feel proud of my accomplishment, and know that each time I do it, it becomes easier and easier.

AZ

From: **Scottsdale, Arizona USA**

Kathleen M, Ph.D..
Very Prolific Member

I'd think about several things:

Is it really true that I never have IBS when I am at home?

Or is it just easier to deal with when I am at home so having an attack at home isn't as scary/potentially embarrassing.

I'd think of the times when I did go out of the house and nothing bad happened, or that something bad happened only because I was so worried about it happening. (The "if I hadn't been so worried I would have been OK").

I'd remember that most places have restrooms and that most people will let me use it if I need it (as everyone's had a GI illness at one time or another and can sympathize with the "I need to go now!"s).

Also, I'd plan ahead so I was prepared for a problem if it did happen. This way I could handle it easily (like have clean undies and baby wipes handy). Prove to myself that I can handle things if the worst were to happen.

K.

From: **Somewhere over the rainbow**

Shyra
Very Prolific Member

Dear Dr. Bolen,

You and Eric have come up with a GREAT idea! Being in CBT myself, this is what my therapist and I are working on, so to be able to practice changing these thoughts right here on the board will be great practice for me. Sometimes I have a hard time changing the irrational thoughts. I'll change them to something that I think is rational, she'll repeat it back to me, and it's still not that rational. And yes, she refers to these thoughts as 'cognitive errors'. I work better with the "What if" statements, so in the same context as the above;

"What if I don't feel well if I go far from home?"

Instead of answering a negative question with a negative answer I find it helpful to answer a negative question with a positive question;

"What if I DO feel well while I'm away from home?"

The answer to that would be: I would feel more confident the next time I travel far from home based on my past positive experience. I hope those were okay! If there are any changes or improvements I can make to those statements I'd be open to opinions. Thanks.

From: **Calga ry, AB Canada**

BQ
Very Prolific Member

"I'm only assured of feeling well if I stay close to home."

New: "I'm never assured of feeling well Anywhere! I choose to go out & live as if I will feel well & prepare for the times I may not feel well. No one is assured 100% of the time that they will feel well if they are away from home. Everyone gets sick. I am better off than others because I will be prepared for that eventuality if it occurs.

Plus I know where most public restrooms are!"

BQ

From: **USA**

Katrinca
New Member

I love this idea!

"I am only assured of feeling well if I stay close to home."

To dispute this irrational thought, I would try and remember that there's no reason why I can't use public restrooms when I'm away from my house. Almost all places have a restroom, they may not be my ideal potty spot, but when it comes down to it, there will be a place to go if need be.

Also, if I limit myself to only going out to places close to my house, am I doing it to avoid being sick while out or am I doing it to avoid the anxiety that I have when I do go out?

From: **Portland, OR USA**

Eric
Very Prolific Member

The anxiety of staying home I believe sometimes adds to the symptoms.

I have also noticed once you go somewhere and get involved and distracted, at least for me, I am not thinking about my IBS. Yes, there are some times where it may get you no matter what, but I think you feel better on the whole when you push yourself to do things and have accomplishments, small or large.

From: **Portland OR USA**

BBolen Ph.D
Prolific Member

Excellent responses! Each of you has offered helpful replacement thoughts that can be internalized by others.

Avoidance of scary things only reduces anxiety in the short run. Each time you avoid facing something; anxiety rises in relationship to that thing. The best way to reduce the anxiety is to face your fears, take small steps, and walk through it. Each time a feared thing is faced; there is a reduction in the associated anxiety.

Restricting yourself to staying home also can contribute to depression, as you are depriving yourself of social contact, pleasurable activities, and as some of you pointed out, the feeling of pride in your accomplishments.

Good work one and all.

From: **Farmingdale, NY USA**

Topic: Irrational Thought—Week 2

BBolen Ph.D
Prolific Member

I have to keep scanning my body (or stool) for symptoms or signs, because maybe there is something more seriously wrong with me.

From: **Farmingdale, NY USA**

BQ
Very Prolific Member

"I have to keep scanning my body (or stool) for symptoms & signs, because maybe there is something more seriously wrong with me."

Replace with: "I have to keep on trusting my doctors & test results, because I don't have a medical degree."

BQ

From: **USA**

Katrinca
New Member

I would replace this one with:

I may have my problems with this condition, but for the most part I'm a healthy person. I may feel bad today, but that doesn't mean there is something seriously wrong with me. Even people without IBS get an attack of D or C every once in a while. Every little ache or stomach cramp I feel isn't necessarily related to my condition. Healthy people sometimes feel nauseated or achy. It's normal to feel sick once in a while.

However, as a disclaimer I'd like to add, that you should talk to your doctor about symptoms that are severe and/or long lasting. I'm not advocating not going to the doctor when you're sick, I'm just trying to help people determine when they are really sick or just interpreting normal sensations as signs of illness.

From: **Portland, OR USA**

Steve
Very Prolific Member

I find this to be a difficult one to change, too. I think in my case, being raised by a registered nurse might have a little something to do with it. Another tricky aspect for this too is that you're encouraged to keep the symptom diaries and look at possible associations with food and stress. When you engage in those activities, it is hard to break the habit and not continue thinking about your problem until you arrive at a "solution."

Maybe there is a better way, but I've used the approach I found Burstall's book about IBS where you explain to yourself that pain can be divided into two groups—the kind that just hurts and the kind that harms. IBS is the former, not the latter. The hurt in IBS does not equal harm.

From: **Illinois**

Eric
Very Prolific Member

This was a tough one for me also—I now no longer do this. I have become more aware of my body's signs of any impending IBS problem since I did the hypnosis.

I would have to say if there are any new physical symptoms I would have them checked out, otherwise due to all the tests I have had, I know I have classic IBS.

After thirty one years of it, if it was something else, it would have gotten me by now, I believe.

From: **Portland OR USA**

Boesie
New Member

I would say:
Since all the tests from different doctors are saying there's nothing physically wrong with me, then it's probably true.

Best regards,

Peter …
(C&D type)

From: **USA**

AZmom1
Very Prolific Member

I would try to under-react to keep the thoughts from spiraling out of control and into panic.

"It's just IBS. I've had all of the tests done, and I know that IBS is not life-threatening. I'm doing what I can to learn how to cope with my symptoms. It's a matter of trying different things to find some strategies that work."

AZ

From: **Scottsdale, Arizona USA**

Eric
Very Prolific Member

AZ, hit a big part of this on the nose with, "thoughts from spiraling out of control and into panic." I think almost every IBSer does this to certain degrees and some of it is not even noticeable to the person. Some of it, I believe, are also unconscious thoughts, as well as conscious ones.

I have seen this myself in almost every IBSer, including myself and it's a big part of the "vicious cycle".

It is a huge problem that I believe all IBSers would be helped by if they recognize it and take measures towards it.

From: **Portland OR USA**

Kathleen M, Ph.D..
Very Prolific Member

Most people have some aches and pains and symptoms on a regular basis, so it is unlikely that every symptom is a sign of something seriously wrong.

And:

I have had my symptoms checked out by the doctor and all the test results indicate that nothing serious is going on.

Also:

I can choose to focus on what is bothering me or what is not bothering me. Focusing on the symptoms gives them my time and energy and keeps me from focusing on the things that are doing well and giving those things my time and energy.

K.

From: **Somewhere over the rainbow**

Collie
New Member

I must keep myself physically challenged (whether it is walking, cleaning, or just moving) and mentally busy with constructive thoughts and deeds!

This keeps my mind, needlessly, off my body.

I've come a long way and hope I can someday feel this way without medication.

From: USA

Ewink
Prolific Member

Gosh, this is one I've been trying to work on, but boy is it tough! Yeah, my doc says it's just IBS, but what if … I think deep down in my brain (the part that can think rationally) I do realize it is only IBS, nothing serious or more harmful. It's just these unconscious thoughts.

At this point I just try to distract that little devil by keeping my mind busy with other things, either working, practicing (I'm a musician), being online, read, go for walks, listen to beautiful music, do relaxation exercises, and recently, listen to Mike's tapes. I seem to be getting a bit better at it slowly.

Best,

Edith

From: **CA USA**

BBolen Ph.D
Prolific Member

Excellent responses. It is interesting how difficult this thought is to replace. I think it has to do with a kind of post-traumatic vigilance that occurs. If a person has been traumatized, their mind scans for cues to the trauma. Unfortunately, in IBS, this vigilance backfires because it can set off the body's alarm system and thus set off symptoms. So instead of checking, scanning, and saying "uh oh", it is much better to work to remain calm and relaxed (using muscle relaxation, deep breathing, distraction, calming self-talk, meditation) sending the message to your body that it is okay to turn off the alarm system.

Your suggestions are so helpful to others, keep up the good work!

From: **Farmingdale, NY USA**

Topic: Irrational Thought—Week 3

BBolen Ph.D
Prolific Member

What if I am out with other people, and I need to keep running to the bathroom? What will they think of me?

From: **Farmingdale, NY USA**

Boesie
New Member

I say:

"I've explained my condition to all my friends and they don't even notice any more how often I go to the toilet. For those that don't know my condition, I'll explain it to them later ..."

Peter ...
(C&D type)

From: **USA**

BQ
Very Prolific Member

Sorry, I'm probably either too old or too "healthy" to care what people say about my frequency of bathroom trips. Anyone I'm out with (when I **get** out) knows I've got IBS. And to be honest I really don't care what others think of me. I'm just happy to be out!!!

BQ

From: USA

Eric
Very Prolific Member

I don't think people pay as much attention to it as we seem to think they do. If they notice, well for me I probably had too much beer if I am out, but also most of my friends know I have IBS.

From: **Portland OR USA**

Ewink
Prolific Member

I don't get that thought very often, but if it would happen, I'd just think, they're probably too busy having fun or thinking their own thoughts to even notice. Everybody goes to the bathroom. I usually don't have the problem of having to go all the time during the day anyway, only in the morning, and usually only once. Only at the beginning of a D flare-up do I spend about 90% of my time in the bathroom, but then I'm so sick, that the remaining time I'm in bed!

Edith

From: **CA, USA**

Sherree
Prolific Member

I used to be very concerned about such thoughts, but no more. My friends all know and are very understanding. Once I realized this, I could relax. I'm much more concerned about actually getting to the bathroom!

From: **Keizer, Oregon USA**

Lilymaid
Very Prolific Member

I just worry about throwing up in front of people, or "What if I carpool and then I feel terrible and have to go home? Will I be able to get home? Will people be mad at me if they have to leave early?" I'm beyond the "won't people look at me" etc. train of thought because I don't care if people see me walk to the bathroom (or run, as the case may be) and I'm quite open about my condition with family, friends, and even acquaintances (if they ask).

Regards, Lilymaid

From: **CA, USA**

Topic: Irrational Thought #4

BBolen Ph.D
Prolific Member

If I am having symptoms, it must be something that I ate. I should avoid this food in the future.

From: **Farmingdale, NY USA**

BQ
Very Prolific Member

Ok Doc, looking back at what I ate is usually where I "go" first. But here I think "first" is the operative word. Because I don't stop there, then I look at my stress management over the last few days, have I been walking through the days with that inner engine running on high rev or with my shoulders around my ears, where I'm sure my Creator never meant them to be? Have I exercised? Made time for myself? Have I "practiced" (hypnotherapy, that is)?

I still think my tendency is to look at me, not my CNS or neurotransmitters/receptors. I used to just look at the food I had eaten & say it was my own fault for eating that & then avoid that food. Which obviously led to more & more food avoidance, which led to a real restrictive diet, which led to under-eating which led me to feeling like ****, which eventually made me desperate enough to visit this Forum.

The rest is history.

I try hard not to "blame" myself anymore, but old thought habits die hard. But I'm trying. Thanks for asking this even though it made me feel uncomfortable to even think about it. Obviously I got work to do.

BQ

From: **USA**

AZmom1
Very Prolific Member

"I have a digestive tract disorder caused by a problem with gut motility. All food and drink will start the digestive process, which can lead to symptoms. It's important that I eat a healthy, well-rounded diet, and approach my IBS symptoms from many sides, including medications, diet, exercise, and stress management/relaxation techniques."

I agree with BQ, that our symptoms could lead us to stop eating properly. There are times when we're having a flare-up that any food will cause symptoms. Obviously some foods are worse than others and should be avoided during a flare-up.

AZ

From: **Scottsdale, Arizona USA**

Kathleen M, Ph.D..
Very Prolific Member

IBS waxes and wanes, and food is not the only thing that sets IBS off.

I may be just having a bad IBS day and any food would set things off.

I should test this food again when my IBS is settled down to see if it really is a trigger food, or I just happened to eat it on a day that anything would trigger symptoms.

Eating a healthy, well balanced diet is important for my overall health. Eating poorly is not likely to make the IBS go away and could cause other problems. Eating so my health is good overall may help me cope with my IBS better. A healthy person can tolerate more things than a sickly person can.

K.

From: **Somewhere over the rainbow**

Ewink
Prolific Member

I am glad you posted this one Dr. Bolen, as I had some questions/thoughts reading this in your book.

While I absolutely, completely, do agree that food is not the only symptom trigger, and certainly not ALWAYS the cause for symptoms, for me, I think that fats are causing problems right now (except for fatty fish). During all the years I have suffered from IBS, I have tested and retested this, and it never misses. Also dietary fiber, e.g. from veggies, fruits and whole wheat. When I am mostly C, I do well on those, but when I am D-type, I have to be very careful or stay away from them when it gets too bad. I have never done any medical tests to confirm this. I do realize that this makes my diet pretty restricted, and that that's not really good.

The way I've been going about it is, in the beginning, when the D was really bad, I got rid of those triggers in my diet, and as I am slowly getting better (with supplements), I am slowly reintroducing little bits of those foods. Is this not the right way to go? I have been improving, slowly but steadily over the last three months or so (when the D flare started), and have been gaining some of the lost weight back as well.

Thanks,

Edith

From: **CA, USA**

SteveE
Very Prolific Member

Yeah, this is one we all struggle with. I'd like to use K's replacement thoughts as an example, because I really like the one she said about testing this food again when my IBS is settled down, but I have a hard time swallowing that this thing almost randomly waxes and wanes. I mean SOMETHING must be responsible for the waxing and waning. I guess I'm perfectly willing to admit that food doesn't need to be the cause, but there has to be a cause, right? Examples of other causes might be: poor sleep or too much activity right after a meal thus interfering with the smooth operation of digestion.

On the other hand, we don't want to ignore the possibility that food is involved, do we? I am 100% certain that a certain symptom that I used to experience has been almost 100% cleared up by avoiding products containing corn sweeteners. If I hadn't kept track of that, I might still be suffering with that one today. Of course, one could argue that corn sweeteners are in no way part of a healthy diet, I guess.

But aren't there numerous other people on the board who have discovered that they are actually celiac or have problems with sorbitol or lactose?

An observation here too—I think when dealing with family/friends/coworkers, who sometimes understand IBS to an even lesser extent than we do, often use this "something you ate" line of reasoning to satisfy themselves. When enough people do that to you, it is hard to ignore, but we must remember that it is based on a lack of understanding.

From: **Illinois**

Kathleen M, Ph.D..
Very Prolific Member

There are definitely times when a particular food or food additive is the suspect, which is why sometimes it takes a bit of testing to see if that was the problem or just random IBS fluctuations or other triggers. The "it did me in today so I'll never eat that again" can get you in trouble (that's the quick and dirty "magical think-ing" that works much of the time, but not all of the time, and if you are a human being you use "magical thinking", it works pretty well, but it isn't good to rely on it 100%) but tracking that food asking: Did it bother me when my IBS was doing pretty good, or while I was already in the middle of a flare-up? Does it bother me each time I eat it, or only sometimes? Does the amount of it I eat make a difference? Does eliminating it for a couple of weeks make any difference in my symptoms? These are the sorts of things that help distinguish food triggers from coincidences.

It's a delicate balancing act and you can err either way, being too cavalier about food and not bothering to avoid problems (although some people, with some foods, feel that the enjoyment of the food is worth the problems it causes—thus the "eat a chili cheese dog at the ballpark and pray there are no red lights on the way home" LOL) and the other side is becoming too fearful of food so that one eats very little and doesn't get enough calories or nutrients to sustain health. For some people some of the symptoms they are having (particularly weakness, fatigue, weight loss etc) may be signs of malnourishment or mis-nourishment rather than the IBS.

After all, the Survivor series has shown that eating nothing but a bit of rice most days makes you tired, weak, lose weight, and have diarrhea when you eat normal food. And in all likelihood they didn't cast all IBSers.

K.

From: **Somewhere over the rainbow**

Lilymaid
Very Prolific Member

I even get freaked out thinking that I might get food poisoning from particular foods. Or even a stomach virus. When my digestive system acts up, I think, "Ugh ... what did I eat? How do I know it's not a virus? How can I tell it's not just IBS? What if it's appendicitis?"

On the food poisoning tip, I'm pretty much suspicious of anything I eat (except for rice, rice cakes, bananas, etc.). And I avoid things that will really set me off IBS-wise. If I know that stewed tomatoes are going to keep me up all night, I'm not going to eat them. No amount of yoga and positive thinking is going to help that. Just trying to stay calm through the ordeal might—but avoiding the ordeal is a much bigger timesaver for me.

I can't think of a more positive way to think of this. If my stomach acts up, it's because I'm nervous, I'm hungry, I ate too much, I drank juice, I ate something non-IBS friendly, I have a stomach virus, I'm pregnant. Those could be the reasons—that's it!!

As for avoiding ... I know that there are so many confounding factors. I could have some grapes and be okay one day, but not on another day. If I really like the food, I'm going to eat it and take a chance.

Regards,

Lilymaid

From: **CA, USA**

Topic: Irrational Thought #5

BBolen Ph.D
Prolific Member

I can't commit to anything. What if I get sick?

From: **Farmingdale, NY USA**

Kathleen M, Ph.D..
Very Prolific Member

What if I am well?

If I am too sick that day I can renegotiate the commitment so that I can take care of my health and have it work for everyone involved.

People understand and I won't be the first, the last, or the only person to have to break or renegotiate because I am sick. After all normal people get sick and can't make it to things.

I know how to control my IBS well enough that, even if I am having a bad day, I can function well enough to go.

K.

From: **Somewhere over the rainbow**

BQ
Very Prolific Member

I can commit to most things. But since I have a definite monthly flare-up & I'm new at this hypno thing, I may have to skip just the most stressful or emotionally charged situations at that time. (And I hope to be able to manage the IBS even better in the future.) But currently, for 75% of the time I can commit & not worry about the IBS because I can manage most situations very well.

BQ

From: **USA**

Sherree
Prolific Member

What if I go nuts?

I CANNOT let this condition ruin my life. I WILL go enjoy and make commitments. I will continue to try and manage the IBS as best as I can. Most of the time I am OK, and on those occasions when I am not, I'll either lay low, or if I'm out, I'll do what I have to do and know that most people can be understanding.

From: **Keizer, Oregon USA**

Eric
Very Prolific Member

The statement itself is negative and hence if I think it, it will cause a negative response in my symptoms.

Better: The more committed I am to understanding and managing my IBS and feeling better, the more committed and free I am to do anything.

From: **Portland OR USA**

MaryBeth
Regular Member

If I am sick, I am sick. I cannot eliminate my IBS—I have to accept that I have this illness. Like other people having heart disease or migraines, there is nothing I can do about it. I will participate as much as I can and take care of myself when needed. I will not feel guilty for being sick with my illness.

From: **Cary, NC, USA**

Topic: Irrational Guilty Thoughts

Clair
Very Prolific Member

I was wondering if anyone else seems to suffer from irrational guilty thoughts when their IBS prevents them from being able to do normal things.

Although hypnotherapy has helped me tremendously, when I go through a bad patch with my IBS—I feel terribly selfish and guilty for taking time off work to try and relax and get well. I feel like a fraud or a cheat, although I know other people would have no qualms about having that time off. Even my doctor is extremely supportive.

I perceive that whether it is real or not I'm being pressured to just live with the pain and deal with it and carry on as normal.

Through my current bad patch, my doctor has been extremely supportive and signed me off for a couple of days to catch up on sleep and try to relax. I must call him tomorrow and let him know if I need more time or whether I'll return to work. I feel really pressured that I MUST be well tomorrow and that I MUST go back to work whatever.

I feel that is what is expected of me—and if I don't do it I'm being a failure and letting everyone down.

Is this common to IBS? And if so, how can I learn to deal with it without turning myself into a quivering wreck?

Any advice/experiences would be useful,

Clair

From: **York UK**

BQ
Very Prolific Member

Clair, I imagine anyone with a chronic illness (especially when one doesn't always 'look' sick) feels this kind of guilt. I know the guilt of which you speak. I struggle with it all the time. I push the negative thoughts out & try to see if I can manage whatever I'm asked to do. Sometimes I can handle it & other times I can't. I know there is value in just not thinking about it & forging ahead. But at times, my physical limitations come up & there is no denying I am not up to the task. This is part of the acceptance of it, I suppose. I don't like it, but then again, so? I can't all of a sudden NOT have IBS can I?

I have found guilt in general, is a waste of my time & emotion. But it is there at times, no denying that either. I'm not perfect, BOY am I not perfect. I have no idea what my future holds. I'm currently a stay-at-home Mom. I have no idea if I can work out of the house & maintain home & hearth & be healthy at the same time. Today, if I was a betting woman, I'd be looking for better odds, if you know what I mean. Right now I dunno how I could work outside the home; I have enough trouble just getting myself to the school to volunteer once in a while. I mean with the amount of days lately that I don't feel well, I'd fire me. I wish I could be more helpful, Clair. I wish I knew the answer. But perhaps someone else can help. Sometimes the guilt doesn't seem all that irrational to me.

BQ

From: **USA**

Shyra
Very Prolific Member

Hi Clair,

Thank you so much for bringing this up. I don't know if I can help you either, but I can say that I can completely relate.

I've lost a few friendships because I'm always bailing out of plans at the last minute.

At this time though, anyone I have any kind of relationship with knows about all my problems (IBS and anxiety). Sometimes I feel extremely foolish when I change plans or just pull out altogether. It does make me feel guilty that's for sure. But just like BQ said, feeling guilt is a waste of energy. Guilt really doesn't serve any purpose except to make you feel bad about something that, for the most part, you have no control over. I've heard plenty of times, "If you're sick, you're sick". There's not much more you can do about it except rest yourself and try to get better.

I just started a new job and have already called in sick once. I've got an advantage there in that my boss is an old friend of my sister who has known of my IBS for years. He'd come visit us out camping and we'd go 4x4-ing and I'd bring the TP with me "just in case". So he knows I'm not making it all up when I tell him I'm not feeling well. At least with that it takes away the stress of thinking I'd lose my job for taking so many sick days.

I can't even count how many times I've been plagued by that feeling of letting others down. Particularly my boyfriend. This may sound sad, but sometimes it surprises me that he's stuck around this long. He's the kind of person that needs to get out, whereas I'm more of a homebody. Lord knows how many times I've turned a weekend that was supposed to be fun and sociable into us ending up sitting at home and watching movies because I'm not feeling well. So along with feeling like I'm letting others down, I also feel like I'm cheating others out of a good time or doing what they want to do.

And of course then I get worried about what other people think (another waste of energy but I'm working on it). I did have a friend who had the nerve to tell me once that I was just being lazy and she was sick and tired of me making "excuses" for not wanting to go out. I think that has stuck in my head and I wonder who else thinks the same thing about me. But again, I have no control over what others think of me.

Sorry if this was a little longwinded but I'm glad you brought it up. This is something that constantly lingers in the back of mind, especially when plans come up in advance—I can NEVER make a commitment. IBS has definitely taken its toll on my social life. I used to go out with friends three or four nights of the week. These days I see my friends once every couple of weeks, if that, and the rest of the time I spend either at home or at my boyfriend's house.

So you're not alone at all in feeling this way. I guess the best thing you can do is take each day at a time. You know what's best for you and over-working yourself or pushing yourself to do too much is only going to cause problems in the long run.

Take good care of yourself.

From: **Calgary, AB Canada**

Maedchen
Prolific Member

Ah, another "SO, I'm not the ONLY one" kind of post.

Clair—I can relate to how you are feeling, and to comments that both BQ and Shrya have made. I just wish I could offer some pearls of wisdom to help all of us. Unfortunately, I am a not too successful, rehabilitating workaholic. I credit most of the aforementioned thoughts to contributing to the IBS. And Shyra's comments about her boyfriend, I have felt that way about my husband. Why, I could have written that paragraph! But they stick with us, heaven only knows why, so there must be something good about us.

You asked if this was common to IBS. I'm not sure, but I have a sneaking suspicion that it is part of the whole IBS/anxiety/depression package. You stated "I feel that is what is expected of me—and if I don't do it I'm being a failure and letting everyone down". I think this is a common comment made by "us" at one time or another. I know I have felt it. In my case, I recognize it as part of the trap of perfectionism. Unlike BQ, I am still having problems accepting the fact that I am not perfect. I should be, why aren't I?! You also commented on feeling like a "fraud or a cheat" though knowing other people would not have qualms about taking off the time. Who is pressuring you to go back to work? Your boss? Your co-workers? Or that steely-eyed guilt demon named YOU? Isn't funny how we can allow others the time off we wouldn't allow ourselves? If your situation were reversed, would you be thinking "oh C is out sick again" or "gee, I hope C is feeling better soon"? Why do we beat ourselves up like this, when we are so understanding of others?

Is there any way you can bring home work with you? That may be defeating the purpose of the time off, but it may help alleviate some of the guilt. At least you will feel like you were contributing still, instead of "being lax"

Now, I'm not sure if this is relative or not, but this thought did occur to me. During the last few years I was still working at my job, when I would find myself getting particularly tense about something needing to be done vs. say, going home or not being about to do anything about the situation; I found myself asking (to myself) the phrase "is it a matter of life or death?" I had taken a course a few years back describing our various international sites (a diversity course). In the section on our site in Israel, the instructor mentioned that the engineers would sometimes say this to each other in meetings when things were getting out of perspective. Considering who said it and where this was being said, it put a different spin on the statement. When I would say it to myself later, I would at the very least stop the onslaught of panicky thoughts and reassess the situation. Things most often would not be a matter of life or death, but it helped me to put things into perspective. I could then ask "Will this matter five years from now? Five days? Tomorrow? If not, go home."

Somehow, someway, we need to learn how to allow ourselves the permission we give everyone else to be imperfect—to be sick, to say no, to make mistakes. If I figure out how, I'll let you know. You do the same, right?! In the meantime, remember, perception is relative and as we all know we can choose our friends but we can't choose our relatives.

From: **Southwest USA**

Clair
Very Prolific Member

It was such a relief reading all your posts … made me feel a little bit more human again.

My IBS seems to be cyclic and when I have a flare-up, I also battle against insomnia and the guilty thought patterns.

Its nice to know I'm not alone struggling with it … I know what I'm thinking when this happens is not rational or productive … but sometimes its difficult to fight, particularly if you have been a perfectionist all your life.

When I go through a good period, I go back to being happy-go-lucky again and I don't worry about the IBS and feeling guilty.

I made myself get up and go to work on Monday and just forcing myself to do that and to concentrate on something else than the flare-up seems to have helped me back into "normality" again.

Next time I get a flare-up I know I'll be straight back to feeling guilty for not having total control over my body … but I guess you're right—feeling guilty is not productive and I have to somehow learn to get over it.

Thanks for all being there for me, you're the greatest.

Clair

From: **York UK**

BBolen Ph.D
Prolific Member

This BB continues to impress me with how hard people work to get better, and how hard people try to make others feel better. This thread is a wonderful example of that. Clair has given us a treasure trove of irrational thoughts, thoughts that are very universal. Before I list these thoughts, I just want to recommend the book "Sick and Tired of Feeling Sick and Tired". It is a good self-help book for dealing with chronic illness.

Here are some irrational thoughts leading to unnecessary guilt. You have already provided some excellent challenges in this thread.

1. It is wrong for me to take time off from work to get well.
2. Other people have more serious illnesses; I am a fraud to be complaining.
3. I should just live with the pain and carry on.
4. I am a failure if I don't do what is expected of me.
5. I am a bad person if I cancel plans because I am feeling sick.

From: **Farmingdale, NY USA**

Clair
Very Prolific Member

Dr Bolen,

I'm sure I've got plenty of IBS related irrational treasures hidden away just waiting to pop out—let me know if you ever run out!

From: **York UK**

Topic: Irrational Thought #6

BBolen Ph.D
Prolific Member

Please take a moment to read the "Irrational Guilty Thoughts". Clair was nice enough to share what she experiences and this provides good material for all.

"It's wrong of me to take time off from work to get well."

From: **Farmingdale**, NY USA

Kathleen M, Ph.D..
Very Prolific Member

That one is tough for me because I come from a family where, for the most part, if you're not in the hospital or throwing-up, you go to school/work (maybe a result of Mom and Dad growing up on homestead farms where the farm animals and crops don't care how sick you are. If you don't feed/milk/plant/weed/clean up after/etc. there will be some major consequences).

My brother has had "interventions" at work when all his co-workers en masse demand that he go home and take a sick day.

That and having had allergies most of my life, if I waited until I felt well to go to work, I never would.

That being said …

What I have found that works for me is that if I take a sick day I get well faster.

So the choice becomes a matter of go to work and be sick for many days or stay home and be sick for one or two days. This at least gets me home for the acute things and the worst of the chronic things.

Also I know that people at work do not want to share in my illnesses. So if it is something infectious, I can usually use the "why get everyone else sick" idea.

K.

From: **Somewhere over the rainbow**

Jane93
Very Prolific Member

This one is tough as I feel guilty taking time off for IBS, because many people think I'm a slacker since IBS is invisible. If it made my skin red and blotchy, I'd feel better about taking time off sick ... even if I didn't feel as bad as I can do now.

The way I have solved this one is that if I'm not too sick I can work at home and my boss is OK with that. I still get the guilt and many who don't know me think I'm a slacker for not sitting in the same spot for 40 hours a week. Little do they know that some people in my office watch TV (yes TV) all day or surf the web.

From: **San Jose, USA**

Clair
Very Prolific Member

This is my toughie ... but I'm trying to work on it.

Like K, I do find that taking a few extra days off does help to get me better faster, and the extra rest helps me become a happier and more productive employee when I return.

So a happy, healthy, and rested employee is a more effective employee than a tired, stressed, unwell employee.

The main crux of this irrational thought is worrying what other people think of you having time off sick ... particularly in an environment where people do not understand how debilitating IBS can be. In my life, this is fueled by personnel staff in my department not believing I have anything wrong, despite the dozens of hospital letters, tests and letters from my doctor to the contrary. I'm trying hard to become less sensitive about what people think … but it is difficult especially if you have always been a perfectionist … *sigh*

Clair

From: **York UK**

MaryBeth
Regular Member

Kmottus, I can completely relate to your story about your parents and not being able to be sick! My parents were the exact same way: I wasn't sick unless I had a fever and if I had a fever, I took an aspirin and went to school anyways! UGH! Even today, I have a hard time just letting myself be sick, thanks to that upbringing.

Clair, I could empathize with your post too. My own FAMILY doesn't even understand what I have to deal with with IBS so I am sure my friends and people at work don't have a clue. Developing a thicker skin is what I have had to do too. It isn't easy, but I found that worrying too much about what other people think of me and my illness would get me all tightened up and I would have an attack … no fun! The way I figure it, I am a very good and conscientious worker and if I need time off to tend to my IBS, I do it. My sick days rarely affect my work to a degree where my boss takes issue. We have people in our office that goof off most of the day too. Guess that just makes me look better … ha ha ha.

Mary Beth

From: **Cary, NC, USA**

Topic: Irrational Thought #7

BBolen Ph.D
Prolific Member

I should just live with my symptoms and carry on without making a fuss about it.

From: **Farmingdale, NY USA**

BQ
Very Prolific Member

Doc, you sure you don't have a "link" into my brain???? I gotta think about it more, but off the cuff, I tried that. It didn't work. To be continued …

BQ

From: **USA**

Sherree
Prolific Member

I will do my best to manage my symptoms, not just live with them, and learn as much as I can. If going to the doctor and complaining some about my symptoms and discussing various treatments until something actually helps is making a fuss, then so be it!

From: **Keizer, Oregon USA**

MaryBeth
Regular Member

Geesh, I never realized that this was an irrational thought! I've always tried to manage my IBS and still maintain a normal life without complaining about it all the time. I just figured that I have it and have to deal with it. Hmmm, let's see,

I guess I would have to restructure this to say that I will take care of myself and fight to minimize my IBS.

From: **Cary, NC, USA**

Shyra
Very Prolific Member

Ummm … I'm with MaryBeth. I'll try my best here:

"These symptoms are very real and if I'm not feeling well and it helps to talk to someone about it then I will. This is *my* health and I'm allowed to fuss about it especially if I'm really not feeling well and must alter plans in order to be comfortable."

Does that work?

From: **Calgary, AB Canada**

BQ
Very Prolific Member

"It's my party & I'll cry if I want to".

Seriously, I own this syndrome. It is mine, all mine. I will do whatever I have to do to live my life functionally, happily, peacefully, etc. And if taking care of myself means I cry sometimes, or I say No to a request, or I make choices that others don't particularly like, etc. that HAS to be okay. This is my life & I want to experience all I can. I can't reach that goal without tending to my symptoms.

From: **USA**

Topic: Irrational Thought #8

BBolen Ph.D
Prolific Member

I am a failure if because of my IBS I don't do all that is expected of me.

From: **Farmingdale, NY USA**

BQ
Very Prolific Member

I've done *more* than what is expected of me despite my IBS. I have a clear picture of what my limitations are, as well as my priorities. I will & have chosen what I can & cannot do. And I have made good choices. I do the best I can and that has to be good enough.

BQ

From: **USA**

Jane93
Very Prolific Member

I'm totally afraid of this thought, so it has become another irrational thought.

I must try to be perfect as I have IBS. I have to show that I am really good otherwise I am letting IBS get the better of me.

I suspect this may be worse … but it is fear of failure that drives me to want to be perfect … I'm not at the point where I would call myself a failure as I try very hard not to be one. I don't think this is any better.

From: **San Jose, USA**

Celticlady
Prolific Member

What a good day for me to read this post!!!! With IBS and also a new diagnosis of fibro (six days ago) and of course I am still trying to be Ms. Perfectionist. I am quite fatigued today, but still trying to clean the house. My hubby wouldn't care if I blew it off, I just have these unrealistic goals sometimes … I think I will lower my expectations, do the little bit I CAN do today, and not fret about the rest … I am NOT a failure, I am another overwhelmed Mom and I am now reminding myself to take care of MYSELF, not just the whole family … Thanks for the posts.

Beth

From: **USA**

SteveE
Very Prolific Member

Hmmm … I guess this one has a great deal to do with what we expect from ourselves. That has changed for me over time. When I first got IBS, my expectations for myself kept going down to the point that I did very little of anything. Gradually, I've been able to do more and expect more. Although, I do wish that I could do some things more regularly—like practice my sax, for example.

But I hold down a job, I climb mountains (well, hike on them anyway) that are over a thousand miles away, I have dinner ready for my wife when she gets home from work every night, and I've even found the nerve to visit a few restaurants every now and then. Just a few years ago, I would've doubted everything on that list.

Making improvements, even if they are small at first, is NOT failure.

From: **Illinois**

Skooz
New Member

This one is tough because we all KNOW that IBS is "all in our heads," right? And therefore, if we cave in to our symptoms we are being "hypochondriacs." Therefore, we have to PROVE that we are not psycho hypochondriacs by FUNCTIONING NORMALLY even if it kills us, right?

Gee, can you tell I've been on the phone with my mom lately? Ha-ha.

From: USA

Clair
Very Prolific Member

I can achieve the realistic goals I set myself, goals that others set are not the be all and end all if I don't live up to them.

Clair

From: **York UK**

MaryBeth
Regular Member

I am not a failure if I keep trying. I have IBS and it is an illness—it is not all in my head. It is not something I can completely control; I can only minimize the triggers and symptoms.

From: **Cary, NC, USA**

Topic: Irrational Thought # 9

BBolen Ph.D
Prolific Member

I can't have a good time if I am going to be physically uncomfortable, therefore I might just as well stay home.

From: **Farmingdale, NY USA**

BR
Prolific Member

Okay, here's my first try at one of these. I should be kind of ready now since I've read Dr. Bolen's book on IBS twice, and also the book she recommended "Feeling Good" by David Burns.

I don't know that I'll be physically uncomfortable and doing something besides focusing on myself may make me feel better and I'll likely end up having a good time.

From: **California**

Clair
Very Prolific Member

If I'm going to be physically uncomfortable, then why waste my time moping at home? I should be out there enjoying myself and making the best of it!

Clair

From: **York UK**

Sherree
Prolific Member

I have always tried not to let this condition keep me at home all the time. And I've learned that more often than not, I DO have a good time and feel OK.

From: **Keizer, Oregon USA**

MaryBeth
Regular Member

If I am going to be physically uncomfortable, I may as well be out doing something that will help me take my mind off of my discomfort instead of staying at home and focusing on it.

However, if I am having a really bad IBS exacerbation then I have to be home, but I don't feel badly when that happens because I know I need to take time to feel better.

Mary Beth

From: **Cary, NC, USA**

Eric
Very Prolific Member

I'm with Mary Beth on this one. Since I have been doing better, I have been more active, and that feels good.

From: **Portland OR USA**

Jane93
Very Prolific Member

This is an easy one ... staying at home will only make me feel negative and increase the negativity spiral and make me feel worse. If I go out it will take my mind off things.

From: **San Jose, USA**

SteveE
Very Prolific Member

Becoming more of a participant in life and less of a victim has improved my outlook tremendously. I will NOT sit here and tell you that making the transition from victim to participant has been an easy one, but it is well worth it!

Concrete example: It used to seem overwhelming to take steps to go on trips. I had to pack so much food because of the various food sensitivities I have identified. Now that I have some "systems" worked out for traveling as comfortably as possible, I not only feel less overwhelmed, but I have gained some significant pride in my ingenuity used to develop these "systems."

Remember ... life is just too short to sit on the sidelines until the clock runs all the way down on you! Get in the game to whatever extent possible & enjoy it!

From: **Illinois**

Topic: Irrational Thought #10

BBolen Ph.D
Prolific Member

I must try to be perfect in all areas of my life to compensate for having IBS.

From: **Farmingdale, NY USA**

BR
Prolific Member

Ho ho ho—I try to be perfect even in spite of IBS! I don't know that I have any answers for this one except perfectionism doesn't exist. Whether you have IBS or not you should only strive to do your best, well, or just good enough depending on the situation. Much better to do SOMETHING then nothing for fear of it not being perfect.

From: **California**

Eric
Very Prolific Member

Nobody's perfect and I agree with BR to do the best you can do, but not to over do it.

From: **Portland OR USA**

Linda2001
Prolific Member

This is one of my biggest irrational thoughts. I try to tell myself that I'm only human and will make mistakes sometimes, and if I do make a mistake I can usually learn from it.

From: **Melbourne, Australia**

Jane93
Very Prolific Member

This is my biggest problem right now. I must be perfect to compensate for the time off for IBS.

I don't see any other way of thinking about it. To not strive for perfection means I'm a slacker taking advantage of this as a disability, doesn't it?

Sure it's easy to say "nobody's perfect", but what is wrong with trying to be the best you can? Where do you draw the line?

Sorry, I don't think I'm helping here.

From: **San Jose, USA**

BQ
Very Prolific Member

Jane, "best you can be" doesn't equal perfect.

BQ

From: **USA**

BBolen Ph.D
Prolific Member

There is a big difference between trying to be the best you can be and expecting oneself to be perfect. It is also a big leap to say that to not strive for perfection makes a person a "slacker taking advantage of a disability." Striving to be perfect causes anxiety and tension that will only serve to exacerbate IBS symptoms. It is much healthier to try to do one's best, but to acknowledge that sometimes there are limitations and that that is okay.

From: **Farmingdale, NY USA**

Jane93
Very Prolific Member

Thank you ... you are right of course, being the best I can be is not the same as perfect.

I guess I need to learn a little self-acceptance and how not to judge. I read books on Taoism now and again, but somehow it's hard not to try too hard and just be. It seems like it should be so effortless.

Jane

From: **San Jose, USA**

Topic: Another irrational thought

BBolen Ph.D
Prolific Member

If I have a bad morning, I am doomed to have a bad day.

From: **Farmingdale, NY USA**

BQ
Very Prolific Member

Yeah, talk about a slippery slope. I used to think this way all the time. I wouldn't necessarily get upset about it, just a frustrated, resignation-type feeling. "It's gonna be one of those days again." Then again, there was a time when this happened every day; in that instance it would be: "It's gonna be another one of those days again." This thought used to set up a BAD chain of events. 'OK, D in the AM. Skip breakfast, because I have to leave the house to get kids to school. Skip lunch, because I gotta go run errands. Wait 'til after I come home from evening meeting at 9:30 PM to eat dinner.' This of course would lead to more D. Vicious cycle. Would go on days at a time. Tried to do most of my eating on the weekends when we had no plans. Whoa, how awful was this??? LOL Then get annoyed at people telling me I was too thin. Well, getting too thin happens … … when one doesn't eat.

I'd try to squeeze in light meals here & there when I had an hour or two to sit by the bathroom. This was a terrible time. If I was too weak from not eating, I could tell by my heart beating way too loudly in my ears. At that point I'd eat something very light and then take Imodium. This pattern continued for years. I was setting myself up for D. No eating or under-eating was only making things worse, not better.

I really thought this is just the way it is. I have to live this way. Did I ever think to call the Doc and let him know how badly I was feeling? Or how severe my symptoms were, to maybe see if there was something I could do to manage them better???? Naaah!!!! Why do that???

When I realized how much I was under-eating, (BTW, this enlightenment came from a post on this Board) I began to slowly increase my caloric intake. Slowly increasing it via the six smaller meals a day. I sucked it up and summoned up the courage & called my Doc. Told him everything. That is when the vicious cycle began to unwind. He helped me manage my pain via meds (sometimes they worked, other times it was as if I had taken nothing), and most importantly, he said he would help me. That gave me some hope that I wasn't in this alone.

I began to eat better and also started increasing my fiber intake. The D was still there, perhaps not as urgent though, and I felt loads better. I began to see it didn't matter whether I ate nothing or next to nothing or a regular meal … the D was the same. So, I might as well eat, I thought. Once I physically felt stronger, that in itself was a positive, and I began to think that maybe I didn't have to live this way. Maybe there was a way to manage these symptoms. Each positive along the way I held up and used to propel myself forward to symptom management. It got to the point where I wasn't saying "it's gonna be another day of D'. I began to think, 'well maybe today I will learn something to help me manage this.' And learn I did. I just kept reading stuff posted here and kept asking questions. I slowly no longer felt like a victim of IBS. My thinking turned more towards, 'okay I have this, but I can manage it.'

I'm sorry this is so long. But Doc Bolen, it was not an overnight process to turn that statement around. It was a long process. I had to educate myself, A LOT. Once I understood certain things, of the science-type variety, I saw a light at the end of the tunnel. I learned about and then made a decision to use hypnotherapy. Well, to be brief, it worked. But not instantly, not overnight. i.e.: No Quick Fix. But a fix nonetheless. I think it was key to build on any positive I saw.

Now when I was going through the hypno, there were days when I had D in the AM. But I began to say, "Okay, so? Doesn't mean the day is wrecked, doesn't mean I can't eat for the rest of the day. I can plan for D, it may not happen, but if it does, I won't let it stop me from doing what I want to do." Of course there were days when I had a slight adjustment of my plans, but I rarely had to cancel anything. Once I saw that, that I didn't have to cancel much, that again was another positive, and then I used that to build upon … and so on.

Do you see what I mean?

It wasn't a simple or brief change in my thinking, but it did happen. I couldn't have changed that thinking without loads of help from the folks here and I'm forever grateful.

BQ

From: **USA**

Discussion: Hypnotherapy

Hypnotherapy has been applied successfully to treat a variety of human conditions, including IBS. Hypnotherapy involves the induction of a naturally occurring altered state of consciousness which is experienced as relaxing and comfortable. Specific thoughts and suggestions are then offered to the subject, becoming imbedded in the subconscious, and leading to a desired goal or a permanent change in behavior.

In this forum, the use of one Hypnotherapy product in particular, the IBS Audio Program 100 (otherwise known as "Mike's tapes", www.ibsaudioprogram.com) generates much discussion. The main reason for the popularity of "Mike's Tapes" appears to be the dramatic results that members who have undergone the program have experienced. As the program is a home course in Hypnotherapy, the Bulletin Board provides an opportunity for individuals who are using the program on their own to get feedback and answer questions about the use of the audiotapes. Their experiences may help you to decide if Hypnotherapy is right for you.

Topic: Would like to hear from D-types how Mike's tapes helped you.

Ewink
Prolific Member

Hi everyone,

I have been on the IBS BB for a little while, but don't think I have posted here. I have had IBS for about four years now, or at least that's when I got the official diagnosis. But really I think I've struggled with it off and on for most of my life. I have been having a D flare-up for a little over two months now, set off by a nasty stomach flu (which my hubby got too, so it WAS the stomach flu). I am getting much better with several supplements, and don't really have D anymore, but my diet is still quite restricted. "Normally" I have been mostly C, but get D flare-ups too.

The thing is, even though my D is mostly better, I still get that terrible anxiety feeling every morning upon awakening, and have an extreme urge to "go". I have been taking very low doses of St. John's Wort and that is somewhat helpful. I do NOT want to go on any real anti-anxiety or anti-depressants! I am also seeing a therapist (Cognitive Behavioral Therapy), and that has been very helpful too, and so are the books I'm reading (relaxation, worry-control, etc.).

I am very seriously considering ordering and doing Mike's tapes, and was wondering if any of you D-types would be willing to share your experiences with the tapes. How they helped you, if the D went away, and how long it took before that happened, etc. Any other info/experiences/opinions also welcome.

Thank you so much in advance,

Edith

From: **CA, USA**

Cookies4marilyn
Moderator

Hi Edith, There are lots of posts here on this forum telling about how the hypnotherapy sessions have helped us. To sum up for you though, I have had IBS for 15 years; D was almost every day, lasting for several hours. After completion of the sessions, I gradually improved to only a few D episodes, now and then, lasting for less time. For me and for many on the BB, the improvement was gradual and subtle, and took place after the sessions were done. For others, they saw improvement within the first few weeks. Everyone is different, but Mike's hypnotherapy has for me been the most successful therapy to date, it has been researched, and he has had over 2000 IBSers do the program with 80–90% improvement or better. Since it is a complementary therapy, it can be used along with other treatments and medications. To find out more, read the other threads in this forum, and you will learn about others' successes.

Hope this helps you a bit. Most people who have completed the program highly recommend it. Good luck to you!

~ Marilyn

From: **Midwest—USA**

BQ
Very Prolific Member

Edith, I'm on day 75 of the program. I'm C/D type. I have seen a great reduction in my pain symptoms & just recently have noticed an improvement with the C/D. It is slight, but I'm hopeful the improvement will continue. The one thing that is a marked change is when I have D; I no longer have the extreme urgency, like I have more time to get to the can.

Hope this helps.

BQ

From: **USA**

AZmom1
Very Prolific Member

Edith, it sounds like you're on track, but I would not dismiss the meds so quickly. For IBS, the dosages are extremely low, and some people have found relief from these meds.

CBT is good, and hypnotherapy is an excellent supplement to CBT. I strongly recommend it.

AZ

From: **Scottsdale, Arizona USA**

Jennifer7
Prolific Member

IBS-D for 11 years. I'm still on Lotronex (I'm so thankful to God) but even on that, I would have "panic attacks" in stores, especially the grocery store. I thought the tapes might improve that. I still have some problems shopping, but since the tapes I'm better able to cope. Sometimes I can get through without any problems. Other times I start to panic and I work through it. I couldn't work through it before. I hope to continue improving. I'm finished with the tapes; however I still listen every now and then as suggested.

From: **Texas**

Eric
Very Prolific Member

Jennifer7, I am glad they helped you out. Success to me means real improvement in IBS, and I believe you will see continued improvement. For me, it is hard to put my finger on everything it helped with, but I am thrilled what it did for my severe IBS personally, and am very happy to see it has had such positive results for so many people. Of course not for everyone, or it would be the cure, but for a lot of people it can do a number on their IBS.

From: **Portland OR USA**

Topic: Mike's tapes help constipation?

Diannie
Regular Member

Has anyone had success with using the tapes to help with constipation and gas? I've noticed that most of the people who have been helped are D types. Don't want to spend the money if the tapes won't help me. Thanks.

From: **Georgia**

Caroline
Prolific Member

I have IBS-C and originally had not noticed an improvement in the pain with anything other than Xanax, but the CDs/tapes put me to sleep, which was a valuable consequence in itself. Now however, 40 days into the program I am starting to see an improvement in pain, though this could be due to the fact that I started using glycerin suppositories regularly. It is a big investment, but if you are not getting sleep I would recommend it as a way to relax. I also was told by members on the BB that it might take a while to see the results. There is some mention of constipation on the tapes, so they don't neglect it as a symptom.

From: **Massachusetts**

Jane93
Very Prolific Member

Yes they helped me a lot ... I rarely get C any more and therefore the gas is reduced ... depending on what I eat. I found relief pretty early on and it's been several years and I still feel good. I believe it helps me relax my belly and so therefore helps get rid of C.

From: **San Jose, USA**

Bada Shanren
Very Prolific Member

I would think the tapes would help with pain as they are a version of hypnosis but I'm not sure they specifically help with constipation as there are so many kinds of constipation?

Tom

From: **Murfreesboro, TN 37130**

Eric
Very Prolific Member

There are quite a few people with C that the tapes have helped over the years. IF the C is in fact caused by IBS, the tapes have a good possibility of helping. Also, they can help other symptoms of IBS, which in turn help the big picture, like pain for example, but there is a lot more to it then that.

It is easier, however, to stop something then to start it, but other factors like total body muscle relaxing can help constipation.

Caroline, hang in there as you're noticing a change in pain at halfway, that is actually good and it will get better. 40 days is perhaps average for starting to notice changes, even though everyone is different, but as has been said before, it's very gradual at first.

It may also have helped your using the suppositories, but I am pretty sure the HT is reducing the pain for you.

Hang in there and let us know how you're doing.

From: **Portland OR USA**

JeanG
Very Prolific Member

Hi Diannie:

Count me as one of those who had constipation that the tapes helped. Prior to doing them I would be constipated 2 to 3 days and then have a day of D. I also had bloating and some pain. Since doing the tapes that is all gone.

C may be a little more difficult than D, but it can be helped.

JeanG

From: **USA**

RitaLucy
Very Prolific Member

I am currently doing the tapes and I am a C-type also. I have noticed that my stomach is much more relaxed and I am much more relaxed in general.

I am able to get through things that before would cause me high anxiety, i.e. medical tests, etc.

I think overall, I am learning how to relax myself, in stressful situations especially.

From: **Houston**

Topic: How gradual are the improvements from the tapes?

Lorraine
New Member

For those of you who achieved a lot of relief from Mike's tapes, would you please tell us how long it took to see effects and what kind of changes you noticed? I have heard people say the changes are gradual, but have no idea whether the reference to "gradual" is a reference to time or whether the changes were hard to notice because they were subtle. Or perhaps both???

Thanks.

From: **U.S.A.**

Spoon
New Member

Hi,

I am on day 48 of Mike's tapes. I have noticed a massive change; this may not be totally attributed to the tapes, as I started taking Elavil around the same time as starting the tapes; however I feel that the tapes have helped me a great deal. They have helped a lot with anxiety, which I suffered with a lot. I would say that I am about 95% better; I can go out anywhere now and not have to worry about a toilet or anything, whereas before I had trouble going to work even.

I live in NZ so the cost of the tapes was considerable, however I wish that I had bought them a long time ago as I believe that they have helped me no end. I totally suggest you try them.

From: **New Zealand**

Eric
Very Prolific Member

Lorraine, basically both as you mentioned. Each person is individual in how fast they respond and what symptoms respond first, etc. The best way is just to finish them and see where you are at, and then try not to think too much about it in the meantime.

Some people respond fast, and a few may even go two times through them, but a lot of people respond roughly somewhere at the half-way point with changes they start to notice. Usually better sleep first it seems, then anxiety reduction, then actually changes in the symptoms themselves. But, everyone is different and this is a therapy, so people respond differently while listening. Hope that helps and if you have more questions let me know.

From: **Portland OR USA**

Kathleen M, Ph.D.
Very Prolific Member

I think most people notice change on a week to week/month to month type of thing, but sometimes changes can be punctuated with a rapid change. Or at least for me with CBT, which seems to affect changes much like hypnotherapy does.

With me, about halfway though the CBT (three months) I saw a fairly major change (I went from 7 Levsin a day to one to two in the space of a week). After that I continued to improve, but gradually. I started not needing the Levsin every day; I remember when I noticed that I wasn't sure the Levsin bottle was IN my purse. When the IBS was bad I knew precisely where the bottle was at all time.

By the end-of-the-year follow-up I did, I was probably down to two to three Levsin a month. Now it is even less than that. I did do Hypnotherapy a while ago and it wasn't enough to get me off of Buspar (which I still take at a low dose to keep the last of the abdominal discomfort at bay), but since then I maybe take four Levsin a year. I keep a script open because I am now a wimp and don't want to deal with even a couple of hours of mild pain.

K.

From: **Somewhere over the rainbow**

Nmwinter
Very Prolific Member

Eric's order of sleep, anxiety, and symptoms is exactly my order. I noticed pretty quickly that nights of waking up with a racing mind were a thing of the past. After finishing the tapes, I thought hmm, doing OK but not great—I went through a bad bout of C (I alternate usually). Then one day a few months later, I thought about how much better I've been. Not perfect—I still get the episode of D occasionally. Most important, I don't feel like I'm on that constant seesaw. And when I do have a bad day or two, I chalk it up to an anomaly rather than a return.

I still have a ways to go. My idea of really being over this will be the time I can travel on a plane without getting hyper about getting sick. I'm better about bad traffic or other situations without access to a restroom, but flying still does me in. But then again, I only finished the tapes a few months ago and plan to go through them again soon.

Nancy

From: **Portland, OR, USA**

Forum VIII: <u>Living with IBS</u>

"Share with everyone how you are living day-to-day with IBS. Share your success with whatever strategy you use to cope with IBS."

Topic: Living with IBS—Instructions—*READ ME*

Jeffrey Roberts
Member # 1
Founder

Welcome!

This forum is intended to be a very positive forum to allow you to **Share Your Success** with whatever strategy you use to cope with IBS. All members will benefit from hearing about your success!!

I invite you to write a sentence, paragraph or story that describes what has been successful for you. Some of your success may include a description of lifestyle changes, diet, medications, clinical experience, behavior modification, etc … Anything that works for you is worth writing about.

Jeff

From: **Toronto, Ontario, Canada**

Discussion: Prolific Members

Prolific Members are the "celebrities" of the IBS Self Help and Support Group. They have given countless hours of their time to offer their knowledge to members in need. You may recognize their names; you will find their stories to be inspirational.

Topic: My IBS Success Story & Food Intolerances

Awcfly
Prolific Member

My IBS-C/D symptoms started in grade school. I was diagnosed at a young age with allergies as a cause of skin rashes, and standard tests were conducted to come up with a list of allergens. I then underwent a long series of allergy shots around age 10.

The allergy shots were successful in the sense that there was no immediate allergic reaction to many of the food items on the list. However, all during my grade school and high school years I experienced IBS-C/D symptoms with lower left abdominal pain, from mild to moderate.

Finally, around the age of 30, the IBS symptoms became progressively much worse. As is typical, my doctor recommended Metamucil fiber supplement. Over the course of one month I took Metamucil, and my health spiraled downhill rapidly, culminating in severe constipation and a trip to the hospital with horrible abdominal pain and chills. Once flushed out, I was OK, but why did the symptoms keep happening?

The reason this crisis occurred is that I was mixing Metamucil with orange juice, one of the food allergens (which I assumed I had not been having much problem with for years). The fiber supplement absorbed the orange juice and transported it farther along the GI tract in an undigested state, producing much worse IBS symptoms.

Over the course of several years, it appears that the allergy shots have "worn off", one food item at a time. Each offending food produces abdominal pain in a different location in the GI tract.

The worst item turned out to be caffeine, which began to produce severe abdominal pain in the upper right abdominal area. (The perplexing and difficult to diagnose aspect of this is that the symptoms occurred 12–18 hours after ingestion of the food, so it was very difficult to pick out which particular items were causing the problem.)

Because of the upper-right location, the pain was misdiagnosed at first as a duodenal ulcer, then as gallbladder disease, and finally as IBS.

I experienced tremendous relief with the anti-depressant amitriptyline [Elavil], 10 mg, as has been reported by many other folks on the bulletin board. This drug appears to work on the autonomic nervous system controlling the GI tract in a way that reduces the occurrence of spasms. In this sense, it is somewhat the opposite of caffeine.

I am happy to report a complete cessation of IBS symptoms after elimination of all offending foods from the diet.

My recommendations are as follows, for people with IBS-C or IBS-C/D:

1. Keep a detailed food journal. Examine the journal, keeping in mind the possibility of a 12+ hour time lag from ingestion to symptoms, to identify foods that aggravate your condition. If you can do so, this self-help may be more valuable than repeated trips to the doctor. (Some people may not have any food intolerances, and will not get useful results from this exercise.) A physician can put you on a more rigorous elimination diet, which may get the same results faster, but with considerably greater inconvenience.

2. Discuss the problem with a good Gastroenterologist, who can properly diagnose GI diseases with similar symptoms: lactose intolerance, celiac disease (gluten intolerance), Crohn's disease, colitis, gynecological problems, etc. This BB may contain recommendations on good GIs in your area.

3. Eliminate caffeine from your diet for a one-month trial period. If this doesn't help, then go back to caffeine. The experiment certainly won't be harmful. This includes all sources of caffeine, including coffee, tea, cola & chocolate.

4. Add greens to your diet, particularly spinach, collards, etc. These seem to have the benefits of fiber supplements without the drawbacks. In my case, they help produce excellent GI system performance. (Some people react to lettuce, so this may be a poor choice.)

Common items which cause problems are as follows:

Caffeine;
Milk & dairy products (may actually be lactose or casein intolerance);
Wheat & gluten products (may actually be Celiac disease);
Alcohol;
Sorbitol (artificial sweetener);
Fructose (natural fruit sugar, especially pears);
Lettuce;
Any foods to which you have known allergies.

PLEASE NOTE: IBS-D, with chronic diarrhea only, may have different causes, often related to gallbladder disease. Treatments may include consumption of calcium carbonate (e.g. Caltrate), or treatment with drugs like Colestid.

Perhaps this information will be helpful to some percentage of IBS sufferers. My best wishes to IBSers in their quest for successful treatment.

From: **USA**

Topic: As close to a cure as I ever hoped to get!

BR
Prolific Member

I was diagnosed with IBS about 15 years ago. The unmanageable problems first started after I spent a day at work pigging out on a bunch of different foods. That night I got the big D and from then on my bowels were messed up. I had a tendency toward loose stools since high school, but it had never affected my life before.

After I was diagnosed, I took Lomotil almost every day because I was so fearful of getting D when I was out. IBS had a big impact on my social life, although now I appreciate the fact that it made me much more independent. Before I was really shy and hesitant to do things on my own, but after IBS I did a lot more on my own in case I had to leave a situation. I decided the Lomotil wasn't good to take so often, so I cut back and then only took it as needed. Then I switched to Imodium and I was to the point where I didn't need it that often. My IBS was definitely D-predominant but I had some cases of C every once in a while.

Then this year I found the IBS BB and the hypnotherapy CDs. I instantly felt a weird sense of calm after I started listening to the CDs. About halfway through, I noticed an improvement in the D, even though I realized from reading the BB that people have it much worse than I did. By the time I finished the series I had improved a great deal, but I had a setback at the end. I went to the BB for advice and found out this is common because those mind armies are trying a desperate attempt to get back to the forefront. This lasted a couple weeks and since then I have only had improvement.

I finished the series in mid-August of this year and now I rarely have D. Maybe two or three incidents shortly after I finished, and no problems for at least a month. I also noticed an improvement in the bloating (a BIG problem for me). As I see it, I will continue to improve and I'm really looking forward to the Beyond 100 series because I'm convinced that hypnotherapy is the only natural way to find such relief. By natural I mean no drugs. This is a big deal to me, because I hate taking medicine if I don't have to. I don't want to rely on it. I needlessly suffered all those years because I didn't know there was help out there that was non-drug related.

I am grateful to this BB, everyone who provides support and to Mike for the IBS hypnotherapy program. Without everyone here, I would have continued need-lessly suffering.

From: **California**

Topic: Had IBS for over 15 years

Cookies4marilyn
Very Prolific Member

Having had IBS for over 15 years, I have been on just about every antispasmodic, IBS medication, antidepressant for IBS symptoms, SSRI, and even a calcium channel blocker, as well as the usual OTC meds for "D". My symptoms have been so severe at times that they leave me incapacitated, curled up in pain for hours with a heating pad, or in the bathroom literally for hours. Travel had become less and less and just going to routine appointments brought on severe attacks of pain and D.

In desperation, I am using Mike Mahoney's IBS Audio Program, which uses gut-specific clinical hypnotherapy techniques. These sessions have taken me from almost daily D attacks lasting several hours with intense pain, to a few attacks a week with much shorter duration. I am still on the road to improvement and hope to continue. I must add here that I am still recovering from surgery, due for another surgery and have recently been divorced. All these things have made IBS go into overdrive. IBS has ruined my life in just about every way. Once I was very outgoing, spoke effortlessly in front of large audiences as part of my profession prior to IBS … I have missed out on many wonderful parenting, travel, volunteer or professional opportunities solely because of IBS. But for me, hypnotherapy has shown to be an effective complementary treatment for my IBS. Also, a dietician who has Crohn's suggested this to me for my nausea … a type of tea called Twig Tea from Japan. I really had to hunt for it, but found it in a health food store … it tastes awful, but after about five sips, it usually stops my nausea.

This is the short version, but I also wanted to mention that I have had four, yes four, colonoscopies, one endoscopy, numerous abdominal ultrasounds, an IVP, bladder scope, barium X-rays, and CAT scans … as well as a partial hysterectomy … all in the effort to find out what this pain was, or to put an end to it … surely something this severe could not be just "functional" … and yes, I was at the Mayo Clinic also …. Some days, I still feel it is more than IBS … the pain can be that bad. But I feel that for the first time in my life, I am finally seeing the light at the end of the tunnel (no pun intended) through the use of hypnotherapy … …

Be well, everyone … Marilyn

From: **Midwest—USA**

Topic: What works for me.

Earthgarden
Prolific Member

I hope that what I write helps at least one person. I am coping with IBS-C. Some days I am very distressed by the condition, some days I am free of symptoms. I definitely believe it is all in the mind; my mental state affecting my physical.

Some years ago, I left my abusive husband, took the children to live in a woman's refuge. It was difficult but a positive experience. However following this, my ex-husband stalked me for about three years. I lived in absolute fear. I thought he would eventually kill me! Anyway, now I am happily settled. The children are doing great and I have been with my present husband for three years. Life is good. Yet at times, my stress/anxiety levels feel at fever pitch! When the stalking was occurring, I would tense up, waiting, ready to run or fight etc., then he would show, I would deal with it and I would feel relief. Now that I am no longer being stalked by him on a daily basis, I feel no relief, the tension mounts and mounts and mounts and mounts! There is no release!

He harassed me recently and for a few days afterwards, I was completely IBS symptom-FREE! I am cured!—Not so … tension mounts, but no relief! I wait for relief.

I thought it was important to give you background.

How I cope:—

I do not overload my digestive system. I have lowered my carb intake, do not over-eat, drink lots of fruit smoothies/juice, take evening primrose oil, and take an herbal preparation of peppermint, fennel and liquorice daily.

If I am really stressed, and my IBS-C is really problematic, I take peppermint oil in a capsule. I get this from my local chemist without prescription. This relaxes the bowel spasms and alleviates the gas. I sometimes use a suppository, just to help things pass along smoothly and calm things down.

It is important for me to feel positive, relaxed and free from fear (fear gives me the runs; tension the constipation) and to do this I meditate, listen to soothing music (wind chimney stuff is nice) do yoga, go swimming and have a sauna twice a week if possible.

I wish everyone out there good will and hope your own worries/stresses/fear/anxieties/phobias lessen. Have faith ... in yourself! Be true to yourself. We are all unique and wonderful.

From: **London**

Topic: Ponderings of an IBSer

Eric
Very Prolific Member

I was just thinking of expressing some of my thoughts on IBS and having it for thirty years. I have pain-predominate IBS and alternating C and D. Although I can say had and really mean it, as I am doing so much better (at about 85%) and I believe I am still improving thanks to this BB and Mike's tapes. I believe my IBS started from a trip to Mexico where I swallowed a small amount of chlorinated water out of a swimming pool and a half hour later, I was very sick with amoebic dysentery and spent the next month seriously close to death. No Joke. They also pumped tons of penicillin into me at this time. However, amoebic dysentery is known to cause inflammation in the digestive tract. I recovered from that and I don't remember when or how soon after I came back from Mexico I was suffering from severe abdominal pain and alternating C and D.

It wasn't too long before they started the first tests on me. The testing would continue on and off for a big part of my life and cost thousands of dollars. The first tests were stool samples and upper GI tests, all negative. The next test was a lower GI, also negative. Blood tests and all the regular tests from a normal MD. I was ten. In those days no one had a clue about IBS and they called it spastic colon or nervous stomach. I missed a lot of school and was always trying to catch up in my school work. Since the good doctors couldn't figure it out, I was sent for therapy and put on Librium and told it was psychosomatic.

I struggled for years through school, some working, and trying to explain to friends why I was in pain a lot and could not do things. Dating was a problem. They thought I had a stomachache and it would go away and I should just quit being a big baby. Funny, because my boss said that to me also ten years later, as well as a lot of coworkers.

More testing. Basically the same kinds of tests over again. When you're in your teens and you're seeing some upstate NY doctor in a small town, in those days, testing didn't amount to much. Still no advice from anyone on what to do.

My parents were very supportive and my mom is a nurse, which was very helpful and supportive. However, sometimes my mom's own concern bothered me as she could not help and I could see that in her eyes while I lay there in complete agony from the knife jabbing sharp pains coming from my gut. When I got these pains I would hyperventilate and all kinds of thoughts raced through my head.

For me, this was already establishing itself into my thought patterns on a day to day basis, and I didn't really know much about living any other way as I hit my late teens. I was having episodes at least two to four times a week and that continued until I join this BB two years ago. Although I would have some remissions, they always came back and for a while my IBS went cyclic and bothered me most in the winter months, but in the summer improved somewhat. But it always came back.

Meanwhile, I continued to try to figure some of it out for myself, in ways I could manage it or do things to reduce it. Late teens to late twenties. More tests. "Maybe an ulcer, but we don't see it." New drugs, and from there Librax, Donnatol, prescription Tagamet, and a few others I don't even remember, but Prozac was one as well. No noticeable long-term improvement. Mid thirties, I got serious and went to the best GI doc in town and told him to test away on everything we could think of that might be applicable. Also worried it could be something else still, although nothing showed up after he tested me. More drugs. Bentyl and Valium. Sent to therapy, told to relieve stress. I knew this wasn't the cause and thought because the pain was so severe that something had to be wrong in there, it just couldn't be possible to have this much pain and not have something physically that they could see wrong.

I just didn't get it. I did know stress aggravated it, but not to the extent I do now, or the kinds of stress, either environmental, physical, or psychological. At the time I did not know how to reduce it enough with the management techniques I was using, and I used a lot of them. I tried all the food aspects and nothing other then some common sense on most things helped. Although it made sense what was going in had something to do with it, but in reality looking back now, it was common sense issues of eating too much too fast, fat, spices, etc., etc..

There were some weird signals before an attack. My skin would turn whiter, my eyes would twitch and my hands would sweat. Sometimes I would get dizzy. My therapist had migraines and knew nothing about IBS, other then realizing some of the symptoms sounded somewhat like some symptoms she would get with her migraines and that it was not in my head (psychosomatic or crazy) and I should go back to the doctor. It wasn't helping me to see her, so I agreed. Although she didn't explain serotonin to me, nor did my doctor take the time to either, I feel if someone would have explained some of the mind-gut connections earlier I could have saved a lot of time and effort. I know some are relatively new, but I think they had some idea and either it was too complicated to explain to me or they just didn't have the time. I think at this point one of the best things a doctor can do is explain some of this to new patients. I didn't have any other issues. I was healthy otherwise and was playing soccer for twenty years and going professional until I blew my kneecap out. I believe I personally have a classic case of IBS. For me, I believe it is faulty neurotransmitters that are not talking right between my brain and my gut.

Thank God for hypnotherapy, which I want to add some of my thoughts on as a side note. Of course most people know I work with Mike Mahoney now, but some probably do not. After meeting him on the BB here and the success I had, I decided to work with him, as I feel he has one of the most effective treatment tools for IBS. I am drug-free and very happy with the results.

I want to say something about hypnotherapy in general, and what I believe and have seen for myself, and these are my own personal comments from my experiences with it, although many others feel the same way now. It is the deepest form of relaxation I personally have ever found. It has tremendously reduced the pain for me, from severe to very mild. I think this has worked two ways. It has steered my thoughts and attention away from the pain and I also believe the relaxation aspect of it is releasing endorphins to my gut. This has been a big achievement and will save me trips to the ER.

When I wake up in the morning I no longer have IBS on my mind first thing.

I no longer dwell on it.

I don't worry too much about going out or bathrooms any more.

I no longer turn white or have my hands sweat.

I can relax my gut at will.

My whole body is more relaxed in general and I didn't realize how tense it was before.

I breathe better and more deeply. Which I have found useful if I feel any twinges of a potential problem.

I sleep better and more deeply.

Day-to-day problems don't bother me like they use to.

I can eat things I couldn't before.

I feel like I have been rewired so to speak.

My BM's have improved substantially.

There are symptoms I don't even remember and that is unbelievable.

Anyway, just some thoughts of an IBSer pondering. I don't know if this helps anyone and I also don't want to say hypnosis is a cure or the only thing people should be doing to manage IBS, but it is one majorly effective tool that isn't understood by a lot of people or used enough by doctors in the IBS world and why I sound like a broken record sometimes.

However, I hope no one gets tired of hearing about something that really works for the majority of people with IBS, as there are just too few of the things that do.

From: **Portland OR USA**

Topic: A breakthrough after years

Kathleen M, Ph.D.
Very Prolific Member

In my twenties I developed a sleep disorder that was not diagnosed until I was about 20 (young, slim, females are not the high risk group for sleep apnea-like disorders). During this time I had mild symptoms of IBS and Fibromyalgia, both of which were probably related to the disordered sleep. I also have a history of severe allergies which developed into asthma as an adult. When my allergies flare up, I have a greater tendency to GI upset.

After the sleep disorder was cleared up and the allergies were getting under control, the IBS symptoms lessened, although I did tend to have some loose stools during times of stress. During this time there was a little bit of cramping, but nothing really bothersome.

In 1997, I was on a field study, camped out along the side of a large hog waste lagoon. I may have picked up something there that didn't agree with me, as when we got back I started feeling bad, ran a low-grade fever for about six weeks, but it wasn't enough for me to go to the doctor over. During this time, the cramps started and continued to get worse. After the fever broke, the pain was still there. The pain was triggered by eating, by walking, and by doing anything (like picking up things off the floor) where I used my abdominal muscles. My allergy shots seemed to be making it worse, so I saw my allergist about that and let him know that an ostomy bag was starting to look really good and I was about ready to remove my own colon by myself, so he got me a referral to Dr. Drossman.

Prior to that appointment, they got me into see another local GI doctor who did a sigmoidoscopy, gave me Levbid and later added Buspar, which got me functional. I wasn't free of symptoms, but they were tolerable, which was a big step up from where I had been.

When I saw Dr. Drossman, he approved the medication and he told me about his clinical trials. I was accepted as a subject and ended up in the Cognitive Behavioral Therapy treatment group in one of his studies. I wasn't able to handle the drug washout, so they kept me on the meds, but monitored my drug use and switched me to Levsin SL rather than the longer acting Levbid. I was taking about seven to eight Levsin to make it through the day, along with 15 mgs Buspar two times a day, at the start of the therapy. Also, I was unable to complete some of the tests done at the beginning and the end of the trial, because they set off my symptoms too badly.

About halfway through the therapy, something happened. I had a breakthrough about some issues, but I don't know how this caused the results. In one week I dropped down to two to three Levsin SL a day, and over the next week or two stopped taking the morning Buspar (it makes me lightheaded in the morning, but doesn't bother me in the evening).

As the therapy progressed, I began taking less and less Levsin, and most of the time it wasn't to be functional, but to get rid of very mild cramping that I just didn't want to deal with. The stool consistency had not improved much, but I didn't care about a few loose stools, given that I was no longer in pain. I was able to complete all the testing at the end of the study.

Since the therapy ended I have continued to improve. The stool consistency went back to normal within three months of finishing the therapy (My internal hemorrhoids let me know about the return to formed stools, but they chilled out after a couple of days) and now I rarely if ever have an attack. I **am** down to 7.5 mgs of Buspar at night, and hope that I may be able to go drug-free soon. I am taking my allergy shots again, and they still upset the GI tract, so I may need to complete those before I can get off of the Buspar entirely.

K.

From: **Somewhere over the rainbow**

Topic: Living With IBS for 26 Years, But No Longer

LNAPE
Very Prolific Member

I started this awful journey at age 26 in 1976, after having my gall bladder removed. Those days it was a major thing to have it removed, with a six-inch scar and a six-week recovery.

Having small children at the time was difficult and not being able to attend many school functions without a lot of planning was painful for me and for the rest of the family.

It was just dumb luck to find what worked for me. I worked in a pharmacy for six years and used to see people come in to get calcium for their bones who also would need some sort of laxative to keep things moving. This connection did not dawn on me at the time. I was young and not worried about bone loss, so I sold them the items and they went their merry way.

Well, time passed and it was my turn to start some calcium to help prevent bone-loss in later years, and from the very first day I felt so much better that I could not explain the difference.

I told no one for three months, thinking like all the other times this could not continue to work. But it did. And for me, I have been able to totally control the urgent attacks of diarrhea, the pain, the cramping the sick feeling when I ate and the "oh no …. I didn't make it to the bathroom on time".

It still amazes me to this day. I have been living a very normal life for more than two years now.

I have the hope that you all can find what works for you, because living a life that makes you a prisoner to the bathroom is not a very happy one.

Take Care,

Linda

From: **Hamilton, OH, USA**

Topic: I used to be chained to the bathroom, then I found this BB

Marianne
Very Prolific Member

I've had IBS since I was a child. It was IBS-C until about 10 years ago when it turned into IBS-D.

It was so bad, and so explosive that there were days I could not leave home. I had to run to the bathroom and always had a wad of toilet paper stuck between my cheeks to prevent floor accidents while I was rushing to the smallest room in the apartment.

Then, about four years ago I found this BB.

I have found many things that helped me. But I have to tell you that I am allergic to many medicines and regretfully had to give up some of the things that were tremendously successful in stopping my diarrhea. But you may not be allergic and I urge you to try them.

Colestid. This is a pill form of cholestyramine, a prescription drug that totally stopped my diarrhea. It is usually given to lower cholesterol. I used it for many months and then had an allergic reaction and had to give it up. If I wasn't allergic, it would still be my #1 choice for stopping diarrhea.

Lotronex. This totally stopped my diarrhea. I had tremendous pain when I took the initial dose and was constipated for four days after taking only two pills. So I reduced the dose to 1/4 of a pill once a day, and had one normal firm bowel movement a day.

Branola Bread—The Original. I eat two slices of this nutritious fiber bread every day. When I don't eat it, no matter what I am taking, my BMs are gummy.

Calcium—Caltrate Plus. Caltrate Plus, recommended by LNape was a Godsend. But I had to take six tablets a day to insure that I only had one firm bowel movement. I took this when Lotronex was not available.

Gas and gut rumbles and intestinal spasms: I had such severe gas that it came out of me every time I walked across the room. I used Jerusalem Artichoke Flour mixed into a small quantity of yogurt and very strong chamomile tea. I rarely have these problems now. When my guts start jumping, I take chamomile extract (it's faster than making the tea). When I have gas, I take the Jerusalem Artichoke Flour.

I have a normal life now. I am always uneasy when I eat out, but this is now based on irrational fear because I have not had a diarrhea attack for almost a year.

Thanks Jeffrey and all of you who helped so much.

From: **New York, New York**

Topic: 8 to 48: Lifelong IBS in Remission-There is Hope

Mike NoLomotil
Very Prolific Member

Started at 8 years old with no specific trauma … intermittent pain and cyclic D and C. Three years of invasive testing and non-invasive testing found nothing, so they actually did an exploratory laparoscopy. Afterwards, surgeon said there was "some mal-rotation" [misplacement] of the small bowel, so that should take care of that, they thought.

Post-surgically after recovery, there was no change. About eight months later, I developed multiple bowel obstructions [adhesions: scar tissue from surgery obstructed bowel in seven different places]. Also had co-morbid onset of salmonella food infection. This was a party I could have done without.

While they postponed surgery trying to eliminate the infection, I slowly got worse and worse and ended up in and out of consciousness for three days, then coma for three or four days, I forget, I was only 11 and when you are in a coma it is hard to mark-off the time. But you do have this weird external perception of what is going on to which you are unable to respond. As least that is how it was for me.

During this time, at some point the bowel perforated, I became septic, went into shock and died temporarily. They resuscitated me and took me to surgery for an emergency laparoscopy at this point, and I had a long recovery period.

The sucky-part was that after all that not only were my original symptoms back again in full force ... they got worse and worse and worse in spite of all possible therapies tried. By my 20's I was almost totally D-predominant and this continued to worsen with the only effective therapy mass-doses of all the various drugs associated with diarrheic and pain management. I had a successful healthcare career for many years working within the hospital as a therapist, then administrator, in some prominent hospitals, so I never lacked for access to the very best doctors in GI disease and the very best ideas and treatments, which did nothing but increase drug sales to me.

By my late 30's I had also developed diverticulosis (20 years of constant spasm-attacks did not let the bowel wall hold up well) and by my early 40's life was one endless D-episode, managed at that point solely by rotating Lomotil and Immodium, sometimes up to 12 to 15 a day. (During the phase I was on Bentyl and Phenobarbitol, before Immodium came on the market as an Rx drug for about $100 for a 100 pills, I reached a point were I was taking about the same dose range, sometimes more, of B & Pheno and walking around completely cogent loaded with phenobarb ... at least I thought I was cogent.)

Facing what all the GI docs told me was certain bowel resection as my only solution, I decided to go in a different direction in the late 1980's. This led me to the group of immunologists and GI docs working on food and chemical intolerance. Their work brought me the first relief of my life by identifying the actual problem (undiagnosed immunologic reactions to certain foods and food additives and colorings). By removing the cause through avoidance, they brought me to my first-ever remission. As long as I remain on my personal dietary plan that eliminates all the food and chemicals I am reactive to immunologically, I remain so.

This is where I remain for about eight years now [did not actually mark the day on the calendar]. My personal goal is to help further the work of these doctors so as many people as possible who are unknowingly suffering from this inscrutable problem can be relieved of it, eliminating the underlying cause/stimulus for their suffering and who at this time have only interventional and alternative therapies to help reduce their symptoms "after the fact".

Eat Well. Think Well. Be Well.

MNL

From: **West Palm Beach, Florida USA**

Topic: I first noticed my IBS when I was 13

WashoeLisa
Prolific Member

I first noticed my IBS (although I didn't know what it was called then or that it wasn't even normal) when I was about 13 in 1980. It first started when I would go to the Mall with friends. I always made the JCPenney's restroom my first stop and then I would be OK to shop for the afternoon. I never considered that it may not be normal; I just figured it was "just me".

Life went on; I went to high school with not many problems and really no class-room disruptions for myself in having to make a bathroom run. I graduated from high school in 1985 and went on to college at UC Irvine. That's when my IBS went from mild to severe. I remember distinctly sitting in class during a lecture (it was a small class that I couldn't leave discreetly) and having cramps so pain-ful that I very nearly passed out. I fought to stay conscious and not let on to my fellow students that I was fighting this, until class let out about 20 minutes later. I struggled to get to a bathroom, trying not to walk completely hunched over and just made it. I was completely emotionally and physically spent for the rest of the day. I would have episodes like that off and on for the next two years or so—always when I wasn't near a bathroom, like in the car or some place like that. I had to make "potty stops" every so often when I just couldn't control the cramp-ing anymore. I also learned where ALL the restrooms were on campus and it just became part of normal life for me. I still didn't feel very well a lot of the time and so my doctor ordered a glucose tolerance test—which was just barely normal. I was told they called it Imitation Hypoglycemia and to treat myself as if I had it even though I was two points above normal.

My IBS was still roaring along and I didn't learn that there was a name for my problem and that it wasn't normal until about 1987 or so. That's when I took myself to the proctologist to get checked. It was a less than glorious exam and he recommended that I take Metamucil daily. That really helped with the D and the overall pain, but it pretty much just took my symptoms to a dull roar instead of an overwhelming thing. But I was happy for the improvement it gave me. After a few months, I experienced more pain on eating and severe fatigue. I went to my college PCP, took a barium x-ray and we found an ulcer and that I was also lac-tose intolerant now. I took Tagamet and was able to control it fairly well. Then, I transferred to UC Riverside and graduated in 1990 with a BA in sociology. I was much more comfortable with my fiber regimen by this point, the ulcer was healed and while I still knew where all the restrooms were on campus, I didn't have to fight that cramping, lose-consciousness type of pain anymore.

I got married in September of 1990 to a wonderful guy, Todd, who understood my need to make sure I knew where all the restrooms were. He got used to me having to make a "right now" potty stop at the grocery store, movies, Costco, church and pretty much everywhere we went. Our oldest daughter was born in December 1991 and my IBS was still a problem in my pregnancy. In fact, it got worse in my last trimester as she grew bigger and put pressure on all my "innards". My PCP was also my OB/GYN and he officially told me what I already knew— that I have IBS. After the birth, my IBS went back to a dull roar and I was happy with that.

Then, in December 1992, I started getting sick with what I thought was the flu. After four weeks, it didn't go away and I got myself to my PCP. He assured me we would get to the bottom of my symptoms which included fever, weight loss, lower right quadrant pain, severe diarrhea at all times of the day and night, and generally feeling yucky. At that time, my childhood best friend and my daughter's godmother passed away unexpectedly. After that, my health took a major turn for the worse. My PCP kept telling me I was just depressed over my friend and I kept telling him that I was sick BEFORE she died. He sent me to a GI to check out Crohn's disease as my sister and two cousins have this as well. The GI told me he saw signs of a mild ileitis (inflammation) but none of the telltale signs of Crohn's. What I had was indicative of, but not diagnostic of, Crohn's. He also found lots of swelling in my terminal ileum and lots of cell changes that indicated an allergic reaction, although we didn't know that part of it then. I only discovered that when I got my records later to take with me to UCLA. So then I went on Asacol, which did help the lower right quad pain but not the fatigue or the fever that peaked at 103 that I had had for four months. I was bedridden at this point and needed help from my parents and in-laws to take care of my toddler daughter. It was horrible to say the least. I also developed major joint pain at this point. My PCP diagnosed CFIDS and put me on Prozac for the fatigue which did help—but I felt he was belittling me by this time, even though he took me a little more seriously when my ulcer flared again which responded to more Tagamet.

So I changed doctors, went to a chiropractor and started in on a one and a half year remission. I felt the chiropractor really changed my life and while I still didn't understand what had happened to me, I was just glad it seemed to be gone. I had to really pace myself and take naps in the afternoon, but I pretty much had my life back.

We decided to have another child during my remission (which we thought was permanent) and our son was born in August 1996. I still had severe IBS in the third trimester but I knew to expect it and it somehow didn't seem as bad.

We moved to Reno, Nevada in December 1996 and I made sure to find a good chiropractor! In the spring 1997, we discovered that I was pregnant again—a wonderful surprise! During this pregnancy, I came out of remission and got the lower right quad pain back, the severe D, fatigue and joint pain. I was so discouraged and upset—especially at how my first doctor treated me—that I decided I would just "ride it out", whatever that meant. I confided in a few close friends, including my best friend's mom, and she made me promise I would get to the bottom of it this time.

I delivered my daughter in December 1997 and after her birth, when I was still not well, I kept my promise. I went to my new PCP and he sent me to a local GI who was no help at all. By this time, I also was getting rashes when I would get the D and the severe lower right quad pain. It helped that there was now something they could see and quantify. That GI did another scope and found while my colon looked fine (no Crohn's), but I had severe blunting in my small intestine which could indicate Celiac Sprue and also explained my lactose intolerance.

He sent me back to my PCP who was pretty angry that he left me hanging with the possible Sprue diagnosis, which is a very serious thing, without doing the tests for them. He did them himself and they came back negative. I did have a flare-up of my ulcer again too—more Tagamet. But by this time, I was patrolling the internet, looking for answers. I started acupuncture and Chinese medicine at this point, as one more avenue to pursue. It helped, but was not the cure-all. So, I went to another GI who pretty much told me that I did have severe IBS and something else that "looked like Crohn's, acted like Crohn's, felt like Crohn's ... but wasn't". He called an expert diagnostician at UC Davis Medical School who was stumped as well. He sent me to a dermatologist to biopsy the rashes I was getting and they were deemed to be "leukocytoclastic vasculitis" which is common in any autoimmune disease. So I went to an allergist who felt I was beyond his abilities in the general, but that he could help my hay fever! I had decided to go to UCLA now and the allergist strongly encouraged it. Last stop before UCLA, a local rheumatologist who examined me for some auto-immunities and declared me free of disease—but a puzzle as I was obviously sick. So off to UCLA I went.

First stop, the GI department. They looked over ALL my records and felt that while I have severe IBS, I needed to be seen by the rheumatologists there to discover the "something else" that plagued me. I went to the rheumys there, was looked over from head to toe, took more blood (I have track marks now from all the blood tests I have had!) and was finally told the "something else"—Fibromyalgia. The rheumy there felt that it still didn't explain ALL my GI stuff but that I definitely tested positive for it.

Now I had something to research!! I found Dr. Jay Goldstein, a premier name in the FM/CFIDS community and went to him. He is only a few miles from where I grew up in CA and so I stayed with my parents when I saw him. I went in three times and was given different meds each time. It was a major success and I felt really pretty good as long as I took my meds. I had to go back each time I developed a tolerance to those meds—which is what brought me back each time. I was happily taking my 20 meds per day, feeling well—more or less, but still struggling with the IBS. He gave me Lotronex samples which I was leery of taking as it was so new to market, so I kept them on my shelf, "just in case".

I went to another rheumy who did a few more blood tests, confirmed my Fibromyalgia diagnosis and put me on physical therapy to help. It did help, along with the meds and I was cruising along, figuring I was on meds for life, OK with that and learning to adjust to life with chronic illness.

Then, the LEAP Program found me on my job as Digestive Conditions Community Leader in the form of MikeNL. I was still struggling with my IBS and some of the GI stuff, including the lower right quad pain, so I checked it out, found it was legitimate, and decided it was one more avenue to pursue and might even help with the rest of my GI puzzle. The science is that IBS and some other illnesses like Fibromyalgia, are the result of delayed food allergies. LEAP had developed a new blood test to find these hidden aggravators.

I took the blood test, the home phlebotomist FedEx'd the sample to Florida and in the ultimate birthday gift—the results in the lab were done on August 1, 2000: my 33rd birthday. I got the pack with all the info a few days later and started the program immediately. I had been told to expect to feel worse on the program at first as my body was cleansing all that gunk out of my system—and boy, did I! It was awful! But I kept telling myself that it was good, that my body was reacting as it should to this new regimen.

After a few days, the pain eased and I started to feel better! The joint pain was disappearing, the lower right quad pain was going away and I just generally felt better! The IBS was even diminishing! I decided to test it and reduce my meds slowly to see what happened. By Day 30, I was pain-free, IBS-free, and off all but three or so of my meds. By Day 45, I was off ALL meds and feeling better than I ever had in my entire life!!

I went to my PCP to show him the incredible results. He had read about LEAP in a journal and was really excited to see how well I was doing and how this program affected me and my life! He took photocopies of my report to refer more patients and was thrilled to know that progress was being made in this area of medicine.

I am now approaching the six-month mark on LEAP and I DO NOT miss any of my reactive foods as I know they are poison to me and I would not trade my hard-fought-for health for anything! And some of those foods include wheat (no more bread, cookies, cakes, bagels, etc.), chocolate, tea, cherries and pears. Not easy to avoid, but well worth it. There have been a handful of occasions where I ate something I was reactive to and didn't realize it until afterwards and I got SOOOO sick. IBS and Fibromyalgia came back with a vengeance for a few days until my body healed again.

This has been the answer to all my hard work, diligence and prayers and I am so grateful that some doctors believe us as patients when we say we hurt and have no life.

I am looking forward to living the rest of my life as pain-free as the first half was painful,

Lisa from Nevada
(Lisa Schultz)

From: **Carson City, NV, USA**

Topic: 62 YEARS WITH IBS!

Verna Eileen
Prolific Member

I've been struggling with excruciating pain and explosive diarrhea in public places for 62 years! My first memory of this disease is fainting on the way to the bathroom from the awful pain. My mother was helping me because I couldn't stand erect, the pain was so bad. She thought I had the flu and I came to with my aunt applying a cold cloth to my head and my mother a warm cloth to the other end, cleaning me up. I was four years old.

During the course of my nearly 66 years I've married (several times), had four children (boys), and now have three daughter-in-laws (who bless me for raising non-helpless men), and seven grandchildren. I started working at the age of 10 cleaning houses and mowing lawns. The remainder of my working life has consisted of waitress, retail, modeling, dental assistant, long distance operator (when they had cord boards and after), teaching, show dog breeder-trainer-exhibitor, and small business entrepreneur. Now I'm a real estate agent in South Western Michigan (whew).

All these years I've struggled with establishing the location of the nearest toilet uppermost in my mind. During the 90's I was blessed with ownership of a 34-foot and a 28-foot completely self-contained motor home. Such joy you can't imagine, and freedom! I carried my toilet with me yet, I STILL couldn't make it sometimes and necessarily opted for the shower instead of the stool. I tried numerous 'special IBS diets' along with walking two miles a day for years, and found only temporary relief for the diarrhea, but not the vague uneasiness in the gut that was my constant lifelong companion. Never in my wildest dreams did I imagine I would be discussing my bowel habits for all the world to see.

I've left enough ruined and soiled underwear in public restrooms to supply the Dallas cheerleaders for life. The driver's seat in every automobile I ever owned has been the cleanest part of the car since it got shampooed so frequently. I went on a trip in '91 up the West Coast from San Diego to Seattle with friends in a van and took so much Lomotil I sounded like I had laryngitis every evening (very sexy). The driver had IBS also, so we stopped frequently and usually at fast-food restaurants where she insisted we buy something in exchange for using their restrooms. Gained weight on that trip.

In addition to IBS, I have FMS/MPS/CFS, Diabetes, Asthma and Hashimoto's Disease. After 24 years my last husband traded me in on a healthier model, same age but anorexic. I'm 5'5" and weigh 200 pounds having gained at least ten pounds with each new medication. My normal weight used to be 125 with an hourglass figure (36-26-36 sigh) until they put me on Prednisone when I developed Acute Costrochondritus (now it's just chronic). But then he's a California native and very concerned with outward appearances (although blind to his own expanding mid-section). I can't complain too much, after all, I picked him.

In February 2000 I was approached to be a subject in a clinical study for Lotronex and I knew within the first 24 hours that I had not been given the placebo. That vague uneasiness in the gut disappeared along with the diarrhea. I realized I was actually becoming constipated! WOW! First time in my life! So all of a sudden I began to eat like a real person! I could even eat all the fruit I so dearly loved! And drink coffee again! And go on trips again (no motor homes anymore since the divorce) … and give up the DEPENDS!! Life was GOOD! Even at 200 pounds!

Of course we all here at the IBS Group know what happened after that Black Day in November 2000 … and I've been collecting and hoarding and using Lotronex along with the rest of you since then. I came to this BB and thus the IBS Group by accident and fervently bless the day. It has filled a need in my life just as it so obviously has for thousands of others.

Verna Eileen in Michigan (without laughter there is no future).

From: **St. Joseph, MI, USA**

<u>Discussion</u>: Survival Guides

Irritable Bowel Syndrome is definitely something that requires survival tactics. Here are some guides, from those who have been in the trenches:

Topic: Almost free

Clarity
New Member

I've had IBS since I was in first grade (at least so I can remember) and now I'm 26. My parents pretty much ignored it, but luckily it wasn't too intense when I was younger, it would come and go. Then in college and after I started working, it became intolerable. Every day. The first time I went to the doctor he gave me Lotronex. As we know, it worked ... but then they took it away. I was devastated. I decided that I can either help myself or stop living ... because every day with this pain and frustration was not worth it to me.

So I found out what triggered it for me. After reading the book "Eating without Fear", I put my diet to the test. I ate nothing that the book said might set IBS off and then gradually started adding things back. This was a year ago and I've only had a handful of bouts and with less cramping.

What did I find?

No milk or ice cream. I found cheese and mayo to be okay, somehow, in small proportions ... but no milk.

Spaghetti/pizza sauce. I think this was my biggie. I ate pizza or calzones for most of college years ... no wonder I was sick everyday. Hard to give up ... but it's worth it. Fresh tomatoes were okay, for some reason ... must have been the spices or the intensity of the acid in the concentrated sauces.

I take calcium ... I know this doesn't help everyone ... but it can't hurt either.

Fried foods. This is no-no. Grilled or bust. I have gotten to the point when I look at a mozzarella stick or French fries … my stomach curdles.

Small amounts of salads. Lettuce and too many greens will upset it.

No caffeine. I gave up coffee (which I love) and soda pop.

A supportive family and boyfriend. Nothing relieves anxiety more when you get into trouble then a person who understands and races you to the quickest bathroom.

Things that **didn't** work: peppermint, Pepcid AC, Imodium (sort of helped), and definitely not fiber.

Sometimes it's hard to go out with people and eat because I get the healthiest thing on the menu or in small portions. Because I'm 26, 5'5" and weigh 115 lbs., they think I'm looking out for my weight or how I look, little do they know that I not only have high metabolism and play sports (which helps, also) but also have IBS.

Anyway, not to digress … every once in a while I have problems, but rare and not as intense. Good luck to all those out there still fighting … my thoughts are with you and hopefully Lotronex will be returned to us. I still have a small stash just in case … but hopefully I'll never need it.

From: **OH**

Topic: My list of helpful things

Gfinster
New Member

Here's my list of things that I do to help me live with IBS:

1. Take deep, slow, abdominal breaths, periodically during the day, instead of chest breathing.

2. Recognize physical tensing of muscles during the day and relax stomach muscles and muscles all over body (15 times a day).

3. Try to remember to chew my food twice as long as I used to (saliva and teeth are first stages of digestion, we eat too fast and ask our bodies to digest whole chunks of un-chewed food!)

4. Eat six times a day (graze). I try not to eat large meals. Our culture has bound us to the three-meals-a-day routine. BREAK OUT! Your gut will thank you.

5. Drink a glass of water after each meal.

6. Drink as much water during the day as I can think about and consume.

7. Minimize as much white sugar and starches as possible (fermenting causes gas, feeds fungus, and spikes blood sugar levels).

8. Try to maintain a steady blood sugar level. (Goes along with frequent eating).

9. Get the right amount of sleep to maintain serotonin level and minimize fatigue.

10. Eliminate as much caffeine as possible and drink herb teas, plum, peppermint, etc.

11. Walk as much as my schedule allows. Regular is best.

12. Eat a bran muffin in AM and PM for fiber (my top advice!)

13. Use Dramamine for nausea during spasms—½ tablet to start, full tab if needed (works better for me than Compazine and Phenergan).

14. Eliminate use of Senna, found it very irritating and caused spasms and episodes.

15. Eliminate alcohol—it really made me sick with D. I do miss good wines but found some great non-alcoholic beers on the market.

16. Use Milk of Magnesia for bad C (more than three days). I try extra-bran muffins, and sometimes three doses of Metamucil a day, first.

17. Quit or scale back working responsibilities. My husband has been supportive, there's more to life than money!

18. Surround yourself with supportive, understanding people. Have at least one personal friend you can talk to about your IBS. I have a friend with Lupus that has similar gut problems. We share farting, C, and D, stories all the time.

19. Stay determined to find a combination of things that will help and believe things can improve.

20. Accept the fact that this is a disability and will intrude on my life at the best and worst times.

21. Maintain a sense of humor about the gas, D, C, and nausea.

22. Monitor diet for foods that trigger attacks. For me, its whey, some preservatives, too much fiber, too much cheese, caffeine, too much sugar, soap, raw onions, alcohol, peppers of all kinds and others yet to be found.

23. Don't use too much dishwasher soap and use the sani rinse to compensate.

24. Rinse my dishes a second time to ensure they are free of dishwasher soap.

25. Be extremely grateful this is NOT a life-threatening disease and remind myself I CAN live a happy life with it.

26. Don't be afraid to change docs until you find one that listens and understands the disease, and will HELP you.

27. Get the colonoscopy! It helped my mental state a great deal knowing there was not something else more serious going on.

28. Read the Bulletin Board on a regular basis and remember I'm not alone.

29. Stay informed on the latest discoveries regarding IBS.

30. Help others by sharing my story on the BB and with people I come in contact with.

I still have episodes, but I know that I have done my best to control the disease, I know what it is and I know what to expect.

From: **Pilot Point, TX**

Topic: My IBS Survival Strategies

Jude_f
Regular Member

I am a 38-year old male who has had chronic illness for approximately the last 11 years, though I had had episodes infrequently before. My primary chronic illness is Irritable Bowel Syndrome (IBS). But I prefer to characterize my illness as a disease-complex that includes other chronic illnesses such as perennial allergic rhinitis, asthma, a bout with functional dyspepsia, a more recently acquired sleep disorder and upper back/neck pain due to compressed disk in spine. I have other periodic, secondary symptoms that are likely a result of these illnesses and include such things as occasional migraine headaches, frequent colds, fatigue, mild "feverish" feeling, back pains, itchy/scratchy tongue, skin rashes, sexual dysfunction, muscle twitches, and other seemingly "random" health problems. Some of these symptoms fall under the umbrella of symptoms of "Fibromyalgia". However, I understand this is a somewhat loosely defined disease.

A summary of my symptoms:

My IBS symptoms can be described as primarily sensitivity to a host of foods. These sensitivities cause a wide range of symptoms including pain, intestinal spasms, diarrhea, constipation, gas, bloating, urgent bowel movements, etc. The actual symptoms vary from day to day, week to week, month to month, or year to year. The symptoms are made significantly worse with stress. My symptoms in the past have also included that of functional dyspepsia in the early stages of the disease. Functional dyspepsia symptoms include frequent stomach acidity, heartburn and potential for ulcers.

How do I cope with my symptoms?

The primary means for coping with symptoms include:

- Identify trigger foods:

Identifying trigger foods is a long, arduous process that is constantly a work-in-progress because trigger foods can change with time. My symptoms and food sensitivities are always worse when my seasonal nasal allergies are worst. One would need to maintain a diary of foods, to track down the culprits—though the general patterns are similar for a lot of IBS patients. For example, dairy products, fried foods, spicy foods, etc. Dairy product sensitivity is commonly attributed to lactose mal-digestion but it could also be due to sensitivity to the milk protein casein. One needs to learn the differences between dairy products: fully cultured yogurt is normally good for most IBSers, but frozen yogurt is only partially cultured so has plenty of lactose.

- Diet control:

Diet control involves controlling one's food intake to avoid or minimize trigger foods, and at the same time getting sufficient calories to maintain a reasonably normal body weight and to provide sufficient nutrients and vitamins needed by the body. Diet control is often made difficult by the fact that one's trigger foods can change with time. Another difficulty is the ability to control one's desire for certain foods and tastes. Also, add supplemental fiber to your diet. Generally, as a matter of policy, eating smaller meals (and maybe eating more frequently) works well.

- Knowledge of disease, symptoms:

Knowledge of the disease and its range of symptoms is a huge factor in decreasing the anxiety associated with the disease/symptoms. The anxiety and stress clearly exacerbate the symptoms of the disease. There is a lot of new research that is being conducted on IBS and information is fairly easy to find on the internet.

- Online Support group

Online support groups are of great value for several reasons:

1) You get to chat with others with similar symptoms, especially symptoms that are awkward and difficult to talk about with most people;

2) Hear other people's approach and solutions to problems;

3) Hear of other treatments, efficacy of herbal treatments;

4) Helps keep you up-to-date on articles and news related to disease.

- Relaxation, Meditation, Alternative medicine, Physical exercise:

Relaxation, abdominal breathing, meditation, massage and other alternative therapies have great value even if they do not offer a cure to the disease. Approaches learned from relaxation, abdominal breathing and meditation helped me to listen to my body better and find simple solutions to ease some of the spasms and pain. I was able to sense the coming of an attack earlier and take some precautions. Overall, I have learned to suffer less with these approaches. Also, this is a constant work-in-progress, always learning new ways to deal with problems, especially because symptoms often change from year to year or season to season. Regular physical exercise also is a great contributor to overall health.

- Lifestyle changes with a goal to reducing stress:

Lifestyle change is another approach that can be beneficial, though is often very hard to do. Especially, for example, changing one's job or career to reduce stress. I have stayed in my somewhat stressful occupation, but I have incorporated some lifestyle changes, such as working regular hours, eating regular hours, taking frequent short breaks in office to relax and breath deeply, letting my co-workers know of my sensitivity to stress, not taking on additional responsibilities (often needed to attain excellence or rapid advancement in career), etc.

- Medications—OTC and Prescription:

I mention this last, but it has been a very critical part of my survival of IBS symptoms. Every time my IBS got really bad, the only way I was able to bring things under control and still go to work every day, was through medication. I have to reluctantly admit that the medicine that helped me the most was the long-term use of low dose antidepressants (amitriptyline, 20 mg/night). I say reluctantly, because there were many a times when I was frustrated with what seemed like very slow effect or some nasty side effects. Other drugs that can be useful include anticholinergics, such as, Levsin (hyoscyamine). Also for me, since my allergies and asthma are almost as bad as the IBS itself, controlling those with drugs has also helped me a great deal.

Several of these coping mechanisms are a constant work-in-progress that needs to be frequently modified or updated.

Miscellaneous Tips:

Consider upgrading health insurance to a PPO to provide flexibility to choose the best doctors;

Find a good gastroenterologist who has significant experience with IBS; one sure place to find that is at a teaching hospital associated with a good university;

Keep a daily/weekly log of health conditions/problems;

Buy books, Search Internet; knowledge is key to symptom management; join Internet bulletin boards/online support groups, chat with other patients.

Books I have found useful:

Irritable Bowel Syndrome and Diverticulosis, Shirley Trickett

IBS and the Mind-Body Brain-Gut Connection, William Salt

Gastro-Intestinal Health, Steven Peikin

The Complete Book of Better Digestion, Michael Oppenheim

Irritable Bowel Syndrome—A Natural Approach, Rosemary Nicol (Not a medical doctor)

Sneezing Your Head Off? Peter Boggs

Allergy Relief & Prevention, Jacqueline Krohn

From: **LA, CA, USA**

Topic: My outlook on IBS

Marredon
New Member

I don't consider myself weak. I, like all of us, have to take a stand on how we treat our illness and how we will allow it to affect our lives. Here are some of the ways IBS (D by the way) affects me:

If I eat this new item what will happen?

No, not traffic. I have to get to ___. I'm safe at ___.

When I go out, the first thing that I do is search for the closest bathroom or 'escape route' just in case.

Is that pain in my gut 'the real deal' or false alarm?

Will I have a normal BM today?

Now, I can only eat the same things every day because they have a 'sure track record'.

I don't like to be away from the house too long.

I can pig out at home because I have 'home field advantage'.

I really don't want to be in mixed company.

This is how I can feel at times and it causes anxiety which only aggravates the situation. In reality, by keeping a daily diary of events, IBS for me is more like this (thinking positively):

I have my good days and bad days. Usually two bad per week (cramps, etc., daily). The odds are in my favor.

I have learned which cramps are the real deal or not. Don't get upset with every gurgle.

I have changed my diet for the better (low-fat, no greasies). I am losing a few pounds!

I have informed my close friends, family and co-workers of my situation (so they will stop asking me to go Mexican for lunch).

I have made peace with myself that this is a sometimes debilitating medical condition for some people and if I have to 'go' I will 'go' anywhere at anytime (trust me on this). I don't care what anyone else thinks. Life happens, and for me right now, this is a part of it.

I still don't pass gas as bad as the dog.

Don't feel sorry for yourself. There are a lot of other people just like you (right here) who, in spirit, are with you.

If there is anyone else out there feeling this way, know that it will get better.

Thanks a lot everyone. Nothing like a little self-affirmation (I look good, I feel good, and darned it, people like me).

Good luck to you.

From: **Portsmouth, VA**

Topic: I feel as if my life has become normal again ...

Nadypoo
New Member

I feel as if my life has become normal again ...

1. I take calcium faithfully ... three pills per day, with meals. This is the biggest success for me! I am able to eat food that I wouldn't touch (yum, yum, Hot Wings!)

2. I drink tons of water.

3. I have really made a conscious effort to keep work at work, and not get stressed about the things I can't control.

4. Telling my friends and family about my problem … this has helped with my anxiousness about socializing. I don't tell EVERYONE, but it really has made a big difference when I feel that my friends understand that I may not feel well after eating out, or I would prefer for them to come over to mine and my hubby's place. I am always amazed at how many others there are out there. I have opened up to some people at work, and there are three other gals that share the same problem! I have shared this web site with them, and the support has helped so much!

5. Seeing a doctor regularly to check up on me and make sure all is OK.

Honestly, I feel as if I've kicked it. With the calcium I am now able to return to a normal life!

The support of the BB has helped so much. Without it, I wouldn't have known how to help myself to feeling well again!

My honest and heartfelt thanks to all of you who have opened your hearts, giving me a glimpse of your hopes and fears … I am so grateful!

From: **USA**

Topic: HELP, SUPPORT, ADVICE! FROM FORMER IBS SUFFERER! READ! STEPS TO GET BETTER!

Roo1029
Regular Member

My name is Amy and I have had IBS for a little under a year. At the lowest point in my life with IBS, I contemplated suicide. I had constant pain, panic attacks, was terrified of leaving the house, going to school, depressed, and just didn't want to live anymore. I thought things could never get better. Boy was I wrong. I am now happy, going to school everyday and having fun, have no panic attacks, and no pain. It took me more pain (both mental and physical) then I have ever encountered to learn what I learned to get to this point, and I figure if what I know now can save someone from what I went through I should tell the world. I have listed steps to getting your life back. Trust me they work. DON'T GIVE UP!

1. TELL YOUR FAMILY! My first mistake was isolating myself and hiding my pain which only served to make me more depressed. Yes its super embarrassing to tell, but after telling, I felt 1000 pounds lighter. My mom has provided me with so much support, that if it weren't for her I would probably be dead by now.

2. MAKE IT A POINT THAT YOU NEED HELP FROM YOUR FAMILY, THAT YOU ARE JUST A TEEN AND CAN'T DO IT YOURSELF. My family didn't believe me at first, they thought I was making it up to skip school, so one night I sat them down and told them everything, all the pain I'd had and how much I NEEDED help from professionals. Don't take any crap from anybody that tells you that its "ALL IN YOUR HEAD" I almost went crazy after hearing that a hundred times. ITS NOT!

3. Make appointments with:

    A) Therapist if you have panic attacks. Mine taught me numerous non-medication methods to deal with panic attacks.

    B) Psychiatrist in order to get antidepressants and anti-anxiety drugs. I recommend Paxil and Clonazepam.

    C) Gastroenterologist to prescribe medication to help with IBS symptoms and to make sure what you have is IBS. I recommend asking about hyoscyamine, an antispasmodic.

    D) School Counselor in order to have your situation understood. Mine gave me a special permanent pass that allows me to go to the bathroom at anytime. My teachers know my problem and let me sit near a door so I can slip out of the classroom without asking and without anybody noticing.

    E) 504 Plan—this plan is in all public schools. It is for people with medical conditions that might hinder them taking tests, such as standardized tests, AP exams, SATs, etc. With it, I can take long tests in a private room with a bathroom nearby. Ask your counselor about it.

4. CHANGE YOUR DIET! This is what really saved me. It turned my life around because it has almost completely stopped my symptoms and pain. I ordered a book called EATING FOR IBS. The book and its sister book, THE FIRST YEAR: IBS, taught me a diet of no fat, dairy, red meat, caffeine, etc. that has completely stopped my symptoms and pain. While this diet may seem insane, the book explains it all and while it's not exactly fun to not be able to eat what I want, who the heck cares if it means not having to sit in the bathroom for three hours in pain? Changing your diet is extremely important in controlling the symptoms of IBS. These two books probably saved my life, written by an almost 30-year veteran of IBS. It explains almost everything you'll ever want to know and has more helpful advice than you could ever want. It's MY BIBLE. I can't stress the importance of a diet change!

5. TELL A FEW EXTREMELY CLOSE FRIENDS. I told my best friend because after rejecting her offer to go out on a Friday night for the billionth time she wanted to know if I hated her. I then explained to her, with some embarrassment, that I simply had a medical problem that made my stomach hurt and that made it not possible for me to go out sometimes. She could tell from my face that it was serious and she was completely supportive and didn't ask questions. I now have someone that I can confide in and I can truly say that she is one of my rocks. You don't have to go into the gory details of diarrhea and constipation, just say gastrointestinal medical condition and stop there. Now almost all my friends know that I eat a weird diet because I have a "screwy stomach" but none of them bug me about it and having them know makes me feel better.

So these are my steps to getting better. IBS is hard, but it can and will get better! You just have to take the initiative.

GOOD LUCK!

From: **MD**

Concluding Remarks

In 1987, when Jeffrey Roberts first decided that he would devote his free time toward educating people about IBS, there was little written about the disorder, very few people talked about their bowel habits, and there were even fewer people who wanted to hear about personal digestive woes. As you can see by the sheer size of *IBS Chat*, look how far things have come! Jeffrey had no idea at the time of the inception of the IBS Self Help and Support Group that his efforts to bring together sufferers would result in the creation of such a prominent, influential entity—one that draws the attention of health care professionals, the media, governmental agencies, and pharmaceutical companies. He is gratified with the knowledge that the group he initiated remains a vital resource for sufferers and serves as a visible reminder of how much work still needs to be done in the search for viable treatment options.

Irritable Bowel Syndrome continues to live in a grey area of medicine, made more complex by the fact that symptoms vary from individual to individual and that true understanding of causation remains elusive. Fortunately, over the last two decades there has been a ten-fold increase in IBS citations in medical literature as research investigators in gastroenterology have focused on improving our scientific understanding of the disorder. This effort has resulted in productive strides in the understanding of the patterns of altered motility, enhanced visceral sensitivity, and brain-gut dysregulation that is seen in the manifestation of IBS. Clinical investigation remains ongoing, particularly in the area of post-infectious IBS and the role of bacteria overgrowth, as well as on the treatment options of probiotics, hypnotherapy, and cognitive behavior therapy and their role in reducing the symptoms of IBS. The pharmeceutical industry continues to maintain a focus on the development of improved pharmacologic agents to provide relief for visceral pain, diarrhea and constipation, including new medications that focus on brain-gut connections.

Jeffrey Roberts plans to continue in his mission to encourage efforts toward further understanding of IBS and to make this information available and accessible to the people whose lives are affected by this challenging disorder. In her work, Dr. Bolen joins Jeffrey in the goal of helping sufferers become educated as to the nature of their distress, to learn to become self advocates in dealing with health care professionals, and to remain aware of new treatment options as they become available.

We actively encourage you to visit the site www.ibsgroup.org and join us in benefiting from the rewards of community membership and support. As has been seen, there is strength in numbers, and together we can continue this odyssey until IBS is fully understood and adequate relief is discovered for all types of IBS sufferers. We look forward to chatting with you.

Jeffrey D. Roberts, M.S.Ed.
President and Founder
Irritable Bowel Syndrome Self Help and Support Group

Barbara Bradley Bolen, Ph.D.
Clinical Psychologist

Signatures

Many members include an inspirational quote at the end of each post. These are some of the best. Enjoy!

Auroraheart
Very Prolific Member

Time is valuable. Waste it wisely.

—Anonymous

From: **Ontario**

Bkitepilot
Prolific Member

Do Not Fear The Winds Of Adversity.
Remember: A Kite Rises Against The Wind Rather Than With It.

—Anonymous

From: **North Georgia**

Bonniei
Very Prolific Member

"You can't buy love ... but you pay heavily for it".

—Henny Youngman

From: **Iowa**

Br-549
Very Prolific Member

The difference between genius and stupidity is that genius has its limits!

—Albert Einstein

From: **The Hills**

Celticlady
Prolific Member

"Hope is the ability to hear the music of the future;
Faith is the courage to dance to it today."

—Peter Kuzmic, theologian and author

From: **USA**

Clair
Very Prolific Member

Even the smallest person can change the future.

—"The Lord of the Rings"

From: **York UK**

Cofaym
Prolific Member

Food for thought: the only kind I can digest.

From: **San Diego**

Feisty
Very Prolific Member

Life is not a journey to the grave with the intention of arriving safely in a pretty and well-preserved body, but rather to skid in broadside, thoroughly used up, totally worn out, and loudly proclaiming:
"WOW—What a Ride!"

—Author Unknown

From: **USA**

GailSusan
Very Prolific Member

"It is the dull man who is always sure, and the sure man who is always dull."

—H.L. Mencken

From: **USA**

IBSsucks
Regular Member

Those with physical differences have experience and knowledge that the average person could not understand.

—Anonymous

From: **USA**

Jazzynala
Regular Member

> Life is not measured by the moments of breath we take,
> but by the moments that take our breath away.

—Author Unknown

From: **Lansing, Michigan**

Lalarainbow
New Member

> God brought me to it; He will get me through it!

From: **Nova Scotia, Canada**

Linda C
Regular Member

> "If four out of five people SUFFER from diarrhea … does that mean that one
> enjoys it?"

—George Carlin

From: **Toronto, Ontario, Canada**

Linda2001
Prolific Member

> "The past is history, the future is a mystery, and now is a gift.
> That's why we call it the present."

—Unknown

From: **Melbourne, Australia**

LyndaG
Prolific Member

"You can't have everything. Where would you put it?"

—Steven Wright

From: **Toronto, Ontario, Canada**

Luna
Very Prolific Member

"Do not fear to be eccentric in opinion,
for every opinion now accepted was once eccentric"

—Bertrand Russell

From: **Ohio, USA**

RitaLucy
Very Prolific Member

"When I die, I hope it's in a meeting. The transition from life to death will be
barely perceptible."

From: **Houston**

Shyra
Very Prolific Member

"I'm not a failure if I don't make it—I'm a success because I tried"

—Unknown

From: **Calgary, AB Canada**

Skye
Regular Member

Stay together cheeks! Stay together!

From: **Florida**

Helpful Resources

The Irritable Bowel Syndrome Self Help and Support Group

1440 Whalley Ave., #145   or   P.O. Box 94074
New Haven, CT 06515   Toronto, Ontario M4N 3R1
USA   Canada
                                     Phone: 416-932-3311

The premier and largest online community for IBS sufferers: the Irritable Bowel Syndrome Self Help and Support Group. This site contains comprehensive IBS information and resources and offers IBS Forums, Blogs, Penpals, and Chats. Selected by The Journal of Consumer Health on the Internet as an Editor's Select Site.

http://www.ibsgroup.org

Irritable Bowel Syndrome Association (IBSA)
(See above for contact information.)

The IBSA offers referrals for treatment and patient support groups, as well as providing accurate information and education about IBS.

http://www.ibsassociation.org

International Foundation for Functional Gastrointestinal Disorders (IFFGD)
PO Box 170864
Milwaukee, WI 53217-8076
Phone: 1-414-964-1799

http://www.aboutibs.org

IFFGD is a nonprofit education and research organization offering assistance to people affected by GI disorders.

The Canadian Society of Intestinal Research
855 West 12th Avenue
Vancouver, British Columbia
Canada
V5Z 1M9
Phone: 604.875.4875
Phone Toll-Free (In Canada): 1.866.600.4875

http://www.badgut.com

The Canadian Society of Intestinal Research (SIR) is dedicated to increasing public awareness, providing patient educational materials, and funding medical research, for a broad range of gastrointestinal diseases and disorders.

University of North Carolina Center for Functional GI and Motility Disorders
CB #7080, Bioinformatics Building
Chapel Hill, NC 27599-7080

http://www.med.unc.edu/medicine/fgidc

Center for Neurovisceral Sciences & Women's Health
GLAVAHS, Building 115/CURE, Room 222A
11301 Wilshire Boulevard
Los Angeles, California 90073

http://www.ibs.med.ucla.edu

http://www.irritablebowel.net

This site discusses IBS causes, symptoms, and treatments and offers the book *Breaking the Bonds of Irritable Bowel Syndrome*, by Barbara Bradley Bolen, Ph.D.

http://digestive.niddk.nih.gov/ddiseases/pubs/ibs/index

A web page provided by the National Institute of Diabetes and Digestive and Kidney Diseases (NIDDK).

http://www.ibsnetwork.org.uk

A website from the IBS Network—the largest UK patient-led charity for individuals with Irritable Bowel Syndrome.

http://www.ibshealth.com

Information for professionals and IBS sufferers in helping to gain a better understanding of Irritable Bowel Syndrome and how IBS sufferers can help to make their lives better

http://www.mayoclinic.com/health/irritable-bowel-syndrome/DS00106

An overview of IBS from the Mayo Clinic.

http://www.helpforibs.com

Information regarding food and diet for IBS. Offers the books *Eating for IBS* and *The First Year: IBS*.

Recommended Reading

Breaking the Bonds of Irritable Bowel Syndrome: A Psychological Approach to Regaining Control of Your Life

Barbara Bradley Bolen, Ph.D. New Harbinger, 2000.

Conquering Irritable Bowel Syndrome: A Guide to Liberating Those Suffering With Chronic Stomach or Bowel Problems

Nicholas J. Talley, M.D. BC Decker Inc., 2005.

IBS for Dummies

Carolyn Dean, M.D. and L.Christine Wheeler. John Wiley & Sons, 2005

√ **A New IBS Solution**

Mark Pimentel, M.D. Health Point Press, 2006.

Irritable Bowel Syndrome and the MindBodySpirit Connection: 7 Steps for Living a Healthy Life With a Functional Bowel Disorder, Crohn's Disease or Colitis

William B. Salt II, M.D. and Neil F. Neimark, M.D. Parkview Publishing, 2002 (2nd edition).

The Second Brain ✗

Michael D. Gershon, M.D. HarperCollins Publishers, 1999.

✓ **IBS—Take Control: Insights into Irritable Bowel Syndrome**

Christine Dancey and Claire Rutter. TFM Publishing, 2005.

The First Year—IBS (Irritable Bowel Syndrome): An Essential Guide for the Newly Diagnosed

Heather Van Vorous. Marlowe & Company, 2001.

Eating for IBS: 175 Delicious, Low-Fat, Low-Residue Recipes to Stabilize the Touchiest Tummy

Heather Von Vorous. Marlowe & Company, 2000.

IBS: A Doctor's Plan for Chronic Digestive Troubles: The Definitive Guide to Prevention and Relief

Gerard Guillory, M.D. Hartley & Marks, 2001 (3rd edition).

IBS Relief: A Doctor, a Dietitian, and a Psychologist Provide a Team Approach

Dawn Burstall, R.D., T. Michael Vallis, Ph.D. and Geoffrey Turnbull, M.D. John Wiley & Sons, 2006 (Revised).

Making Sense of IBS: A Physician Answers Your Questions about Irritable Bowel Syndrome

Brian E. Lacy, Ph.D., M.D. The Johns Hopkins University Press, 2006.

Romance, Riches, and Restrooms: A Cautionary Tale of Ambitious Dreams and Irritable Bowels.

Tim Phelan. iUniverse, Inc., 2006.

Irritable Bowel Syndrome (Food Solutions): Recipes and Advice to Control Symptoms

Patsy Westcott. Hamlyn, 2002

Gastrointestinal Health: Completely New and Revised

Steven R. Peikin, M.D. Perennial Currants, 1999 (Revised).

Sick and Tired of Feeling Sick and Tired: Living with Invisible Chronic Illness

Paul J. Donoghue, Ph.D. and Mary E. Siegel, Ph.D. Norton, 2000.

Feeling Good: The New Mood Therapy

David D. Burns, M.D. Avon, 1999 (Revised).

About the Authors

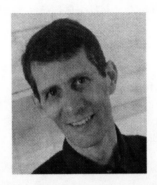

Jeffrey D. Roberts, M.S.Ed.

Jeffrey Roberts is recognized world wide as the voice of the IBS community.
In addition to running the Irritable Bowel Syndrome Self Help and Support Group web site, Jeffrey works tirelessly as a patient advocate, in close collaboration with sufferers and health care professionals. His work includes encouraging regulatory agencies and pharmaceutical companies to fund research into, and access to, new treatments for the disorder. He has provided testimony to the United States Food and Drug Administration (FDA) on several occasions in support of treatment for IBS sufferers, most notably of Lotronex for the treatment of diarrhea-predominant IBS and Zelnorm for the treatment of chronic idiopathic constipation and constipation-predominant IBS. He has been interviewed on the topic of IBS in numerous media venues, including the Discovery Channel, the CBS Evening News, National Public Radio, the Washington Post, the New York Times, USA Today, and the major national news services. He annually attends Digestive Disease Week (DDW), the World Congress of Gastroenterology and the American College of Gastroenterology's Annual Scientific meetings, and serves as the coordinator for the IBS Patient Action Group. He holds a Master of Science in Education degree from Medaille College, located in Buffalo, New York.

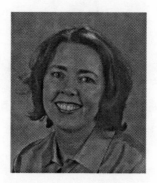

Barbara Bradley Bolen, Ph.D.

Dr. Bolen is a Clinical Psychologist with a private practice on Long Island, New York. She received her doctorate from Hofstra University and has over twenty years of experience treating adults who suffer from depression, anxiety disorders, and chronic health problems. In her work, she utilizes a Cognitive Behavioral (CBT) treatment approach, an approach that has empirically been demonstrated to be effective in reducing symptoms of a variety of disorders, including IBS. The astonishing fact that there was no self help book offering a CBT approach to managing IBS symptoms prompted her to write her first book, *Breaking the Bonds of Irritable Bowel Syndrome: A psychological approach to regaining control of your life*, which was published in 2000 by New Harbinger Publications.

978-0-595-39827-0
0-595-39827-8

Printed in the United States
74798LV00003B/8